TRIGEMINAL NEURALGIA

TRIGEMINAL NEURALGIA

Edited by

Peter J. Jannetta, MD
Drexel University College of Medicine
Department of Neurosurgery
Allegheny General Hospital
Peter J. Jannetta Center for Cranial Nerve Disorders
Pittsburgh, PA

OXFORD
UNIVERSITY PRESS
2011

OXFORD
UNIVERSITY PRESS

Oxford University Press, Inc., publishes works that further
Oxford University's objective of excellence
in research, scholarship, and education.

Oxford New York
Auckland Cape Town Dar es Salaam Hong Kong Karachi
Kuala Lumpur Madrid Melbourne Mexico City Nairobi
New Delhi Shanghai Taipei Toronto

With offices in
Argentina Austria Brazil Chile Czech Republic France Greece
Guatemala Hungary Italy Japan Poland Portugal Singapore
South Korea Switzerland Thailand Turkey Ukraine Vietnam

Published by Oxford University Press, Inc.
198 Madison Avenue, New York, New York 10016
www.oup.com

Oxford is a registered trademark of Oxford University Press

Library of Congress Cataloging-in-Publication Data

Trigeminal neuralgia / edited by Peter J. Jannetta.
p. ; cm.
Includes bibliographical references and index.
ISBN 978-0-19-534283-3 (alk. paper)
1. Trigeminal neuralgia. I. Jannetta, Peter J.
[DNLM: 1. Trigeminal Neuralgia. WL 544 T8275 2011]
RC412.T392 2011
616.8—dc22

2010002202

ISBN-13 978-0-19-534283-3

The science of medicine is a rapidly changing field. As new research and clinical experience broaden our knowledge, changes in treatment and drug therapy occur. The author and publisher of this work have checked with sources believed to be reliable in their efforts to provide information that is accurate and complete, and in accordance with the standards accepted at the time of publication. However, in light of the possibility of human error or changes in the practice of medicine, neither the author, nor the publisher, nor any other party who has been involved in the preparation or publication of this work warrants that the information contained herein is in every respect accurate or complete. Readers are encouraged to confirm the information contained herein with other reliable sources, and are strongly advised to check the product information sheet provided by the pharmaceutical company for each drug they plan to administer.

9 8 7 6 5 4 3 2 1

Printed in the United States of America
on acid-free paper

To my teachers at every level: Parents, brothers and sister, professors, colleagues, residents, fellows, students, patients, children, and my dear wife.

Thank you to Michele Birgelen and Lynn Fletcher, RN, for administrative and research work and to my superlative editor, Craig Panner.

Foreword

I am extremely honored and pleased to write the foreword to this long-expected, and much needed, book. I congratulate my dear friend Peter Jannetta on this wonderful achievement and to express my deep admiration to his great achievements and his personality.

Trigeminal neuralgia is one of the most severe and incapacitating pain syndromes. This, along with its relatively high incidence in the population, makes it the focus of, and interest of, generations of scientists and physicians for the last century. The first mention of the features of trigeminal neuralgia can be found in Avicenna's book "Qanun" (or The Cannon of Medicine) in 1025. Johannes Bausch described it from a patent's point of view in 1671, while Locke provided the first complete description in the medical literature in 1677. Some 55 years later – in 1732 - Nicolaus André described several cases and gave it the name "tic douloureux".

In the 10th century, the recommended treatment for "tic douloureux" corresponded to the level of the scientific knowledge of the times: begin by drinking wine and then rest in a darkened room as suggested by Avicenna. In the 17th century John Fothergill proposed that the extract of hemlock of, the ferrous carbonate of Hutchinson and Davidoff, as well as multiple other therapies, be attempted.

The modern therapy of trigeminal neuralgia started with the application of Phenytoin in 1942 by M. Bergouignan. The most popular and effective medication turned out to be Carbamazepine, introduced by S. Blom in 1962. Currently, various medications are available, such as valproate, gabapenthin, lamotrigine and oxcarbazepine, which possess similar efficacy but have less severe side effects. Still, a considerable number of patients are either refractory to medical treatment or experience severe side effects.

The attempts at operative treatment of trigeminal neuralgia paralleled the developments of medical therapy. Initially, and for a prolonged period of time, destructive procedures – the partial or complete intracranial trigeminal rhizotomy - were popularized. In 1934 Dandy was the first to observe and describe a case of vascular compression of the superior cerebellar artery but did not treat it as such. In 1959 Gardner and Miklos proposed vascular compression theory as a mechanism for pain generation in trigeminal neuralgia.

The real breakthrough in the treatment of trigeminal neuralgia, however, happened in 1967 with the development of the microvascular decompression concept by Peter J. Jannetta. The central issue of his concept was that a vessel chronically compressed the nerve and lead to a cascade of events that ultimately resulted in pain. Consequently, the most rational treatment, consisted of decompressing the nerve. Thus, Jannetta's truly pioneering work on the mechanisms of pain generation, the type and location of the neurovascular conflict, and the most safe and reliable technique for nerve decompression, turned out to be one of the revolutionary developments in neurosurgery in the last century.

The predominantly conservative medical society frequently needs time to accept new ideas, as shown throughout the history of science. Likewise, the majority of neurosurgeons could not accept the concept of microvascular compression and even regarded it as ridiculous. I will never forget my initial impressions when I first met Peter Jannetta at a neurosurgical meeting in the early seventies: there was a young man standing in front of an auditory of neurosurgeons, among them several of the most respected and well-known, who, despite his very logical and convincing presentation, were unable – or unwilling - to understand or accept his ideas. I remember clearly the tears I saw in the eyes of Peter. Once created, revolutionary ideas need a man of big capacity, intellectual strength, and endurance that will put them into practice. Peter Jannetta was just that person.

Microvascular decompression became the most efficient treatment in the treatment of trigeminal neuralgia and hemifacial spasm. It was also applied with varying success in cases of tinnitus, vertigo, glossopharyngeal neuralgia, spasmodic torticollis and even essential hypertension. I have always regarded microvascular decompression as one of the most elegant and effective neurosurgical operations.

I, myself, started to perform this operation in 1970 on patients with trigeminal neuralgia. The initial success rate was, however, less than optimal: in some cases no compressive vessel was seen. Discussing the issue with P. Jannetta, I realized that the root entry zone is the most sensitive portion of the trigeminal nerve and the neurovascular conflict is usually located at, or proximal to, the junctional area of central and peripheral myelin. Other important lessons that I learned over the years are that veins are frequently the responsible vessels and that more than one compressive vessel might exist. Thus, the nerve should be inspected over its entire length. If these concepts are followed and combined with a good microsurgical technique, the outcome is most favorable and the complication rate is minimal. Over the last 38 years I have performed more than 1000 microvascular decompressions in various compressive syndromes with excellent results.

I am absolutely convinced that the current book that summarize a lifelong experience and includes the lessons learned from 4500 cases of neurovascular decompression procedures will be a must for every neurosurgeon, neurologist, otolaryngologist and dentist; indeed for all practitioners who see patients with face pain.

M. Samii MD, PhD

Preface

I came into my neurosurgery residency during the time when carbamazipine was being studied under stringent conditions. It was found to be a potent medication with serious side effects which could be mitigated or avoided if the drug were monitored carefully. This medicine, to my mind, brought forth unprecedented new interest in trigeminal neuralgia (TN). The reader may recall, if long in the tooth, that in 1963, the year of which I speak, the best drug used for TN was phenytoin, the effect of which lasted at best 12 to 18 months in most patients and could not be repeated with good effect once it was discontinued. Medical treatment has evolved considerably as have diagnostic techniques over this period. We now have a number of drugs, some useful, some not, in our armamentarium. The medical treatment of TN will be discussed in great extent and with, we hope, some essence of profundity and clarity in the book before you.

Also in 1963, operative treatment was generally restricted to alcohol injections into a proximal trigeminal nerve branch or middle fossa retrogasserian section. The observations of Dandy including porto major section at the pons (Dandy 1925, 1934) had not been brought to fruition by subsequent generations and were largely ignored. The cerebellopontine angle was a dangerous place, a terra incognito. As the Romans said, "There are dragons here." Few surgeons were able to operate safely and effectively in the cerebellopontine angle. The morbidity rate of a mere cerebellopontine angle exploration was 10 percent; the mortality rate, one percent.

Along with the new interest in TN came an era of analysis of the symptom-complex and the development of new treatments, both medical and surgical. Medical treatments evolved considerably as other new drugs, primarily anticonvulsants, were developed and applied to patients. Concomitantly the undertaking of variations on the theme of TN was broadened and deepened by various investigators. As frequently occurs, new ideas develop only if the technology is present to prove or disprove them. If the technology is inadequate to do this, the new idea lies fallow or dies. The application of two technological advances enabled neurosurgeons to have new ideas and to develop them into useful therapies.

The first advance was the application of carefully modulated heat in the tip of an electrode placed with radiographic guidance in the trigeminal ganglion. This work by Sweet and Wepsick (Sweet and Wepsick 1974) using radiofrequency lesions refined the attempts by Kirschner (Kirschner 1942, 1963). The second, beginning earlier but slower in acceptance, was the application of the binocular dissecting microscope to the treatment of TN focusing on the nerve in the cerebellopontine angle (Jannetta 1963, 1977). The first application of the microscope to neurosurgery was by Kurze in 1957. The first publication concerning use of the microscope in neurosurgery was by Rand and Kurze (1960), both of whom were my teachers. Kurze thought wonderfully well, spoke lucidly but wrote sparingly. He contributed major constructive ideas to neurosurgery and, with his interest in vestibular schwannomas, contributed great technical improvements and new concepts to the surgery of these tumors. Rand, to a degree, became Kurze's Boswell, writing papers derived from Kurze's observations and ideas. All this was important and useful but we are speaking here specifically of trigeminal neuralgia, a specific area of interest, and an area the treatment of which began a yeasty and surprisingly rapid development. Radiofrequency rhizotomy (RFL) was accepted rapidly as an important treatment. Microvascular decompression took much longer for generalized acceptance and utilization. Why the difference? RFL was a newer, easier way to impair trigeminal nerve function as treatment and was introduced by a distinguished senior professor from a distinguished old institution. Microvascular decompression (MVD) was a new treatment dependent upon clear observation and understanding of anatomy and pathology in the cerebellopontine angle (terra incognito) and developed by a junior person from a new institution with no reputation; in short, a possible heretic. The subsequent development of importance of the new paradigm of vascular compression causing cranial nerve, and more recently brainstem dysfunction, is the type of sequence described in detail in Kuhn in his benchmark treatise, The Structure of Scientific Revolutions (Kuhn 1962).

Radiofrequency percutaneous rhizotomy and microvascular decompression were soon accompanied by other techniques, percutaneous glycerol rhizotomy, focused irradiation (gamma knife and linear accelerator techniques) and percutaneous balloon compression. These will be dealt with in depth in this volume by authorities in the various areas.

Understanding of the epidemiology and demographics of TN as a disease entity has not kept pace with advances in definition and treatment of the entity. We still do not truly know the real incidence and prevalence of TN in the United States, for example. Understanding of the various types of TN and the effects of duration, medical and operative treatment upon TN are developing rapidly as more investigators study facial pain. I gave the authors free reign so that the material would be seen from various perspectives. It will be noted that there is redundancy in our chapters. This is deliberate, as repetition is useful and so is continuity when one is reading and studying any subject.

When doing my reading on preparation for the organization of this volume, not to mention the historical "vignettes" above, I began by reading several of the old books concerning trigeminal neuralgia. Following the Oslerian precept that young men should read old books and that old men should read new books, I started with the contemporary literature. I soon discovered that although my knees are very old, I am young after all, as I felt myself progressively drawn to the old literature. Although the early contributions are often quaint, verbose and in error, they are just as often full of incisive and perspicacious observations. Clear thinking was often based on inadequate information, but the best available at the time.

The reader will accompany us from the old to the new in scholarly and sometimes didactic descriptions of TN, its variations and treatments. We will even peer at possibilities for future understanding and treatments. All of us, patients and their families, physicians and surgeons look forward to the Edenic era when there is no TN or it can be cured by simple means. We have attempted to make available to the reader a compendium of contemporary information and practice based on both the old and the new information available to us. As the editor, author and co-author, I have tried throughout to bring to you insights from various authors in this area of face pain with new materials which we hope will stimulate the next generation, the young, bright and dedicated neuroscientists, men and women of today to work for tomorrow.

One cannot change thought for the better without a knowledge base. You can think clearly without the old information. You can work effectively without knowing the status of prior knowledge. Indeed, the development of new paradigms is mostly due to young naïve, interested people doing and thinking the impossible (Kuhn 1962). But you cannot transmit it clearly to others without the old, classical information. In essence, you cannot convince unless you speak a common language.

And so, we have attempted to blend old anatomy and physiologic concepts with contemporary modes of thought and observations. Similarly, we have brought the patients (and you, gentle reader) from the earliest beginnings of recognition of the face pain syndromes through the various medical therapies and then a detailed review of operative techniques, their pros and cons with a look at tomorrow.

I speak for all the authors in saying we hope we have succeeded in this endeavor.

Peter J. Jannetta, MD

Contents

Contributors

Ronald I. Apfelbaum, MD
Department of Neurosurgery
University of Utah
Health Science Center
Salt Lake City, Utah

Jeffrey A. Brown, MD, FACS
Neurological Surgery, P.C.
Great Neck,
New York

Kenneth F. Casey, MD
Department of Neurological Surgery
Michigan State University School of Medicine
Trenton, MD

Jeffrey Cohen, MD, PhD
Albert Einstein College of Medicine
Department of Neurology
Beth Israel Medical Center
New York, New York

Andrew Grande, MD
Department of Neurosurgery
University of Cincinnati
Cincinnati, Ohio

George J. Hadeed, DMD
Prosthodontic consultant
Pittsburgh, Pennsylvania

David Halpert, MD
Horseheads Neurology Associates
Horseheads, New York

Paul A. House, MD
Department of Neurosurgery
University of Utah
Health Science Center
Salt Lake City, Utah

Peter J. Jannetta, MD
Drexel University College of Medicine
Department of Neurosurgery
Allegheny General Hospital
Peter J. Jannetta Center for Cranial Nerve Disorders
Pittsburgh, Pennsylvania

David H. Jho, MD, PhD
Department of Neurosurgery
Massachusetts General Hospital
Harvard Medical School
Boston, Massachusetts

Diana H.J. Jho, MS
Jho Institute for Minimally Invasive Neurosurgery
Department of Neuroendoscopy
Allegheny General Hospital
Drexel University College of Medicine
Pittsburgh, Pennsylvania

Hae-Dong Jho, MD, PhD
Jho Institute for Minimally Invasive Neurosurgery
Department of Neuroendoscopy
Allegheny General Hospital
Drexel University College of Medicine
Pittsburgh, Pennsylvania

Douglas Kondziolka, MD, MSc, FRCSC, FACS
Department on Neurological Surgery
Center for Brain Function and Behavior
Center for Image-Guided Neurosurgery
Pittsburgh, Pennsylvania

Mark E. Linskey, MD
Department of Neurological Surgery
Neuro-Oncology Program
University of California-Irvine Medical Center
Orange, California

L. Dade Lunsford, MD
Department of Neurological Surgery
University of Pittsburgh
Pittsburgh, Pennsylvania

Mark R. McLaughlin, MD, FACS
Princeton Brain & Spine Care
Princeton, New Jersey

Chad J. Morgan, MD
Springfield Neurological and Spine Institute LLC
Springfield, Missouri

Toba N. Niazi, MD
Department of Neurosurgery
University of Utah
Health Science Center
Salt Lake City, Utah

Majid Samii, MD, Dr. h.c. mult.
International Neuroscience Institute Hannover
Otto-von-Guericke-University
Magdeburg, Germany

Raymond F. Sekula, Jr., MD
Department of Neurosurgery
Drexel University College of Medicine
Peter J. Jannetta Center for Cranial Nerve Disorders
Allegheny General Hospital
Pittsburgh, Pennsylvania

John M. Tew, Jr., MD
Department of Neurosurgery
University of Cincinnati Neuroscience Institute
University of Cincinnati College of Medicine
Mayfield Clinic
Cincinnati, Ohio

Joanna M. Zakrzewska, MD, FDSRCS, FFDRCSI, FFPMRCA, FHEA
Division of Diagnostic, Surgical and Medical Sciences
Eastman Dental Hospital
UCLH NHS Foundation Trust
London, United Kingdom

TRIGEMINAL NEURALGIA

1

History of Trigeminal Neuralgia

Kenneth F. Casey and Peter J. Jannetta

False facts are highly injurious to the progress of science, for they often endure long; but false views, if supported by evidence, do little harm, for everyone takes a salutary pleasure in proving their falseness; and when this is done, one path toward error is closed and the road to truth is often at the same time opened

Charles Darwin, *The Descent of Man*

There is considerable controversy, in the various source books, as to whom and when the first description of trigeminal neuralgia (TN) is attributed. Many credit Aretaeus of Cappodocia with this distinction, based on his second-century description in *Cephalaea*. Other authors, including Stookey and Ransohoff (1959), believe no real distinction was made in that account between migraine headache and TN. Aretaeus was a Greek physician from Cappodocia who practiced in Rome and Alexandria and led a revival of Hippocrates' teachings. He wrote a four-volume work in which he described diabetes and differentiated spinal from cerebral palsy; however, his references to cephalalgia are too vague to be considered definitive descriptions of TN:

> If the head be suddenly seized with pain from a temporary cause, even it (sic.) should endure for several days, the disease is called cephalalgia. But if the disease be protracted for a long time, and with long and frequent periods, or if greater or more intractable symptoms supervene, we call it cephalea… . In certain cases, the parts on the right side, or those on the left solely, so far that a separate temple, or ear, or one eyebrow, or one eye, or the nose divides the face into two equal parts… the pain does not pass this limit, but remains in the half of the head. This is called Heterocrania. (Aretaeus 1856, 2)

In reviewing the works of Arab physicians of the 10th and 11th centuries, it is apparent that the recognition and treatment of various pain conditions and of painful conditions of the teeth and face was a common part of medical practice (Avicenna 1999). A foremost physician of the time, Avicenna (980–1037) was also a philosopher, poet, and statesman. He was referred to by his peers as the "second teacher," Aristotle being "the first." He began his investigations into the field of medical science at age 18; his *Canon of Medicine* (the *Law of Medicine* is perhaps a more correct translation, as the word *quaqanun* means "law"), written in 1012, had a major influence on medical education up until the 17th century. The tremendous popularity and impact of the *Canon* in Europe can be best judged from the fact that its Latin translation, by Gerard, was reissued 16 times during 1470–1500, and it went through 20 further editions during the 16th century, thus becoming the medical "bible" of all major universities in Europe. According to the *Canon,* "Medicine is a science by which we learn the various states of the human body, in health, when not in health, the means by which health is likely to be lost, and when lost, is likely to restore to health." Thus, when Avicenna discusses types of pain, he states: "Stabbing pain… this is the result of transverse stretching of the membranes as if their continuity was being separated… throbbing pain… the cause in an inflammatory process… (arising) if the adjoining member is sentient and has pulsating arteries around it" (Avicenna 1999).

In describing various other conditions of the head and neck, he later states, "That the patient can blow only with one side of his face and spit from one side… if it is of spasmodic type, he may have pain in his face and head… the skin of the forehead is bowled (sic.), and the muscles of the face are hard, and the part of the face affected is pulled down toward the neck." This description is clinically in line with that of hemifacial spasm, and Avicenna makes a distinction between this painful condition and pain due to abnormalities in the teeth. "In spasmodic *levqet*… there is not much change in power and sensation… the other sign of disease is pain in the face… if the pain is not too deep and affects the jaw; and if the teeth should feel a little numb, then it is due to disease in the nerve… ."

Despite Stookey and Ransohoff's assertion that Avicenna was describing only facial palsy, these paragraphs may support the contention that he was describing a range of syndromes involving both the fifth and seventh nerves. His description of the tonus in hemifacial spasm is clear, and readily distinguishes it from facial palsy. His assertion that pain in the teeth, accompanied by numbness, is nerve-based provides clear evidence for the distinction that we continue to struggle with today. Odontalgia and TN both involve the trigeminal pathways, but involve different pathophysiology. Avicenna went on to suggest many remedies for this type of pain, and we will return to look at these remedies—along with others described in greater detail.

Jurjani (1066–1136) was 44 when he penned the most famous medical dictionary of his time, *The Thesaurus of the Shah of Khwarazm* (Al-Jurjani 1110). Therein, when discussing pains of the head and neck, he noted "There is a type of pain which affects the teeth on one side and the whole of the jaw on the same side which is painful. With the pain, there is severe spasm of the face and severe anxiety. It should be known that the pain is from the nerves which are attached to the root of the teeth. The cause of the spasm and anxiety is the *proximity of the artery to the nerve* [italics added]." Jurjani's work drew from that of his predecessor, Avicenna, and he continued the distinction that pain in the nerve was caused by an artery.

These two physicians paint a clear clinical picture of the different types of face and tooth pain, and a hypothesis of the pathophysiology also begins to emerge.

Although it is disputed whether doctors Johannes Michael Fehr and Elias Schmidt, secretaries of the Imperial Leopoldian Academy of Natural Sciences, described a case of face pain or TN in 1688, their story is compelling. Their colleague, Johannes Laurentius Bausch, was stricken by an intense, unexpected pain in the right maxilla, which left him mute and unable to eat. The pain was variable: It was noted to be absent in the fall of 1665, but present again later that year, but more intense than before. Bausch became emaciated and bedridden, and he eventually died from the circumstances associated with the pain (Lewy 1938). It seems likely that the infliction may have been TN, but the present nomenclature did not become widely utilized until the work of Charles Bell and Francois Magendie in the 1820s. These researchers separated the functions of the cranial nerves and described the distinction of the sensory function of the fifth nerve, thus describing an anatomic locus for the pain.

John Locke (1632–1704) is widely known as a philosopher, but he became interested in medicine while studying at Christ Church in Oxford. He obtained his Bachelor of Medicine in 1674, and worked with such noted scientists and thinkers as Robert Boyle, Thomas Willis, Robert Hooke, and Robert Lower. He also spent a great deal of time with Thomas Sydenham, who was widely regarded for his diagnostic acumen, in which he placed great emphasis on observation. At the same time, the school of experimental philosophy was in its infancy, and Locke joined this group of modern philosophers, which included Descartes, who was a force in the empiricist school. According to Locke's philosophy, what we know is always properly understood as the relation between ideas, and he devoted much of his work (Locke 1690) to an extended argument that all of our ideas, simple or complex, are ultimately derived from experience. One consequence of this empiricist approach is that the knowledge of which we are capable is thus severely limited in its scope and certainty. He opposed the rationalist belief in innate ideas, holding that the mind is born blank, and all knowledge is inscribed upon it in the form of human experience. For him, multiple observations allowed for the recognition of concepts, ideas, and ultimately syndromes.

Ongoing political upheaval and loss of his sponsors' protection forced Locke to leave England. While traveling through France, he had a chance encounter with the wife of the English Ambassador, the Countess of Northumberland. His classical background in experiential thinking and medical training resulted in a lucid, concise description of her affliction: "Whom I found in a fit of such violent and exquisite torment that it forced her to such cries and shrieks as you would expect to come from one upon the rack, to which I believe hers was an equal torment which extended itself all over the right side of her face and mouth. When the fit came, there was… as if a flash of fire all of a suddaine [sic] shot into all those parts… .

Her mouth was constantly drawn on the right side towards the right ear by repeated convulsive motions… which were consistently accompanied by her cries. These violent fits terminated on a suddaine and then my lady seemed perfectly well, excepting only a dull pain which ordinarily remained in her teeth on that side… . She usually had a presentiment of the fit. In all of this time of her being ill, she has not found the least pain in all of the other side. Speaking was apt to put her into these fits, sometimes opening her mouth to take anything, or touching her gums… ." (excerpts from a letter to Dr. Mapletoft 4 December, 1677).

This account is remarkable for its detailed description of the paroxysmal nature, the inter-attack interval with its seemingly normal exam, and the secondary symptoms of TN, including the fullness, sense of pulling, and the like. In this case, the description of the residual pain in the teeth "a dull pain which ordinarily remained in her teeth on that side and an (uneasiness) in that side of her tongue" suggests that he was describing type 2 TN (Burchiel 2003). Thus, we have the evolution of a more complete picture of this pain syndrome, one that adds to the previous clinical details and expands the exam features. These clinical contributions continued to gain clarity, and produced new treatment options through the remainder of the 18th century.

Samuel Fothergill (1711–1780), nephew of the more famous John, opined regarding the cause of TN: "I do not even hazard a conjecture, but wait until greater information experience should throw some light on a subject which opinion cannot explain nor hypothesis prove" (McMurtry 1969). Interestingly, a large number of neurologists hold this to be true today, suggesting that the pathophysiology and causative agents in TN remain unknown.

Nicolas André coined the descriptive term *tic douloureux* (painful twitch) in 1787 (André 1688). His first case appears to be one of a TN injury with subsequent pain. Pujol describes his first account with this clinical problem thusly: "It is surprising how often *tic douloureux* is confused with toothache. Unfortunate and useless extraction of an entire row of teeth has usually followed that diagnostic blunder" (Pujol 1787). As this clinical picture now became clearer to diagnosticians, subsequent authors began to add detail and other clinical observations to those cases subsequently termed TN. Oppenheim noted the association with multiple sclerosis, and bilateral pain, either in multiple sclerosis or independently, was first described by Harris (Oppenheim 1904). This clinical diagnosis of TN and its variants is best made by hearing a patient's own description:

A remarkable document from the archives of a hospital in Italy, penned by an Italian attorney who suffered from facial pain, has provided a detailed insight into both the diagnosis and the state of Italian medicine in the early 1800s. His description of the condition leaves little doubt as to the diagnosis of TN. The attorney wrote of "excruciating, paroxysmal pain in the region of the left nose, upper lip and upper gum." He referred to the concept of the pain as occasionally penetrating and as a sense of heat. He described the paroxysms as being related to "eating, chewing, talking, blowing the nose, and washing his face." His paroxysms were intermittent at first, but as time progressed became more constant. The manuscript serves as a remarkable record of the treatments that he was offered, including volatile oils, blood letting, purgatives, and a fonticulus—a wound made to allow for the application of topical irritants (presaging some of the topical applications used at the current time). The patient saw a number of eminent physicians, including A.G. Testa, Scarpa, Luigi Barra, and Tomasini. He underwent electric therapy and mustard treatments, but refused a suggestion from Andre and Tomasini for peripheral neurectomy. In the paper, the results of his autopsy are detailed and the entire autopathograph makes fascinating reading (Govoni & Granieri 1996).

A family with trigeminal and glossopharyngeal neuralgia, which affected several individuals over three generations, was described by Knuckey and Gubbay (Knuckey & Gubbay 1979). Familial incidence of TN is estimated at 5%; it is suggested that when the initial presentation includes bilateral pain, the incidence may be higher.

In 1912, Osler described TN as follows: "In patients with advanced TN, the paroxysms follow one another rapidly without any assignable cause, and in the intervals the patient may never be quite free from pain. They are initiated by almost any form of external stimulus, for example by a draught of air; movement of the facial muscles or tongue while speaking; touching the skin, particularly over those points from which the pain seems to take its origin; and the act of swallowing, especially when pain involves the mucus membrane field and distribution of the nerve. It is not a self-limited disease. In some instances, the neuralgia reaches such a frightful intensity that it renders the patient's life unbearable. In earlier times, suicide was not an uncommon consequence" (Osler 1913). This description is consonant with our current appreciation of so-called classic or type 1 TN. Burchiel (2003) suggests that TN can be divided into several subcategories.

The physical examination between paroxysms is reported to be normal. However, in 1938, Lewy and Grant reported that 25% of patients with TN had sensory abnormalities on exam (Lewy & Grant 1928). This figure was confirmed in several additional studies. The sensory examination did not receive much further focus until Bennett and Jannetta reported on trigeminal-evoked potentials. In that setting, the nerve received an electrical stimulus, utilizing a small current passing above the canine teeth, and recordings were made from the classic sites for sensory-evoked potentials. The trigeminal-evoked potential paradigm was developed by Bennett (Bennett & Jannetta 1983). Bennett and Jannetta (1983) reported that 86% of patients with TN had abnormal potentials.

This extends the observation made by others that, in intervals between attacks, a careful sensory exam using a light touch or even pinprick will show sensory loss in the central area of the face. This is in contradistinction to the common reports and descriptions in neurology literature, which state that finding sensory abnormality or loss of the corneal reflex excludes the diagnosis of TN. Such statements include the following: "The diagnosis of idiopathic TN is tenable only if no physical findings of fifth-nerve dysfunction are present."

Recent presentation examining all five sensory modalities in the face (light touch, pressure, pinprick, hot/cold, vibration) demonstrated similarly that 80% of patients with type 1 TN had abnormalities in one or more modalities. In this study, subsequent evaluation of the subgroups did not disclose a correlation between the length of time from diagnosis and the finding of sensory modality changes (personal communication, Kenneth F. Casey and Peter J. Jannetta).

Fromm reported on an interesting subgroup of patients who have had prodromal pain, which he termed "pre-trigeminal neuralgia" (Fromm et al. 1990). These patients described their pain as a toothache or sinusitis-like pain lasting up to several hours, sometimes triggered by jaw movements or drinking hot or cold liquids.

PATHOPHYSIOLOGY

So, the clinical picture, with all its variations, has become nearly complete—but what of the pathophysiology? In recent years, as physicians have become enamored with confirmatory testing for many conditions, the diagnosis of various forms of face pain has become seemingly more difficult. In the diagnosis of cranial nerve afflictions, such as TN, however, a complete history and appropriate examinations will yield a correct diagnosis in well over 90% of patients.

Love and Coakham examined trigeminal nerve dorsal roots from patients with compression of the nerve root by an overlying blood vessel. Focal demyelination was seen in the region of compression, with close apposition of demyelinated axons and an absence of intervening glial processes. Similar foci of nerve root demyelination in juxtaposition with axons have been demonstrated in multiple sclerosis patients with TN (Love & Coakham 2001). Experimental studies indicate that this anatomical arrangement favors the ectopic generation of spontaneous nerve impulses and their ephaptic conduction to adjacent fibers, and that spontaneous nerve activity is likely to be increased by the deformity associated with pulsatile vascular indentation.

Kerr and colleagues (Kerr 1967; Kerr & Miller 1966), Beaver, Moses and Ganote (1965, 1967) and Kruger and Maxwell (1967) almost simultaneously provide the first detailed descriptions of ultrastructural abnormalities in the nerve root. They observed focal loss of myelin and close apposition of demyelinated axons. There were few residual oligodendrocytes and no inflammatory cells. They used electron microscopy and immunological staining of glial fibrillary acid protein (GFAP) to show that astrocytic processes were largely confined to the periphery of the lesion Jannetta extended the observations of Dandy and Gardner at the dissecting-microscope level and added some histological details. Using intraoperative microscopy, he confirmed the nature of the vessels, their origin, and site of compression. Jannetta described the incidence of arterial, venous, and mixed vascular compression; heretofore, the assumption was that only arterial compression could produce symptoms. His group catalogued the source of the arteries and veins, listing the superior cerebellar as most common in venous compression, with components of the cerebellomedullary vein as the next most common.

Vascular compression of the nerve root entry zone causes demyelination and secondary ephaptic transmission. Alternatively, it may cause repetitive activation of primary afferens in the nerve, causing hyperexcitability in the central neurons. Activation of N-methyl-D-aspartic (NMDA) acid receptors has been invoked as a possible additional factor. The conventional view in contemporary modeling is that TN is the result of an irritative lesion of the nerve causing secondary hyperexcitability and mixed signaling leading to pain. However, a central and peripheral mechanism has also been postulated, describing abnormal impulses arising from the demyelinated axons, with secondary activation along peripheral and central cores of the gasserian ganglion fibers leading to increased nuclear activity. (Rappaport and Devor 1994)

Kerr's group discusses in detail a transitional zone of the fifth cranial nerve called the *Obersteiner-Redlich zone* (Kerr, Fraher, & Delanty 1987). The two Austrian neurologists who named this eponymous zone describe it as one of transition from the central to the peripheral myelin-producing cells; namely, the oligodendrocytes and Schwann cells, respectively. The Obersteiner-Redlich zone or root entry zone is the putative site at which pulsatile compression affects nerve function and can result in clinical hypo- or hyperactivity. Other observers have noted that compression can occur at multiple sites along the course of the nerve and cerebellopontine angle, but it is generally accepted that the initial point of contact in the root entry zone produces the classic syndrome.

Devor had opined that "the hypothesis states that trigger stimuli set off bursts of activity in the small cluster of trigeminal ganglion neurons that have been rendered hyperexcitable as a result of ganglion or trigeminal root damage" (Devor, Amir, & Rappaport 2002). Activity then spreads from this ganglion ignition focus to encompass more widespread portions of the ganglion. After a brief period of autonomous firing (seconds to minutes), the activity is quenched and a refractory period is initiated by an intrinsic suppressive (hyperpolarizing) process, which was engaged as a result of the rapid firing. The primary abnormality resides in the trigeminal root ganglion and the trigeminal root, rather than in the skin or central nervous system. Because of this, sensation is essentially normal between periods of ectopic paroxysmal trigeminal root ganglion discharge.

TREATMENT

As we've seen, the roll call of physicians and clinicians who observed and described facial pain, especially trigeminal pain, extends over several centuries and many physicians. Each contributor added an essential element to the clinical description; many confirmed symptoms coincident to the pain and signs that might be found to help secure the diagnosis. The distillation of this research brings us to the present, wherein the vascular compression theory, as well as various clinical presentations and their evolution over time appear to have a reasonable pathophysiologic explanation.

But what of treatment? Trigeminal pain syndromes are diagnosed by history and physical examination, and the examination can tell us something about the stage of nerve dysfunction and, perhaps, something about selecting the appropriate therapy.

Although nonoperative treatments for trigeminal pain have been used for over a millennium, we have a relatively scant list to document. A review of the current literature shows that only a few medications have been subjected to a randomized controlled trial. Therefore, we have very little evidence-based pharmacological data on which to base the care of our patients. Rushton summarized the problem well: "A detailed review of the medical literature concerning nonsurgical treatment of trigeminal neuralgia… would be arduous for the author, tedious to the reader, and profitable to neither" (Rushton & Macdonald 1957). The uncertainties of response to recurrence, as well as the clinical presentation of the patients in pain, may help explain the myriad number of substances, topical agents, and medicines that have had some transient, but mostly insubstantial, effect. We will not explore each blind avenue, but we will review some of these agents to give the reader a sense of the range of options pursued.

Early Treatments

First, let us take a look at the treatments proposed by Avicenna (1999): Anethum linseed poultice, gold salt, and inebriants, *aqua dolcis* (sweet almond water), and oils. *Anethum gravolens*, dill, is an antiflatulent with some lipid-lowering properties. Linseed (flaxseed) is an antioxidant in its seed form, but not as an oil; linseed poultice is used around the world for headaches and for superficial pains.

Gold salt, in reality gold compound, is proposed to be linked to antimitochondrial activity and thus induces cell apoptosis. It is thought that gold affects the entire immune response (phagocytes, leukocytes and T cells), reducing the potency of the response and limiting its oxidizing nature, and thus ending the cycle of inflammation. Three to 6 months are often required before gold treatment noticeably improves pain in general and this is similar to the time course for some of our more modern treatments; gold compounds remain a good treatment option for arthritis.

Aqua dolcis is most likely sweet almond oil. This is still in use today as a topical applicant for skin irritation and orally as a laxative. Taken together, Avicenna's remedies seem designed to treat both the patient's psyche and pain, as well as to assuage the psyche of the physician dealing with this recalcitrant and painful disorder—an approach that persists today: "Even up to the present moment, the medical journals teem with fresh contributions to the overgrown and redundant accumulation of remedies" (Rushton & Macdonald 1957).

Other traditional remedies included poison hemlock (*Conium maculatum*), which Fothergil, as well as many others of his time, used (Stookey & Ransohoff 1959). Poison hemlock has sedative and antispasmodic properties; it contains compounds that relieve pain. It is a dangerous agent; the difference between lethal and therapeutic dose is quite narrow.

The list of treatments continues with quinine, muriate of mercury, histamine (intravenously), arsenic, hydrocyanic acid, antimony tartrate, and phosphorus with peppermint oil. The first forays with these various treatments produced dismal results, with little lasting improvement, and so they were largely abandoned. Thompson (1867), however, reported a series of 12 patients who improved with the use of peppermint oil—an enviable result.

Ball (Brown 1999) produced relief by using *fever therapy*, which was induced by injecting boiled milk. He and several other physicians found that the introduction of mild toxins that induced fever could produce pain relief while the patient was recovering from the fever. The pain cycle can be nicely disrupted by the introduction of mild protein denitration through the medium of heat. At most physiologic temperatures, tertiary protein structure loss probably requires a concomitant change in pH as well, so it is difficult to ascertain the exact method of action (protein denitration vs. pH change) in these cited treatments.

Two other agents— trichloroethylene and stilbamidine—used in the early treatment approach to TN demonstrated good results, and good science supports their initial use. Trichloroethylene was used in Germany as a solvent and was noted to cause trigeminal neuropathy. Plessner was the first to pursue this treatment, and he reported its efficacy in 1915 (Plessner et al. 1915). Oppenheimer and Plessner together continued to use trichloroethylene to treat TN, despite the fact that it was primarily known as a grease remover. Its action on the patient produced vomiting, optic disc swelling, vertigo, and the bilateral loss of sensation in the distribution of the sensory portion of the trigeminal nerve, but total sparing of the motor root (Oppenheimer 1904). In 1918, Plessner reported on an additional 17 patients, all of whom felt that the side effects of the nausea, occasional ventricular tachycardia, and unconsciousness were preferable to the face pain and continued to endure treatment. Nonetheless, it seems an early instance of substituting one toxicity for another, a strategy that continues to be employed in some aspects of pain management today.

Stilbamidine, a treatment for parasites, was utilized in 1942 by Napier and Sen Gupta (Napier & Sen Gupta 1942). They used the agent NA 4, 4-dicarbonamidine to produce bilateral trigeminal neuropathy. In 1955, 41 patients treated with stilbamidine were reported Woodhall and Odom 1955). The side effects included bilateral facial numbness, paresthesias in the face, and discomfort in the eyes, but also included irreversible hepatic and renal damage. Patients appeared to be especially sensitive to these effects if exposed to ultraviolet light. Despite the fact that subjects saw a decrease in facial pain, it was a delayed effect occurring 40 to 150 days after the initial 10-day treatment. Smith and Miller, also in 1955, reported excellent results for stilbamidine with TN. They described a resultant neuritis, which resembled deafferentation pain in many ways (Smith & Miller 1955).

VITAMIN THERAPY

One area of therapy with continuing impact is the use of vitamins, especially the B series. The use of B vitamins for relief from painful neuralgic states ranging from alcoholic neuropathy to TN has been generally fruitful. Zimmerman's group looked closely at the physiologic underpinnings of these effects, concluding that B_6 has the greatest effect on spinal cord nociception and attributing to B_{12} an additive effect (Fu, Carstens, Stelzer, & Zimmerman 1988). In addition, data suggest that B_{12} (in either its methyl or cyanocobalamin forms), an essential component of myelin repair, may play a role in the regenerative process that appears to be in a dynamic cycle in cases of vascular cross-compression causing TN (Caram-Salas, Reyes-Garcia, Medina-Santillán, & Granados-Soto 2006). Additional work suggests that this is a class of agents useful for the adjunctive treatment of neuropathic pain. B vitamins appear to diminish the nociceptive response evoked in individual neurons in the rat thalamus when electrical stimulation is applied to the afferent C-fibers (Caram-Salas et al. 2006). Additionally, in phasic analgesic models (such as the writhing test and the heat coil test) the administration of fixed, proportioned doses of B_1, B_6, and B_{12} have been shown to provide both an analgesic effect and an improvement in pain when added as an adjunct (Jurna, Carlsson, Kömen, & Bonke 1990). Additional studies show that the use of thiamine and pyridoxine with dexamethasone reduces tactile allodynia in rats.

ANTICONVULSIVE THERAPY

The paroxysmal nature of TN attacks, with their intervening periods of relative calm, prompted may clinicians to consider anticonvulsants to treat this condition. Armand Trousseau described the syndrome as *névralgié epileptiform* (Trousseau 1877). Bergouignan reported phenytoin as an effective agent in reducing some degree of complaints in patients (Bergouignan 1942).

Sweet (1985) reminds us that, within his group of patients, the use of anticonvulsants produced remissions lasting for up to 1 year in one-quarter of these patients.

Do anticonvulsants have a role in the treatment of TN? Scientists began to address that point as early as 1962. Blom utilized several clinical guidelines to detail the use of carbamazepine in patients with face pain, and he demonstrated good results (Blom 1962). Since that time, a variety of anticonvulsants have been used in TN, each with modest success. Nonetheless, few if any evidence-based guidelines for the management of TN exist due to the paucity of information regarding Class 1 evidence for these agents.

In a most recent edition of *British Medical Journal* guidelines for the treatment of TN, the summary concludes:

> Carbamazepine: One systemic review of three crossover randomized control trials (RCT) found that carbamazepine had much increased pain relief compared with placebo, but also increased adverse effects (drowsiness, dizziness, constipation, and ataxia). One retrospective cohort study suggested that in the long term (5 to 16 years) only about one-third of the people who initially responded to carbamazepine continue to find it effective. One small RCT found insufficient evidence to compare carbamazepine versus tizanidine.
>
> Baclofen: We found no systemic review or RCTs of baclofen in people with trigeminal neuralgia.
>
> Lamotrigine: One week crossover RCT identified by systemic review provided insufficient evidence about the effects of lamotrigine in people with trigeminal neuralgia.
>
> Other drugs (phenytoin, clonazepam, sodium valproate, gabapentin, mexiletine, oxcarbazepine, and topiramate): We have found no systemic review or RCTs of sufficient quality of the antiepileptic drugs with the antiarrhythmic drug mexiletine in patients with trigeminal neuralgia.

One other antiepileptic agent, pimozide, has some Class 2 evidence. Pimozide, a neuroleptic, has had a narrow application in patients who fail carbamazepine therapy (Lechin et al. 1989). This drug was successful in a blinded crossover study in a large cohort of patients.

Thus, an algorithm for the medical management of a newly diagnosed case of TN would look like this:

- Carbamazepine as the initial choice (unless the patient is anemic or had a previous reaction)
- Oxcarbazepine as an effective alternative to first-line treatment if carbamazepine is contraindicated or not tolerated; the incidence of cross-reactivity between the two drugs is low
- Gabapentin as a third option, if the sedating effects of the two first-line drugs preclude effectiveness

- Aim to control the pain until remission occurs, as drug treatment does not prevent future attacks or alter the disease process. Start with a low dose and titrate slowly upward until the pain settles or adverse effects limit further dose increases.

Typically, carbamazepine is initially dosed at 100 mg three times daily, with increases by 200 mg/day every week until a maximum dose of 2,000–2,500 mg/day is reached. Patients have reported relief without toxicity at all of these levels. The occurrence of toxicity does not appear to be related to the measured blood levels.

The initial dose for oxcarbazepine is 300 mg twice daily over the first 7 days. The dose may be escalated to 900–1,800 mg/day, with the latter being the most common effective dose in a cohort of American patients.

Gabapentin can be started at 200 mg twice daily, increasing up to 1,800 mg/day in the second week. This drug has a maximum recommended dose of 3,600 mg/day, although instances of higher doses with little or no toxicity or organ effects have been documented.

Careful documentation of dose and effect is essential:

- A pain diary is useful to assess the frequency of the attacks and response to treatment. A pain diary can help adjust the timing of the dose(s) and, if needed, allow for extended-release preparations to be introduced to cover sleep periods and other periods between doses.
- When pain is in remission, reduce the dose of the drug, but avoid totally withdrawing the drug while the patient remains pain-free. An ideal baseline dose is 25% of the treatment dose used to obtain pain relief.
- If the pain recurs, restart a maintenance drug at a higher dose before adding a second agent.
- If first-line drug treatment is ineffective, or cannot be tolerated, first refer for neurosurgery and second, consider additional medications while awaiting referral. Options at this point include adding a tricyclic antidepressant (amitriptyline, nortriptyline, imipramine) rather than a selective serotonin reuptake inhibitor (SSRI) or baclofen. (Gronseth et al. 2008)

Zakrewska and colleagues have emphasized our gaps in both knowledge and evidence in the medical treatment of TN (Spatz, Zakrzewska and Kay. 2007. They remind us that "trials of nonepileptic drugs for treating trigeminal neuralgia have all been limited by poor methodological quality or poor reporting."

OPERATIVE TREATMENT

The history of operative TN treatment offers important insights into both the evolving field of pain management and the pathophysiology of TN.

With Bell and Magendie's separation of the functions of the fifth nerve, the path to a direct attack on the problem was open. Prior to that, however, Avicenna had suggested alcohol for peripheral pain: an early attempt at a chemolytic solution. More attempts at chemoneurolysis followed. Maréchal, surgeon to Louis XIV, attempted to cut the infraorbital nerve of André's patient in 1756, but failed; however, chemoneurolysis was uses by André with good success (André 1688). The procedure was repeated in 18 months, again with success. This mimics our present experiences with some of the percutaneous chemical procedures using agents such as glycerol and alcohol. Sweet detailed how André was careful to include an unbiased audience to his surgery. The criticism of his initial procedures was blunted by this testimony of his peers: "He was perfectly cured by an operation which André performed" (Sweet 1985). This unbiased assessment created a climate for continued work in the area of chemoneurolysis.

In the 1904 edition of the *Therapeutic Gazette*, Neuber was credited with the first use of osmic acid for nerve pain (Wright 1904). He used as many as 20 percutaneous injections, suggesting that this was a difficult technique with which to achieve success, at least at the peripheral level. Eulenberg recorded very little success with his series using the same technique; however, Schapiro had five of eight cases do well. Schapiro was using 1% osmic acid dissolved in glycerin. It may well be that the glycerin was the active agent, as we see later with the work by Hartl (1913) and Håkasson (Håkasson 1981); Williams reported a case series that started in 1897, using osmic acid with continued success in patients up to 2.5 years after the first injection. Chemoneurolysis became a focal part of the treatment for TN in the late 1800s. Both Barthlow in 1876 and Neuber in 1883 determined that the treatment of chemoneurolysis had beneficial effects, but suggested different agents and anatomic loci for use. Barthlow used chloroform, Neuber used osmic acid, but both made injections in the vicinity of the nerve trunk. This led to further experimentation, finally culminating in the use of a gasserian alcohol injection for TN in 1904 by Schloesser (Horrax 1952). However, alcohol was not without its side effects, including weakened muscles and sensory loss. Even with the use of alcohol, TN eventually reappeared, presumably through nerve regeneration and recovery.

This did not stop the investigation into peripheral treatments, however. Instead, new areas for application were explored. In 1907, Wright injected the gasserian ganglion with osmic acid using an open transcranial approach, and in 1910, Harris used the percutaneous approach (Harris 1950; Wright 1904). By 1937, Harris, with a series of 1,433 patients, demonstrated that multiple injections would likely be needed before relief from pain occurred. However this technique (multiple injections) had a lower recurrence rate. With the use of these varied agents, the complications were still formidable: paresthesiae, activation of herpes, hyperesthesia, neuroparalytic keratitis, unilateral loss of taste, and paralysis of mastication were seen in many subjects. Despite this, the main limitation of the treatment was the occurrence of multiple nerve palsies. Many thought this was related to the operative approach, and Hartl was credited with defining an alternate approach through the foramen ovale, which is widely used today (Hartl 1913). Through that approach, Harris completed a series in which patients experienced sustained relief for as long as 3 years, accompanied by complete facial anesthesia. Harris reported a series of alcohol injections in 316 patients, given during 1910–1947.

Alcohol remained in use until the mid 1970s, but gradually has been replaced by aliphatic alcohol (glycerol). The use of glycerol became quite popular after Håkanson's initial report using Hartl's transforaminal approach (Håkanson 1978, 1981). Glycerol remains a popular option primarily for gasserian ganglion use at the current time (Lunsford, Bennet and Martinez 1985). A series of papers have discussed its use in more peripheral locations.

In the later 19th century, Winternitz and Walker used ice for peripheral pain control (Winternitz 1873). They reported reasonable time-limited success, and cryotherapy continues to be utilized in small series, with reasonable success. Zakrewska followed 145 patients after peripheral cryotherapy, with a median time to pain recurrence of 14 months in the infraorbital location, less for the mental nerve (Zakrzewska & Nally 1999). The results of cryotherapy seem more durable than peripheral neurectomy.

Unfortunately, Pujol's warning notwithstanding, patients continue to experience the removal of a large number of teeth, in the name of "curing" facial pain. In 1999, correlating data from the Trigeminal Neuralgia Association database, an average of 9.2 teeth were removed in patients prior to their diagnosis with TN. Fifty percent of the patients with TN had had extensive dental work, and 100% of those surveyed reported no lasting relief from the tooth extractions, whereas 44% of the group reported that the dental work made the pain worse (personal communication, K. Casey).

Nerve avulsion was revived after Putnam and Waterman indicated an average relief of 10 months with their 43 cases as cited by Murphy and Neff (1901). However, other reports followed that showed the duration of success with peripheral procedures was more short-lived and rather disappointing. Thus, in 1844, John Mears suggested a gasserian ganglion resection for trigeminal pain, and Rose performed the first successful procedure in 1890 (McKenzie 1934; Rose 1907). Rose commented, "the main trunks should be attacked as they emerge from the cranium, and success depends on the amount resected… ." He had quite durable results lasting up to 6 years, but other practitioners noted that the approach had significant hazards, especially those related to bleeding. Frank Hartley then chose an extradural temporal approach. After further description of this approach, Krause reported a successful total ganglionectomy utilizing an extradural intracranial approach. Following more widespread application of that approach, Rose demonstrated a high likelihood of bleeding from the middle meningeal artery and therefore proposed a retrogasserian approach.

Frazier did this procedure successfully in 1901. Tiffany then emphasized the importance of preserving the motor branch to reduce some of the complications related to the procedure, as detailed by Stookey and Ransohoff (Stookey & Ransohoff 1959). Frazier subsequently suggested the idea of subtotal sectioning of the nerve, specifically sectioning only the fascicles of the sensory root in the outer two-thirds of the ganglion and sparing the motor root on the inner third. Attempting to reconcile these methods, Cushing (who coined the term *tic convulsif*) commented, "The methods proposed by Doyen, Quénu, Poirier, and the French school utilizing an approach known as the combined temporosphenoidal route, still possesses some of the disadvantages of the method Rose . . for though the exposure is better, the ganglion is approached from below through the bloody area of the pterygoid plexus with the necessary ligation of the internal maxillary artery, and after location of the inferior maxillary nerve, the nerve mandibularis, the roof of the zygomatic fossa is rongeured away to the foramen ovale and an attempt is made to remove the ganglion by utilizing this nerve as a guide to its position" (Cushing 1900).

In view of some of these issues, Doyen, in 1917, employed an endoscope during a suboccipital craniectomy to perform a trigeminal rhizotomy (Doyen 1917). Dandy extended this approach using a horseshoe incision and a generous retromastoid craniectomy to approach the nerve more directly. Dandy emphasized the importance of the junction of the transverse sinus/sigmoid sinus transition and dural opening exposure to approach the fifth cranial nerve. He felt that this approach more easily preserved the motor branch, as had been previously advocated by Tiffany. It was Dandy who first observed in his patients that the nerve seemed to be compressed by a vascular loop (Dandy 1934).

However, Dandy's insight and success were overshadowed by Cushing's, already a giant among his peers, who felt that the total ganglionectomy as performed by Spiller and Frazier was the proper route to follow. Due perhaps to the dominance of the Philadelphia School of Neurosurgery, posterior root section was the predominant procedure for some 50 years (Spiller & Frazier 1901). Although relief was afforded to 95% of the patients initially, long-term success was incompletely documented and not durable. The 3-year results for many patients included partial or complete return of the pain in the affected distribution. This may be related to the observations of Cajal and Beyers regarding the mixed sensory and motor nerve fibers in the portio minor or motor portion of the fifth nerve (Byers et al. 1986; Cajal, Pasik, & Pasik 2000). The presence of these sensory fibers, 30% of the nerve by most accounts, may allow for persistent pain signaling to the abnormal trigeminal nuclear complex despite sectioning of the main nerve.

Other approaches were sought to reduce the morbidity of ganglionectomy and nerve section. Galvanism swept through medicine in the 1870s and 1880s, producing all varieties of electrical applications, especially to the face of patients with TN. Blunt reported the use of electricity in 1786, following his failure with hemlock. His approach was to apply sparks and shocks to "the part which had been uniformly the seed of pain" twice daily. He did this for consecutive days of treatment and found that this caused the patient's pain to subside for a sizable interval, by his account. Keen, who codified the approach, reported it to be very useful in cases of neuralgia and neuritis. However, in 1931, Kirschner described his elaborate operative setup that included a specially designed head frame to guide the insertion of an insulated needle through the foramen ovale to perform electrocoagulation to the gasserian ganglion (Rushton & Macdonald 1957). In these techniques, monopolar Bovie-type current was used for the coagulation. With only modest technical advances over the next few decades, electrocoagulation continued to have a relatively high application, but also relatively high complication rate. Kirschner reported that, in 10% of his cases, the needle did not enter the foramen ovale, and pain relief was transient. Electrocoagulation remained somewhat of a secondary procedure until Sweet reintroduced the lesioning procedure by combining electrophysiological localization and a thermistor tip to guide the lesion site (Sweet 1985). Cosman and his collaborators refined the lesion generator to produce discrete, well-controlled lesions with additional refinements to the thermistor tip (Cosman, Nashold, & Bedenbaugh 1983). Tew further developed the procedure, later producing specific root lesions with his directional tip method (Taha and Tew 1996).

In 1896, Louis Tiffany had noted the importance of sparing the ophthalmic division to maintain corneal protection. With Tew's directional electrode, this has become the standard for the technique. Corneal complications, however, have remained at between 2% and 14%. Electrocoagulation utilizing radiofrequency lesioning produces durable relief, as reported by Taha and Tew (1996).

The previously reported neuroablative approach, using glycerol, was enhanced by Håkanson's report of transovale cysternography in 1978 (Håkanson 1978). Transovale trigeminal cysternography offered the possibility to control the position of the tip of the needle relative to the various portions of the nerve at the level of the trigeminal ganglion. Håkanson also commented that cysternography "may also be used for target localization and stereotactic radiosurgery in the treatment of trigeminal neuralgia." In fact, it was in the latter situation, in the clinic of Lars Leksell, that Håkanson first reported the use of glycerol and tantalum dust and its serendipitous effect on pain relief. Glycerol has remained a part of armamentarium of neuroablative procedures. It is used preferentially in patients with multiple sclerosis and TN, with an initial success rate of approximately 80%; however, 50% of these patients experience recurrent pain within 18 months. This is true for patients with classic type 1 TN.

Mullan had an interest in treating head and neck pain in cancer patients. In 1980, he described some of the uses of a balloon technique in neurosurgery.

This included "a compression balloon to treat trigeminal neuralgia [with] a dilating balloon to release the web obstruction in the internal carotid artery, a detachable balloon to seal carotid cavernous and vertebral venous fistulas,... a temporary occlusive balloon to aid in the thrombogenic treatment of giant aneurysm, and... a temporary occlusive balloon with a double or triple lumen capacity to assist in the angiographic diagnosis and to provide reversible carotid occlusion in those settings" (Mullan 1980). Mullan saw great applications for temporary balloon occlusion in neurosurgery. Teaming up with Lichtor, they reported success with balloon compression of the fifth nerve in a large cohort of patients (Mullan & Lichtor 1983). Subsequently, these authors and others have gone on to detail the effects of balloon size, time of compression, and the amount of pressure delivered. The initial success rate of balloon compression is generally reported at 80%–85%, with a robust 66% of the patients remaining pain-free at 4 years; the incidence of permanent numbness hovers at 5%–7% (Skirving 2001).

Irradiation originated as a treatment when, in 1897, Gocht introduced the use of radiotherapy for the treatment of TN. He treated a patient who had failed other therapies over the previous 10 years (Calchi-Novati 1937). The patient was treated daily for one-half hour with the newly described Roentgen ray. The patient experienced little pain from the second day onward, although his cheek and facial hair showed evidence of radiation changes.

Subsequently, the value of this technique was widely recognized by radiologists and neurosurgeons, and is still acclaimed as a brilliant intuition. Gocht's pioneering work led to the concept of radiosurgery to treat TN (Bongiovanni 1907; Rand et al. 1993). Leksell treated three patients with an orthovoltage stereotactic technique, which provided long-term relief of TN symptoms. With the introduction of the gamma knife, a series of 46 patients were treated in Stockholm, but had less encouraging results; the target in these cases was the gasserian ganglion, and targeting was by bony landmarks or cysternography. The dosages reported were 16.5 GY and 22 GY, and the length of relief was recorded as 1 and 5 months, respectively. The re-entry zone was later suggested as the target for radiosurgery following case reports in which 12 patients were treated with 57–75 GY. Seven of the 12 reported relief; the interval to continued relief was not specified, however (Leksell 1971).

A multi-institutional study authored by Kondziolka confirmed the utility of this latter target (Kondziolka et al. 1996). Currently, radiosurgery, whether linear accelerator or gamma based, provides relief in 88% of patients; 30%–45% report themselves to be pain free and utilizing no further medications. Sixty percent report a decrease in the pain by 50% or better. At 2 years, 15%–18% of these patients have developed paresthesia in the irradiated areas, and recurrence rates range between 18% and 22% or higher.

The use of balloon, glycerol, radiofrequency, and radiosurgery treatments have sought to relieve pain using neuroablation or a controlled injury to the nerve (Abdennebi, Mahfouf, & Nedjahi 1997; Caram-Salas et al. 2006; Fisher, Zakrzewska, & Patsalos 2003; Meglio 1987); however, the difficulty of controlling the extent of nerve injury in some cases and the problem of recurrence prompted a different approach, based on the observations of previous surgeons. Following Jurjani's hypothesis, Dandy observed that some patients undergoing operation for TN appeared to have vessels lying across the nerve (Dandy 1934). Gardner and Miklos (1959) extended this observation by suggesting that decompression of the sensory root would result in pain relief, but were limited by poor magnification tools. Gardner's thinking was superb but his findings and results were handicapped by limited technology.

Jannetta introduced the operating microscope to this problem and, using a variation of Dandy's approach, characterized and quantified the steps in the vascular decompression technique (Jannetta 1967, 1975; Jannetta et al. 1977; Barker et al. 1996; McLaughlin et al. 1999). Jannetta offered the operation as an alternative to ablative procedures, opening an era in which neuromodulation gained promise over neuroablation for pain management, especially in the central nervous system. Microvascular decompression (MVD) has emerged as the first approach for the healthy patient with classic type (or type 1) TN. The concerns regarding the risk of this procedure have yielded to accumulated data showing its safety and efficacy. Death (0.4% or less), stroke (0.1% or less), hearing loss (0.8%), cerebrospinal fluid leaks (3%), and infection (1%) occur at an acceptably low rate with careful attention to detail, knowledgeable posterior fossa operative techniques, and intraoperative electrophysiologic monitoring.

In the early 21st century, five standard modalities exist with which to treat TN: glycerol, radiofrequency, balloon compression, radiosurgery, and MVD. Comparison data among the procedures exist, (Lopez et al 2004) although, in general, Class 1 data on the combined effects of different procedures in one patient are difficult to obtain, despite larger databases (i.e., the effect of a previous glycerol procedure on the subsequent success rate of MVD). Several analyses exist to offer comparisons across the spectrum of procedures (Ong & Seng 2003).

Sindou and colleagues (2007) recently compiled a review in which they stated:

> Twenty-eight studies, mostly including microvascular decompression (MVD) and radiofrequency thermal rhizotomy (RF-TR) that met the inclusion criteria are included in the review. The efficacy of MVD and percutaneous balloon compression (PBC) were similar (odds ratio = 0.15 $p > 0.05$), and their effects were superior to the other modalities ($p < 0.001$). Although RF-TR provided a high initial pain relief, its average pain free rate was 50.4% for a mean follow up of five years. Recurrence rate was high after RF-TR (46%) while the lowest recurrence rate (18.3%) was

> after MVD ($p < 0.001$). Within the long-term follow-up period, recurrence of pain affects at least 19% of the patients who undergo any surgical treatment for TN… . (Sindou et al. 2007)

This review suggests that each operative technique for the treatment of TN has merits and limitations. However, MVD provides the highest rate of long-term patient satisfaction with the lowest rate of pain recurrence and better quality of life. Nonetheless, Class 1 data are still lacking.

Zakrewska and her group from London have pointed out the inconclusive nature of many surgical papers covering the treatment of TN (Zakrzewska & Lopez 2003), and they have outlined potential directions for future work (Zakrzewska 2006). There is, however, bright light at the end of the tunnel of clinical work: Patients are reporting improved quality of life following all types of operative therapy. Using a questionnaire to measure disease-specific satisfaction, Zakrewska and colleagues reported that patients' outcomes were uniformly high for MVD (Spatz, Zakrzewska and Kay 2007). In addition, the Trigeminal Neuralgia Association/Facial Pain Association have established a registry in which patients report both medical and surgical use and outcomes; evaluation of the resulting database demonstrates that operative therapy is preferred to medical therapy by patients, especially as regards their improved quality of life. Patients persist in choosing operative therapy over medication, even when repeat surgical procedures are required following a classic pain occurrence.

Future trends in pain-related surgery are directed at neuromodulation and nanotherapy (Al Malyan et al. 2006; Brown & Pilitsis 2005; Leary, Liu, Yu & Apuzzo 2005; Leary, Liu, & Apuzzo 2006a, 2006b) (Rasche et al 2006). Neuroablative procedures are becoming less attractive due to some of the effects on redundant pain systems. Thus, motor cortex and deep brain stimulation, direct gasserian stimulation, and novel analgesic delivery systems are some of the current applications being explored in the field of TN treatment Rappaport and Devor 1994). Among these new technologies are nanoscaffolds to aid in nerve repair, and Apuzzo and colleagues have outlined an early map in the as-yet uncharted territory of nanoneurosurgery for less invasive, more correlative pain procedures.

Pain control is an important goal since 21% of the world's population experience some form of chronic pain. Trigeminal neuralgia, as a prototypical example of neuropathic pain, can offer both historical precedence as well as valuable future signposts for neurosurgeons to continue in their role as preeminent clinicians in the diagnosis and treatment of pain.

REFERENCES

Abdennebi B, Mahfouf L, Nedjahi T. Long-term results of percutaneous compression of the gasserian ganglion in trigeminal neuralgia (series of 200 patients). *Stereotact Funct Neurosurg* 1997;68:190–195.

Al Malyan M, Becch C, Nikkola L, et al. Polymer-based biodegradable drug delivery systems in pain management. *J Craniofac Surg* 2006;17:302–313.
Al-Jurjani. *Zayn al-Din al-Jurjani* (The Thesaurus of the Shah of Khwarazm). 1110.
André N. Observations pratiques sur les maladies de l'urethre et sur plusieurs faits convulsifs, & la guérison de plusieurs maladies chirurgicales, avec la decomposition d'un remède proper à réprimer la dissolution gangréneuse & concéreuse, & á la réparer; avec des principes qui pourront server à employer les differens caustiques.
Paris: Delaguette (1756). *J Neurol Neurosurg Psychiatry* 2003;74:1688; doi:10.1136/jnnp.74.12.1688.
Aretaeus AF. *The extant works of Aretaeus, the Cappadocian.* London: Sydenham Society, 1856.
Avicenna GO. *The canon of medicine of Avicenna,* adapted by Laleh Bakhtiar. Chicago: Kazi Publications, 1999.
Barker FG, Jannetta PJ, Bissonnette DJ, et al. The long-term outcome of microvascular decompression for trigeminal neuralgia. *N Engl J Med* 1996;334(17):1077–1083.
Beaver DL, Moses HL, Ganote CE. Electron microscopy of the trigeminal ganglion. II. Autopsy study of human ganglia. *Arch Pathol* 1965;79:557–570.
Beaver DL, Moses HL, Ganote CE. Electron microscopy of the trigeminal ganglion. III. Trigeminal neuralgia. *Arch Pathol* 1965;79:571–582.
Beaver DL. Electron microscopy of the trigeminal ganglion in trigeminal neuralgia. *J Neurosurg* 1967;26(Suppl):38–150.
Bennett MH, Janetta PJ. Evoked potentials in trigeminal neuralgia. *Neurosurgery* 1983;13:242.
Bergouignan M. Cures heureuses de neurologies essentielles par le dephenyl hydantoinate de sounde. *Rev Laryngol Otol Rhinol* 1942;63:34–41.
Blom S. Trigeminal neuralgia: its treatment with a new anticonvulsant drug (G-32883). *Lancet* 1962;1:839–840.
Bongiovanni A. Alcune applicazioni pratiche della radium terapia alla cura delle paralisi periferiche del faciale e nevralgie del trigemino. Nuovo apparecchio. (Some practical applications of radium therapy in the treatment of peripheral paralysis of faciale and trigeminal neuralgia. New equipment). *Gazz Osp Clin* 1907;93:962–964.
Brown D. *Encyclopedia of herbs & their uses.* London, New York: Dorling Kindersley, 1999.
Brown JA, Pilitsis JG. Motor cortex stimulation for central and neuropathic facial pain: a prospective study of 10 patients and observations of enhanced sensory and motor function during stimulation. *Neurosurgery* 2005;56:290–297.
Burchiel K. A new classification for facial pain. *Neurosurgery* 2003;53:1164–1166.
Byers MR, O'Connor TA, Martin RF, Dong WK. Mesencephalic trigeminal sensory neurons of cat: axon pathways and structure of mechanoreceptive endings in periodontal ligament. *J Comp Neurol* 1986;250:181–191.
Cajal SR, Pasik P, Pasik T. Texture of the nervous system of man and the vertebrates, volume 2. Wien: Springer, 2000.
Calchi-Novati G. La roentgenterapia nelle nevralgie del trigemino (The roentgen therapy in trigeminal neuralgia). *Rivista di Clinica Medica (Firence)* 1937;38.
Caram-Salas NL, Reyes-García G, Medina-Santillán R, Granados-Soto V. Thiamine and cyanocobalamin relieve neuropathic pain in rats: synergy with dexamethasone. *Pharmacology* 2006;77:53–62.
Cole C, Liu J, Apfelbaum R. Historical perspectives on the diagnosis and treatment of trigeminal neuralgia. *Neurosurg Focus* 2005;18:E4.
Cosman ER, Nashold BS, Bedenbaugh P. Stereotactic radiofrequency lesion making. *Appl Neurophysiol* 1983;46(1–4):160–166.

Cushing H. A method of total extirpation of the Gasserian ganglion for trigeminal neuralgia. By a route through the temporal fossa and beneath the middle meningeal artery. *JAMA* 1900;34:1035–1041.

Dandy W. Concerning the cause of trigeminal neuralgia. *Am J Surg* 1934;24:447–455.

Devor M, Amir R, Rappaport ZH. Pathophysiology of trigeminal neuralgia: the ignition hypothesis. *Clin J Pain* 2002;18(1):4–13.

Doyen E. Surgical therapeutics and operative techniques. London: Balliere, Tindall, Cox, 1917.

Fisher A, Zakrzewska JM, Patsalos PN. Trigeminal neuralgia: current treatments and future developments. *Expert Opin Emerg Drugs* 2003;8:123–143.

Fromm GH, Terrence CF, Chattha AS. Baclofen in the treatment of trigeminal neuralgia: double-blind study and long-term follow-up. *Ann Neurol* 1984;15: 240–244.

Fromm GH, Sweet W, et al. Pre-trigeminal neuralgia. *Neurology* 1990;40:1493.

Fu QG, Carstens E, Stelzer B, Zimmerman M. B vitamins suppress spinal dorsal horn nociceptive neurons in the cat. *Neurosci Lett* 1988;95:192–197.

Gardner WJ, Miklos MV. Response of trigeminal neuralgia to "decompression" of sensory root. *JAMA* 1959;170:1773–1776.

Govoni V, Granieri E. The history of the *tic douloureux*: autopathograph of an Italian lawyer. *J Hist Neurosci* 1996;5:169–189.

Gronseth G, Cruccu G, Alksne J, et al. Practice parameter: the diagnostic evaluation and treatment of trigeminal neuralgia (an evidence-based review). Report of the Quality Standards Subcommittee of the American Academy of Neurology and the European Federation of Neurological Societies. *Neurology* 2008;71(15): 1183–1190.

Håkanson S. Transovale trigeminal cisternography. *Surg Neurol* 1978;10:137–144.

Håkanson S. Trigeminal neuralgia treated by the injection of glycerol into the trigeminal cistern. *Neurosurgery* 1981;9:628–646.

Harris W. Rare forms of paroxysmal trigeminal neuralgia. and their relation to disseminated sclerosis. *Br Med J* 1950;2:1015–1019.

Hartl F. Die Leitungsanaesthie und Ijektionsbehandlung des Ganglion Gasseri und der Trigeminusstamme Arch. *Klin Chir* 1912–1913;193.

Hilton D, Love S, Gradidge T, Coakham H. Pathological findings associated with trigeminal neuralgia caused by vascular compression. *Neurosurgery* 1994;35: 299–303.

Horrax G. *Neurosurgery: an historical sketch*. Springfield, IL: Charles H. Thomas, 1952.

Jannetta PJ. Structural mechanisms of trigeminal neuralgia. Arterial compression of the trigeminal nerve at the pons in patients with trigeminal neuralgia. *J Neurosurg* 1967;26(1 Pt. 2):159–162.

Jannetta PJ. Trigeminal neuralgia and hemifacial spasm: etiology and definitive treatment. *Trans Am Neurol Assoc* 1975;100:53–55.

Jannetta PJ, Abbasy M, Maroon JC, et al. Etiology and definitive microsurgical treatment of hemifacial spasm. Operative techniques and results in forty–seven patients. *J Neurosurg* 1977;47(3):321–328.

Jurna I, Carlsson KH, Kömen W, Bonke D. Acute effects of vitamin B6 and fixed combinations of vitamin B1, B6 and B12 on nociceptive activity evoked in the rat thalamus: dose-response relationship and combinations with morphine and paracetamol. *Klin Wochenschr* 1990;68:129–135.

Kerr FLW. Correlated light and electron microscopic observations on the normal trigeminal ganglion and sensory root in man. *J Neurosurg* 1967;26(Suppl): 132–137.

Kerr FLW. Pathology of trigeminal neuralgia: light and electron microscopic observations. *J Neurosurg* 1967;26(suppl):151–156.

Kerr F, Fraher J, Delanty F. The development of the central-peripheral transitional zone of the rat cochlear nerve. A light microscopic study. *J Anat* 1987;155: 109–118.

Kerr FWL, Miller RH. The pathology of trigeminal neuralgia. Electron microscope studies. *Arch Neurol* 1966;15(3):308–319.

Knuckey N, Gubbay S. Familial trigeminal and glossopharyngeal neuralgia. *Clin Exp Neurol* 1979;16:315–319.

Kondziolka D, Lunsford LD, Flickinger JC, et al. Stereotactic radiosurgery for trigeminal neuralgia: a multi-institutional study using the gamma unit. *J Neurosurg* 1996;84:940–945.

Leary SP, Liu CY, Yu C, Apuzzo ML. Toward the emergence of nanoneurosurgery: part I—progress in nanoscience, nanotechnology, and the comprehension of events in the mesoscale realm. *Neurosurgery* 2005;57:606–634.

Leary SP, Liu CY, Apuzzo ML. Toward the emergence of nanoneurosurgery: part II—nanomedicine: diagnostics and imaging at the nanoscale level. *Neurosurgery* 2006b;58:805–823.

Leary SP, Liu CY, Apuzzo ML. Toward the emergence of nanoneurosurgery: part III—nanomedicine: targeted nanotherapy, nanosurgery, and progress toward the realization of nanoneurosurgery. *Neurosurgery* 2006a;58:1009–1026.

Lechin F, van der Dijs B, Lechin M, et al. Pimozide therapy for trigeminal neuralgia. *Arch Neurol* 1989;46:960–963.

Leksell L. Stereotactic radiosurgery in trigeminal neuralgia. *Acta Chir Scand* 1971;137:311–314.

Lewy F. The first authentic case of major trigeminal neuralgia and some comments on the history of the disease. *Ann Med Hist* 1938;10:247–250.

Lewy F, Grant F. Physiopathologic and pathoanatomic aspects of major trigeminal neuralgia. *Arch Neurol Psychiatry* 1928;40:1126–1134.

Locke J. An essay concerning human understanding. London, 1690.

Lopez BC, Hamlyn PJ, Zakrzewska JM. Systematic review of ablative neurosurgical techniques for the treatment of trigeminal neuralgia. *Neurosurgery* 2004;54: 973–982.

Love S, Coakham HB. Trigeminal neuralgia pathology and pathogenesis. *Brain* 2001;124(12):2347–2360.

Lunsford LD, Bennett MH, Martinez AJ. Experimental trigeminal glycerol injection. Electrophysiologic and morphologic effects. *Arch Neurol* 1985;42:146–149.

Maxwell DS. Fine structure of the normal trigeminal ganglion in the cat and monkey. *J Neurosurg* 1967;26(suppl):127–131.

Maxwell DR, Kruger L, Pineda A. The trigeminal nerve root with special reference to the central-peripheral transition zone: an electron microscopic study in the macque. *Anat Rec* 1969;164:113–126.

McKenzie KG. Operative treatment of trigeminal neuralgia. *J Nerv Mental Dis* 1934; 79(5):579.

McLaughlin MR, Jannetta PJ, Clyde BL, et al. Microvascular decompression of cranial nerves: lessons learned after 4400 operations. *J Neurosurg* 1999;90:1–8.

McMurtry III J. The history of medical and surgical interests in facial pain. *Headache* 1969;9:1–6.

Meglio M. Percutaneous microcompression of the gasserian ganglion: personal experience. *Acta Neurochir Suppl (Wien)* 1987;39:142–143.

Mullan S. Some examples of balloon technology in neurosurgery. *Neurosurgery* 1980;52:321–329.

Mullan S, Lichtor T. Percutaneous microcompression of the trigeminal ganglion for trigeminal neuralgia. *J Neurosurg* 1983;59:1007–1012.

Murphy JB, Neff JM. Excision of the Gasserian ganglion. With reports of the cases operated upon by the Hartley-Krause Method. *JAMA* 1901;39(16):981–987.
Napier L, Sen Gupta P. A peculiar neurological sequel to administration of 4:4á;-diamidino-diphenyl-ethylene (M & B 744). *Indian M Gaz* 1942;77:71–74.
Ong J, Seng SB. Evaluation of surgical procedures for trigeminal neuralgia. *Anesth Prog* 2003;50(4):181–188.
Oppenheim H. Diseases of the nervous system: a text-book for students and practitioners of medicine (trans. Edward E. Mayer). Philadelphia: J.B. Lippincott, 1904.
Osler W. *The principles and practice of medicine*. New York: D. Appleton, 1913.
Plessner W. Uber Trigeminuserkrankung infolge von Trichlorathylenvergiftung (On trigeminal disease due to tricloroethylene intoxication). *Neurol Zentr* 1915;34:916–918 (Ger).
Pujol A. Essai sur la maladie de la face, nommée le tic douloureux. (Essay on the disease of the face, called tic douloureux). Paris: Barrois, 1787.
Rand RW, Jacques DB, Melbye RW, et al. Leksell gamma knife treatment of tic douloureux. *Stereotact Funct Neurosurg* 1993;61:93–102.
Rappaport Z, Devor M. Trigeminal neuralgia: the role of self-sustaining discharge in the trigeminal ganglion. *Pain* 1994;56:127–138.
Rasche D, Ruppolt M, Stippich C, et al. Motor cortex stimulation for long-term relief of chronic neuropathic pain: a 10 year experience. *Pain* 2006;121:43–52.
Rose W. Practitioner. In Keen WW, ed., *Surgery, its principles and practices.* Philadelphia: WB Saunders, 1907.
Rushton JG, Macdonald HN. Trigeminal neuralgia; special considerations of non-surgical treatment. *JAMA* 1957;165(5):437–440.
Sindou M, Leston J, Decullier E, Chapuis F. Microvascular decompression for primary trigeminal neuralgia: long-term effectiveness and prognostic factors in a series of 362 consecutive patients with clear-cut neurovascular conflicts who underwent pure decompression. *J Neurosurg* 2007;107:1144–1153.
Skirving DJ. A 20-year review of percutaneous balloon compression of the trigeminal ganglion. *J Neurosurg* 2001;94:913–917.
Smith G, Miller J. The treatment of tic douloureux with stilbamidine. *Bull John Hopkins Hosp* 1955;96:146–149.
Spatz AL, Zakrzewska JM, Kay EJ. Decision analysis of medical and surgical treatments for trigeminal neuralgia: how patient evaluations of benefits and risks affect the utility of treatment decisions. *Pain* 2007;131:302–310.
Spiller WG, Frazier CH. The division of the sensory root of the trigeminus for the relief of tic douloureux. *Univ Penn Med Bull* 1901;14:341.
Stookey B, Ransohoff J. *Trigeminal neuralgia: its history and treatment*. Springfield, IL: Charles C. Thomas, 1959.
Sweet WH. The history of the development of treatment for trigeminal neuralgia. *Clin Neurosurg* 1985;32:294–318.
Taha JM, Tew JM Jr. Comparison of surgical treatments for trigeminal neuralgia: reevaluation of radiofrequency rhizotomy. *Neurosurgery* 1996;38:865–871.
Thompson H, Cheadle H . Reports of Medical and Surgical Practice in the Hospitals of Great Britain. *The British Medical Journal* 1873;1:88–89.
Trousseau A. Clinique medicale de l'Hotel Dieu de Paris. Paris: J.B. Bailliere, 1877.
Woodhall B, Odom GL. Stilbamidine isethionate therapy of tic douloureux. *J Neurosurg* 1955;12:495–500.
Winternitz W. Tic douloureux treated by local application of ice. *Am J Med Sci* 1873; 65:262.
Wright F. Trigeminal Neuralgia. *Therapeutic Gazette* 1904;18:254.

Zakrzewska JM. Robust randomised control trials needed for drug treatments for trigeminal neuralgia. *Evidence-based Dentistry* 2006;7:107.

Zakrzewska JM, Lopez BC. Quality of reporting in evaluations of surgical treatment of trigeminal neuralgia: recommendations for future reports. *Neurosurgery* 2003;53:110–120.

Zakrzewska JM, Lopez BC, Kim SE, et al. Patient satisfaction after surgery for trigeminal neuralgia: development of a questionnaire. *Acta Neurochir (Wien)* 2005;147:925–932.

Zakrewska JM, Nally FF. The role of cryotherapy on paroxysmal trigeminal neuralgia: a six year experience. *Br J Oral Maxillo Surg* 1999;29:1–4.

2

Anatomy and Physiology

Kenneth F. Casey

The trigeminal nerve is the largest of the cranial nerves. It takes its origin in the cell bodies located in the gasserian ganglion. The ganglion is located in the dural fold labeled the cave of Meckel. The semilunar ganglion (*ganglion semilunare* [*gasseri*]; *gasserian ganglion*) occupies a cavity (*cavum Meckelii*) in the dura mater covering the trigeminal impression, near the apex of the petrous part of the temporal bone. It is somewhat crescent shaped, with its convexity directed forward: medially, it lies in relation with the internal carotid artery and the posterior part of the cavernous sinus. The anatomy of the region of the gasserian ganglion was extensively measured and described by Kanavel and Davis (1922). They found the gasserian ganglion to be immediately subjacent to the foramen lacerum, separated by a fibrous membrane. In 40% of cases, this was quite thin, and in a minority, contained some thin bone. These data were from 60 cadaver dissections. The dimensions for the ganglion were 1.0 cm width (W), 0.8 anterior-posterior (AP) (range W 0.41.0, AP 1.4–2.2 cm). The authors also noted that the motor branch was usually easily separated from the sensory root, and lay superomedial to it in the posterior portion of the fossa of Meckel. Cushing and many previous authors described it as coursing medial to the ganglion in the midportion, and exiting by angling toward the mandibular branch in the foramen ovale. The root was described as "somewhat whiter… and more compact, about the size of the lead of a pencil." Medially, this is bounded by the internal carotid artery; inferiorly by the motor root of the greater petrosal nerve; and inferomedially and superiorly by the foramen lacerum.

The motor root, the portio minor, which also carries proprioceptive fibers, is frequently double and splays out at the pons. Fascicles on the portio major separate out from the coalescent area as the nerve nears the pons. This portio intermedius (Jannetta 1966, 1967) appears to carry mainly proprioception, including the stretch receptors in the masticatory muscles (Carpenter 1976). One cannot differentiate the portio intermedius from the portio minor (motor-proprioceptive) fascicles proximally. This anatomy was partly described by Dandy (1929, 1945) and subsequently, and more comprehensively, by Jannetta and Rand (1966) and Jannetta (1967), using a binocular dissecting microscope. The nerve has about 100 fascicles just inside Meckel's cave. These fascicles enter individually into the cone of central myelin, the coalescent area, which can extend nearly to Meckel's cave (the so-called "fibrous cone"), with others entering separately at the brainstem (portio minor, portio intermedius) (Jannetta and Rand 1966, 1967). One can count about 65 fascicles near the pons. The number of fibers found in the motor root of the human trigeminal nerve is estimated to be 8,100, of which 20% carry sensory information as well, whereas the sensory root (portio major) has approximately 140,000 fibers, 20% of which are classified as unmyelinated C fibers.

The trigeminal nerve root arising from the gasserian ganglion travels to the brainstem and enters on the lateral aspect of the pons in the anterolateral quadrant. The trigeminal nerve maintains somatotopic order during its course from the side of brainstem. In the region of the ganglion, the maxillary fibers lie between the ophthalmic fibers medial and the mandibular fibers laterally. Rotation occurs as the root goes toward the root entry zone (REZ), thus causing the ophthalmic fibers to lie caudally and the mandibular fibers cephalad, with the maxillary fibers sandwiched between. It penetrates through the middle cerebral peduncle, with approximately 50% of the fibers dividing and the remaining 50% ascending and terminating in the nucleus of the trigeminal nerve. This is of note in that these purely sensory nerve endings have their cell bodies lying within the central nervous system. The ascending fibers go to a principal sensory nucleus and the descending fibers, especially the longer segments, terminate in the uppermost cervical segments of the spinal cord. The fibers entering the spinal trigeminal nucleus have topographical organization as described by Kerr. (1966) and Jacquin et al (1982) The V_1 fibers are most ventral and the V_3 fibers are most dorsal, with the V_2 fibers in between. This spatial orientation is reflected in the well-known onion-skin pattern on the face, as projections from the upper spinal nucleus represent the central area of the nose, whereas the lips are seen in the peripheral portion of the lower nucleus of the brainstem.

Several studies have suggested that the fibers from the three divisions do not intermingle as they pass through the spinal trigeminal tract and spinal trigeminal nucleus. In addition to the sensory fibers, the spinal trigeminal tract has general somatic afferent fibers, which come from the facial, glossopharyngeal, and vagus nerves. These ascending fibers carry the sensory modalities of fine touch and two-point discrimination, and from here the proprioceptive information goes to the mesencephalic nucleus. The mesencephalic nucleus also receives muscle spindle-fiber efferent information, as well as afferent information from the facial muscles and extraocular muscles, and from the two special receptors. Those fibers form the first afferent arc of the trigeminal reflex arc, which goes to the motor nucleus via the spinal trigeminal tract. The descending fibers from the brainstem synapse in the spinal trigeminal nucleus, with some fibers going to the solitary tract. The spinal trigeminal nucleus is itself divided into the nucleus oralis, interpolaris, and caudalis.

The nucleus caudalis is found at the level of the obex to approximately C4, and has fiber synapses of A-delta and C fibers, as well as interaxonal connections. In addition to fifth nerve, input from cranial nerves VII, IX, and X; the medial and lateral cuneate nuclei; and the nucleus caudalis in the upper level of the cervical spinal cord also go to the nucleus caudalis. It is in the nucleus caudalis that nociception as a primary event occurs in the trigeminal nerve, integrating information from the upper neck and entire head and neck ipsilaterally. In the same region of the brainstem, the motor nucleus lies in the upper pons of cranial nerves IV and V. It receives afferent input from the corticonuclear tracts and local sensory nuclei, including the locus caeruleus, medial longitudinal fasciculus, and nuclei of cranial nerves IX and X. It is through these pathways that mastication is coordinated, as well as integrated with the need for salivary secretion.

Cranial nerve V also projects fibers to the contralateral ventral posteromedial nucleus of the thalamus using the trigeminal lemniscus. This in turn sends fibers to the sensory cortex both in the S1 and S2 areas. Trigeminal nuclei in the brainstem project to the nucleus centralis, which is medial to the ventral posteromedial nucleus and to the contralateral superior colliculus. Fibers running in the nucleus caudalis also project to the periaqueductal gray in the midbrain and other elements of the limbic circuit, which are less well defined.

HISTOLOGY OF THE TRIGEMINAL NERVE AND GANGLION

Ultrastructure of the Trigeminal Ganglion

Within the trigeminal ganglion, neuronal cell bodies tend to occur in clusters separated by myelinated and unmyelinated fibers, capillaries, fibroblasts, and collagen fibrils. The cytoplasm processes of surrounding satellite cells and Schwann cells engulf each neuron. Most commonly, the satellite cells project microvilli into the small intercellular space between the neuronal membrane and the satellite cell. These spaces are devoid of a basement membrane. The cytoplasm of ganglion cells contains varying amounts of Nissl substance, Golgi vacuoles, mitochondria, pigment (remarkably lacking in melanin), and small dense bodies. The nuclei are central in position and exhibit an irregular nuclear membrane shape. The nucleolus exhibits two portions: An osmiophilic granular cortex and a finely granular, less–electron-dense eccentric area. Within the nucleoplasm are aggregates of irregular electron-dense particles, 20–30 mμ in diameter, and prominent 300–400 mμ diameter spheroids (Beaver, Moses, & Ganote 1965; Moses, Beaver, & Ganote 1965).

The trigeminal ganglion in trigeminal neuralgia (TN) has ultrastructural findings of note. The cytoplasm of trigeminal ganglion cells in patients with TN exhibit a peculiar vacuolization, giving the cells a fenestrated appearance. This appears to be unrelated to mitochondrial swelling or Golgi apparatus dilation. The satellite cells also exhibit irregular cytoplasmic vacuolization, but to a lesser degree. Aside from vacuolization, both the neuronal cell bodies and satellite cells appear unaltered from normal. The Schwann cells investing myelinated axons in the trigeminal ganglia of TN patients, however, appear markedly different. In some areas, the Schwann cells appear degenerated, often preceding the loss of myelin. In other areas, there is evidence of marked and disorganized hypermyelination. In areas of severe degeneration, nerve axis cylinders appear folded, tangled, or plicated (*plexiform microneuroma*) (Beaver et al. 1965).

Central Myelin–Peripheral Myelin Transition Zone

The vascular compression theory of TN proposes that compression of or proximal to the central–peripheral myelin transition zone (TZ; the Obersteiner-Redlich line) of the trigeminal nerve by a vessel is the central cause of TN. In general, there is a very sharp demarcation between central and peripheral myelin in the trigeminal nerve. The distance from the pons to the TZ is shorter on the medial aspect of the nerve than on the lateral aspect (mean 1.13 mm medially vs. 2.47 mm laterally). The zones themselves vary in shape between blunt/short (46%), gradually tapered (49%), and sharp/long (6%). The average length of central myelin is 2.55 mm, whereas the mean cisternal portion of the nerve is 12.3 mm, so that the average proportion of centrally myelinated cisternal nerve is 23%.

The nerve is organized into three branches (ophthalmic, maxillary, mandibular) to and from the facial structures; the ophthalmic and maxillary branches consist exclusively of sensory fibers; the mandibular branch is joined outside the cranium by the motor root. The ophthalmic nerve carries sensory information from the scalp and forehead, upper eyelid, conjunctiva and cornea of the eye, nose (including the tip of the nose), nasal mucosa, frontal sinuses, and parts of the meninges (the dura and blood vessels). The ophthalmic branch is a 2.5 cm long, flat band as it leaves the gasserian ganglion; it passes forward along the lateral wall of the cavernous sinus, below the oculomotor and trochlear nerves. The ophthalmic nerve then divides to supply sensation to the eyeball, lachrymal glands, and conjunctiva; part of the nasal mucosa; and skin of the nose, eyelid, and forehead. Prior to entering the orbit, through the superior orbital fissure, it divides into three branches, lachrymal, frontal, and nasociliary.

The maxillary nerve carries sensory information from the lower eyelid and cheek; nares and upper lip; upper teeth and gums; nasal mucosa; palate and roof of the pharynx; maxillary, ethmoid, and sphenoid sinuses; and parts of the meninges. The maxillary nerve is the intermediate branch; it begins at the middle of the semilunar ganglion as a flattened plexiform band, and, passing horizontally forward, it leaves the skull through the foramen rotundum, where it becomes more cylindrical in form and firmer in texture. It then crosses the pterygopalatine fossa, inclines laterally on the back of the maxilla, and enters the orbit through the inferior orbital fissure; it traverses the infraorbital groove and canal in the floor of the orbit, and appears upon the face at the infraorbital foramen.

The mandibular nerve carries sensory information from the lower lip, lower teeth and gums, chin and jaw (except the angle of the jaw, which is supplied by C2–C3), parts of the external ear, and parts of the meninges. The mandibular nerve is the largest of the three divisions of the fifth nerve, and is made up of two roots: a large, sensory root proceeding from the inferior angle of the semilunar ganglion, and a small motor root (the motor part of the trigeminal), which passes beneath the ganglion and unites with the sensory root, just after its exit through the foramen ovale. It divides into several sensory branches to supply sensation to the lower third of the face and the tongue, floor of the mouth, and the jaw. The motor root of the mandibular nerve innervates the four muscles of mastication (masseter, buccinator pterygoids, temporalis), then the mylohyoid, anterior belly of digastric, tensor muscle of the tympanic membranes, and tensor muscle of the velum palatinum.

The intermediate root (occasionally present) will emerge between the principal sensory root and the motor root, which is more rostral and composed of two to three rootlets. The mandibular nerve carries touch/position and pain/temperature sensation from the mouth. It does not carry taste sensation, but one of its branches, the lingual nerve carries multiple types of nerve fibers that do not originate in the mandibular nerve.

The nerve endings on the afferent side are located in the skin of the face, sinuses, mucosa, mouth, middle ear, tympanic membrane, teeth, tongue. The nerve is served by modality receptors for pinprick, touch, pressure, temperature, and vibration. In general, touch/position information is carried by myelinated (fast-conducting) nerve fibers, whereas pain/temperature information is carried by unmyelinated (slow-conducting) nerve fibers. The primary sensory receptors for touch/position (Meissner's corpuscles, Merkel's receptors, Pacinian corpuscles, Ruffini's corpuscles, hair receptors, muscle spindle organs, Golgi tendon organs) are structurally more complex than the primitive receptors for pain/temperature, which are bare nerve endings. Proprioceptive receptors exist in the periapical portions of the teeth, as well as in the mandible. There are afferent fibers from the muscles of mastication (masseter, buccinators, pterygoids), as well as from the tensor tympani and tensor palatini.

The sensory distribution has several variants described, and of particular note to the surgeon would be the sensory distribution within the ear canal with the fifth nerve subserving sensation in the anterior portion of the external auditory canal, as well as in the tympanic membrane. Cranial nerves IX and X overlap at the region of the posterior aspect of the tympanic membrane and along the posterior aspect of the external acoustic wall and to a lesser extent the pinna. The fifth nerve also supplies the mucosa of the oral and nasal cavities and the dura mater, as well as supplying the major blood vessels up to the first major branches from the circle of Willis.

Motor Root

The fibers of the motor root arise from two nuclei, a superior and an inferior. The superior nucleus consists of a strand of cells occupying the whole length of the lateral portion of the gray substance of the cerebral aqueduct. The inferior or chief nucleus is situated in the upper part of the pons, close to its dorsal surface, and along the line of the lateral margin of the rhomboid fossa. The fibers from the superior nucleus constitute the mesencephalic tract: they descend through the mid-brain, and, entering the pons, join with the fibers from the lower nucleus. The motor root, thus formed, passes forward through the pons to its point of emergence. It is uncertain whether the mesencephalic root is motor or sensory (Jannetta & Rand1966, Jannetta 1967). Two to three rootlets emerge rostral to the sensory portion of the nerve, leaving the posterior fossa through the porous trigeminus. This may be the explanation for the clinical experience in which a complete dorsal root sensory section will be followed by retained sensation in the face. This may reduce the expected efficacy of partial nerve section for persistent pain.

The motor branches of the trigeminal nerve control the movement of eight muscles, including the four muscles of mastication (the masseter, temporalis, medial pterygoid, and lateral pterygoid). The remaining four muscles (tensor veli palatini, mylohyoid, anterior belly of digastric, tensor tympani) contribute to the other phases of mastication (bite, swallow, chew). All have bilateral cortical representation. Thus, lesions affecting unilateral cortex will not affect the muscle function.

The somatotropic organization of the sensory nuclear group is discussed in Carpenter (1976). Of interest to the surgeon is the three-dimensional location of the nuclear components. The atlas proposed by the group headed by Ashfar (Ashfar and Dykes 1984) shows in detail the surface locations and external landmarks for such targets as the nucleus caudalis. These data allow for precise lesioning in the tract, one of the main targets in the dorsal root entry zone (DREZ) procedure. The depth of the target allows the surgeon to reduce, or avoid, morbidity related to tracts en passage to the target nucleus (Ashfar and Dykes 1984).

The arterial supply to the nerve is from the trigeminal arteries. These were most often noted to arise from the superolateral pontine branch of the basilar artery (89%) and from the peduncular cerebellar branch of the anterior inferior cerebellar artery (75%). The trigeminocerebellar artery supplied two roots (6%) of the trigeminal nerves. The number of trigeminal arteries ranged from two to six, and their diameters ranged from 100 to 510 microns. Anastomoses among them were seen in 37.9% of specimens.

The arteries formed vascular rings around 58.6% of the roots. The motor portion of the trigeminal nerve most often received blood from the superolateral pontine artery (79.%). The same artery most commonly supplied the rostral part of the sensory portion, which corresponded to the ophthalmic division of the trigeminal nerve. The superolateral artery, together with the inferolateral pontine artery and the peduncular cerebellar branch of the anterior inferior cerebellar artery, irrigated the middle part of the sensory portion, which corresponded to the maxillary division. The caudal part of that portion, which corresponded to the mandibular division, was commonly perfused by the peduncular cerebellar branch of the anterior inferior cerebellar artery in one of its two forms, while the venous drainage is supplied by anastomoses of the cerebellar–medullary vein.

The remainder of the cerebellopontine angle has relatively constant arterial relationships. The arteries crossing the cerebellopontine angle, especially the anterior inferior cerebellar artery, have a consistent relationship to the facial and vestibulocochlear nerves, foramen of Luschka, and flocculus. The anterior inferior cerebellar artery originates from the basilar artery and encircles the pons near the pontomedullary sulcus. After coursing near, and sending branches to the nerves entering the acoustic meatus and the choroid plexus protruding from the foramen of Luschka, it passes around the flocculus to reach the surface of the middle cerebellar peduncle and terminates by supplying the lips of the cerebellopontine fissure and the petrosal surface of the cerebellum. The anterior inferior cerebellar artery usually bifurcates near the facial and vestibulocochlear nerves to form a rostral trunk and a caudal trunk. The rostral trunk courses along the middle cerebellar peduncle to supply the upper part of the petrosal surface, and the caudal trunk passes near the lateral recess and supplies the lower part of the petrosal surface.

An intriguing study was performed concerning the vasa vasorum of nerves sectioned during TN procedures. The authors concluded that the peripheral and intraneural vessels showed pathological changes, including basement membrane thickening and apoptotic cell states. They speculated that the pathophysiology of TN might be related to nerve ischemia, as well as to demyelination.

The metencephalic vein (ventral metencephalic vein) is the first to drain the infratentorial structures during embryonic development. This vein drains the anterior aspect of the brainstem and cerebellum and, at a later stage, becomes the vascular channel familiar to neurosurgeons under the name "superior petrosal vein". The tributaries of the superior petrosal vein constitute one of the largest infratentorial venous channels, the superior petrosal venous complex (SPVC). The sinus is located in the attachment of the tentorium at the petrous ridge. It runs laterally from the transverse and sigmoid sinuses, ending medially in the cavernous sinus. The cerebellum and brainstem contribute veins along its course, many emanating from the surface of the superior and lateral cerebellum. There are several patterns;

the most common tributaries of the SPVC are the transverse pontine and pontotrigeminal veins, the veins of the cerebellopontine fissure, and the middle cerebellar peduncle (Rhoton 1990). There are no supratentorial cerebral veins contributing to the superior petrosal sinus (SPS). The average distance between the midpoint of the roof of the Meckel cave and the site of entry of the SPVC into the SPS was 10.05 mm (range 3.39–27.34 mm). It is commonplace to attempt to spare these bridging veins while approaching the trigeminal nerve. Occasionally, it is necessary to section a single vein or a trunk made from two veins. In the latter instance, there is a minimal risk of cerebellar infarction. Experimental models have demonstrated that when a vein is sacrificed along with brain retraction, it is more likely to induce brain damage than either vein sacrifice or brain retraction alone. Our experience also finds that altering pontine surface venous anatomy through coagulation and division may lead to recurrent venous compression caused by reconstitution of the collateral veins.

The veins on the medial side of the brainstem are the vein of the pontomedullary sulcus, which courses transversely in the pontomedullary sulcus; the lateral medullary vein, which courses longitudinally along the line of origin of the rootlets of the glossopharyngeal, vagus, and accessory nerves; the vein of the cerebellomedullary fissure, which passes dorsal or ventral to the flocculus before joining the other veins in the cerebellopontine angle; the vein of the middle cerebellar peduncle, which is formed by the union of the lateral medullary vein and the vein of the pontomedullary sulcus and ascends on the middle cerebellar peduncle to join the vein of the cerebellopontine fissure; and the vein of the cerebellopontine fissure, which is formed by the union of the veins that arise on the petrosal surface of the cerebellum and converge on the apex of the cerebellopontine fissure. All of these veins course near the lateral recess and the junction of the facial and vestibulocochlear nerves with the brainstem.

The work of Matsushima and Rhoton (Matsushima and Rhoton 1983) affords the reader meticulous detail on the venous anatomy in the area of the trigeminal nerve. For surgeons using a supralateral cerebellar approach to the nerve, the work of Ueyema, (Al-Mefty and Tamaki 1998) details the number and location of the lateral bridging veins. All these researchers caution that the sacrifice of these veins may be hazardous, as these are terminal veins from the surface with few anastomoses.

The nerve is often partially covered by the bony entrance to the cave of Meckel. In rare instances, however, the exposure of the trigeminal nerve may be hindered by a prominent petrous tubercle (suprameatal tubercule). This can be addressed by drilling off a portion dorsal and lateral to the nerve. Care must be taken to protect the superior petrosal complex and bridging veins during this maneuver. The limits of the drilling of the suprameatal tubercule relate to the intraosseous landmarks: posterior wall of superior semicircular canal, superior portion of the posterior semicircular canal, and the crus. Once the drilling is successfully completed, additional access to the nerve is afforded for Meckel's segment. This averages 10.3 mm (range 8.0–13.0 mm); the porus trigeminus marks the transition from the posterior fossa to the intracanalicular portion of the nerve. The cisternal portion of the trigeminal nerve has a mean length (6 standard deviation) of 9.66 +/− 1.71 mm. The mean length of the nerve varied between the sexes: 9.15–1.52 mm in women and 10.27–1.57 mm in men (significant difference between sexes, $p < 0.0001$) (Kakizawa et al. 2008). The trigeminal nerve has a segment in the cave of Meckel (Meckel's segment); this averages 3.1 mm. The nerve narrows in this portion, widening as it approaches the ganglion. The ganglion is contained within the split dural fold of the middle fossa, at the anterior edge of the trigeminal depression in the bone. The nerve runs at a slight angle to the tentorial edge. Although there are no reported changes in nerve angulation or position with aging, the trigeminal nerve was found to be significantly longer in older individuals (Kakizawa et al. 2008). The temporal bone forms the ventral wall of the cerebellopontine angle. This posterior portion of the bone has three margins: the petrous ridge, the sphenopetrosal suture inferiorly, and the sigmoid groove medially. The distance from the midpoint of the internal auditory canal (IAC) to the trigeminal notch averages 10.5 mm (range 7.2–12.5 mm). The caudal border of the nerve can be found at the notch.

TRIGEMINAL NERVE REFLEXES

The evaluation of the physiology of the nerve involves testing the modalities of its function: light touch, pinprick, proprioception, vibration, temperature, and deep pressure.

To test light touch, use a small shred of cotton to lightly touch and stroke each division, varying the initial side of contact. Diagram each division, paying special attention to the area around the vermillion border. This is often affected in cases of TN, creating an "onion-skin" effect between the second and third divisions. Temperature is tested with two small tubes of warm and cold water. Each division is tested, in turn, and comparison between divisions ipsilaterally can be useful in cases of suspected TN.

The use of reflex and sensory exam findings to distinguish the pathophysiology of the fifth nerve can be supplemented by electrophysiological testing.

The neurons in the trigeminal nerve have been classified into three types, using the afore-mentioned mechanical stimuli: wide dynamic receptors (WDR), nociceptive sensitive (NS), and low-threshold mechanoreceptors (LTM). Trigeminal brainstem reflexes, such as the masseter inhibitory reflex and the blink reflex, are mediated by central multireceptive neurons that are also involved in trigeminal nociception. Trigeminal axons, via the trigeminal ganglion, synapse on second-order cells in the principal sensory nucleus (PSN), the spinal trigeminal nucleus (STN), the mesencephalic nucleus (MNu), and the interstitial nucleus of the spinal trigeminal tract (ISVT). From there, they project to various cortical (S1, S2) and subcortical regions.

Several reflexes involve more complex arcs. The masseter reflex (jaw jerk) tests both sensory and motor portions of the nerve. Use a reflex hammer to tap the mandible along the anterolateral edge, near the mentalis nerve exit. The resulting contraction is observed on both sides. The jaw will deviate ipsilaterally to the side of a lesion. This arc does not have bilateral efferent representation. Proprioception is elicited by passively opening the jaw, in a fashion similar to small-joint testing in the limbs.

To test the corneal reflex, touch the cornea, not the conjunctiva, with a shred of cotton. This will induce a blink, bilaterally. This reflex tests the fifth and seventh nerves. With a fifth-nerve lesion, the bilateral blink reflex will be lost. With a seventh-nerve lesion, only the ipsilateral blink reflex will be lost, while preserving the consensual side.

The trigeminocardiac reflex (trigeminal depressor response), first described in 1908 by Aschner, is related to, and may indeed be, the oculocardiac reflex (Aschner 1908)). It is theorized that the reflex mechanism consists of sensory nerve endings of the trigeminal nerve sending impulses via the gasserian ganglion to the sensory nucleus of the trigeminal nerve. This forms the afferent pathway of the reflex arc. These neurons continue in the reticular formation to connect with the efferent pathway in the motor nucleus of the vagus nerve. Cardio-inhibitory efferent fibers come from the motor nucleus of the vagus nerve and terminate in the myocardium (Naccarti 1921, Lang et al 1991, Paton et al 2005). The effector site in the heart is the sinoatrial node. It can be avoided through the use of atropine as a premedicant in at-risk cases. However, releasing the mechanical traction on the fifth nerve during an open surgical procedure will have the same terminating effect.

SURGICAL PATHOPHYSIOLOGY

The prevailing theory that explains the success of microvascular decompression (MVD) postulates arterial cross-compression. This pulsatile compression results in metabolic derangements in the nerve. This results in alterations in the extent and degree of the normal repair process. Proof of concept is offered in multiple series of operative and cadaver observations.

Devor, Govrin-Lippmann and Rappaport (2002) obtained specimens from compressed nerves in patients with type I TN. They endeavored to include tissue taken from the site of cross-compression, but did not have specimens from other sites. They observed that "in areas of the most severe damage, few axons remained and nearly all that did were demyelinated. Adjacent areas contained more surviving axons, including a significant proportion having a residual myelin sheath, albeit disrupted. We refer to these areas as zones of "demyelination" and "dysmyelination," respectively". The most severe injury was not usually observed in a single contiguous region, but rather interdigitated with areas of less severe damage. There were also areas of collagen overproduction in the extracellular matrix; this has been described as commonplace following compression injury in spinal roots. Additionally, the myelin sheath is particularly sensitive, and undergoes graded changes from minor dysmyelination to frank disintegration as trauma becomes more severe. Devor and colleagues (2002) noted that the trigeminal nerve appeared to have a less-robust mechanism for clearance of injury debris. This may factor into the cycle of symptoms with interspersed quiescence, but a gradual loss of the asymptomatic baseline between attacks.

The location of the superior petrosal vein (SPV) can be an issue. A preoperative magnetic resonance (MR) venogram can sometimes delineate the overall types of SPV (i.e., types I, II, III). Normally, the caliber of the SPV varies between 1.5 and 3.0 mm. There are three named tributaries of the SPV: mesencephalic, cerebellar, and pontine. If the complex is found to enter the sinus in what has been referred to as the type II pattern (Rhoton lab), then the surgeon will have reduced visibility during the initial approach to the nerve. A short and superficially placed SPV can be easily avulsed during initial retraction. A long and deeply placed SPV, on the other hand, can have predominant drainage from the pontine area and, by virtue of its proximity to the REZ, is sometimes implicated in causing TN. Matsushima (Matsushima et al 1983) has reported that the more deeply situated transverse pontine vein is frequently part of venous compression in TN. We have noted a relatively higher incidence for the type II pattern, which might be a related factor in TN. A recent review of patients with second-division pain found a large proportion of women patients with venous compression affecting the maxillary segments of the nerve (Sekula & Jannetta 2009). In addition, there is a higher likelihood that the SPV will need to be partially or completely sectioned with this pattern. The SPV can be absent: when this is the case, every attempt should be made to preserve any other venous structures traversing the cerebellopontine angle (CPA). If multiple SPV trunks are present, it is usually possible to preserve some of them.

When sectioning the SPV, the surgeon would be well served to have a good three-dimensional image of the length and angle of the entry point of the SPV to the sinus. During low-wattage coagulation (15–20), care is taken to avoid traction at an angle to the entry point, to avoid shearing the vessel prior to complete coagulation. Once a blanched vessel is noted, a partial cut through the SPVC, until the lumen can be visualized, is done. This allows for a second round of coagulation of both ends of the lumen. The discerning surgeon will frequently note that the lumen is still partially open, and the second period of coagulation allows for more secure closure. Then the final portion of the vein can be cut, leaving a stump of the SPV. To minimize the damage to the sinus by heat, while allowing for a more complete closure, it is best to work as near as possible to the cerebellar surface. In the event that the vein is sheared off near its junction with the sinus, the best maneuver is to raise the head slightly (10–15 degrees), place a small rolled surgical sponge or similar agent parallel to the course of the sinus and then a micro-cottonoid. If this results in hemorrhage control, one can often proceed with the case. Resist the urge to look beneath the cottonoid, as it takes a good 10 minutes or so for firm coagulation at the entry point to the sinus. Vigorous attempts at suctioning are to be avoided, as these can result in additional damage to the cerebellar surface. Coagulation on or near the sinus usually results in a larger rent, since the walls of the sinus are held immobile.

When approaching the trigeminal nerve, the initial view should be caudal to rostral, allowing for visualization of the caudal and ventral surface of the nerve. Subsequently, the scope can be positioned in line with the entry from the cave of Meckel, assuring a clear view of the rostral ventral border. Some surgeons report that the use of the endoscope facilitates this inspection (Rak et al 2004). An angled mirror suffices for this view. The preoperative imaging studies can add some information as to the orientation to best visualize the fifth nerve. The angle between the tentorium and a line drawn from the hard palate defines the tentorial angle. This averages 45–55 degrees. When the angle is steep (>51 degrees) this limits the operating field between these cranial nerves when reaching the petroclival or the superior CPA regions through the retrosigmoid approach. The operating surgeon should bear in mind the reduction in the distance between the tentorium and the acoustic nerve complex. (Rusu 2009, Sade 2007).

The ideal amount of polytetrafluoroethylene (PTFE) felt is not known, but a thickness of at least 1 mm in the transverse dimension of the vessel seems to suffice in the series from Jannetta. In general, the larger the blood vessel, the larger and thicker the felt that should be interposed. The felt must also be placed to avoid kinking the vessel, be it arterial or venous. It is helpful to visualize both ends of the felt after placement, to assure complete interposition between the vessel and nerve. There is a sparse literature regarding the degree of pulsation dampening by PTFE, however.

The use of a 2–3 mm curved tip retractor, such as a Jannetta 3 (KLS Martin Instruments), or a Rhoton 6 (Codman) ventral to the nerve, allows the operator to palpate and move the arterial loop(s) rostrally and ventrally. It is important to visualize all the motor branches (1–4) and include them against the sensory root. If they are displaced rostrally, the patient will complain of aching jaw pain, even when not present preoperatively.

These anatomic points will aid in MVD. Knowledge of the three-dimensional anatomy of the nuclear complex is useful when performing a DREZ lesion of the nucleus caudalis. The nucleus extends from the tuberculum cinereum to C3. At its rostral end, the fibers decussata from the medial surface of the tract. The somatotopic orientation, with the mandibular fibers and nuclear connections most ventromedial, aids the surgeon in identifying the target site(s). We use a stimulating electrode sited on the affected division(s), and record from the dorsal surface of the brainstem to maximize lesioning.

Many of the pain and temperature fibers (C and A-delta) enter the brainstem from the ganglion cell bodies and descend into the most caudal portion of the spinal nucleus of the fifth nerve. The nucleus is referred to as the "spinal" nucleus due to its caudal extent to the upper three cervical segments. The pain fibers synapse here in the substantia gelatinosa of Rolando, mimicking the dorsal root ganglion fibers from the body dermatomes. Since touch and two-point discrimination are handled by the parasympathetic nervous (PSN) system, lesions of the nucleus caudalis do not alter tactile sensitivity. Sjoqvist described the effects on pain relief and decreased thermal sense following trigeminal tractomy in this nuclear region (Sjoqvist 1938). Grant reported on mild tactile loss, with preserved corneal sensation in patients so lesioned (Grant 1938). The observation that lesions of the nucleus caudalis produce facial analgesia supports the notion that the nucleus is entirely concerned with pain transmission.

REFERENCES

Aschner B. Ueber einen bisher noch nicht heschriebenen reflex vom auge auf kreislauf und atmung: Verschwinden des Radialispulses bei Druck auf das Auge. Wein Klin Wochenscr 1908;21:1529–30.

Ashfar F, Dykes E. Computer generated three-dimensional visualization of the trigeminal nuclear complex. *Surg Neurol* 1984;22:189–196.

Beaver DL, Moses HL, Ganote CE. Electron microscopy of the trigeminal ganglion. 3. Trigeminal neuralgia. *Arch Pathol* 1965;79:571–582.

Carpenter MB. *Human neuroanatomy*, 7th ed. Baltimore: Williams and Wilkins, 1976.

Cha ST, Eby JB, Katzen JT, Shahinian HK. Trigeminocardiac reflex: a unique case of recurrent asystole during bilateral trigeminal sensory root rhizotomy. *Craniomaxillofac Surg* 2002;30(2):108–111.

Cruccu G, Biasiotta A, et al. Diagnostic accuracy of trigeminal reflex testing in trigeminal neuralgia. *Neurology* 2006;66:139–141.

Dandy W. *Lewis's practice of surgery*, Vol. 12, Chap. 1. Hagerstown, Md.: Hoeber Medical Division, Harper and Row, Publishers, Incorporated, 1945.

Dandy WE. An operation for the cure of tic douloureux. Partial section of the sensory root at the pons. *Arch Surg* 1929;18:687–734.

Devor M, Govrin-Lippmann R, Rappaport HZ. Mechanism of trigeminal neuralgia: An ultrastructural analysis of trigeminal root specimens obtained during microvascular decompression surgery. *J Neurosurg* 2002;96:532–543.

Grant FC. Results in operative treatment of major trigeminal neuralgia. *AnnSurg* 1938;107:14–19.

Jannetta PJ. Anatomy of trigeminal ganglia: gross (mesoscopic) description of the human trigeminal nerve and ganglion. *J Neurosurg* 1967;26(1-Suppl):109–111.

Jannetta PJ, Rand RW. Transtentorial retrogasserian rhizotomy in trigeminal neuralgia by microneurosurgical technique. *Bull LA Neurol Soc* 1966;31:93–99.

Jaquin MF, Semba K, Rhoades RW, Egger MD. Trigeminal primary afferents project bilaterally to dorsal horn and ipsilaterally to cerebellum, reticular formation and cuneate, solitary, supratrigeminal and vagal nuclei. *Brain Res* 1982;246: 285–291.

Kakizawa Y, Seguchi T, Kodama K, et al. Anatomical study of the trigeminal and facial cranial nerves with the aid of 3.0-tesla magnetic resonance imaging. *J Neurosurg* 2008;108(3):483–490.

Kanavel A, Davis R. Surgical anatomy of the trigeminal nerve. *Surgery, Gynecology, and Obstetrics (SG&O)* 1922;34:357–366.

Kerr FWL. The ultrastructure of the spinal tract of the trigeminal nerve. *Exp Neurol* 1966;16:359–376.

Lang S, Lanigan DT, van der Wal M. Trigeminocardiac reflexes: maxillary and mandibular variants of the oculocardiac reflex. *Can J Anaesth* 1991;38(6):757–760.

Marinkovic S. The trigeminal vasculature pathology in patients with neuralgia. *Headache* 2007;47:1334–1339.

Matsushima T, Rhoton AL Jr., de Oliveira E, Peace D. Microsurgical anatomy of the veins of the posterior fossa. *J Neurosurg* 1983;59(1):63–105.

Matsushima T, Rhoton AL Jr., Lenkey C. Microsurgery of the fourth ventricle: Part 1. Microsurgical anatomy. *Neurosurgery* 1982;11(5):631–667.

Moses HL, Beaver DL, Ganote CE. Electron microscopy of the trigeminal ganglion. I. Comparative ultrastructure. *Arch Pathol* 1965;79:541–556.

Naccarti S. The oculo-cardiac reflex (Dagnini-Aschner phenomena): its use in medicine and psychology. *Arch Neurol Psych* 1921;5(1):40–57.

Paton J, Boscan P, Pickering A, Nalivaiko E. The yin and yang of cardiac autonomic control: vago-sympathetic interactions revisited. *Brain Res Brain Res Rev* 2005; 49(3):555–565.

Rak R, Sekhar LN, Stimac D, Hechl P. Endoscope-assisted microsurgery for microvascular compression syndromes. *Neurosurgery* 2004;54(4):876–881.

Reed H, McCaughey T. cardiac slowing during strabismus surgery. *Br J Opthalmol* 1962;46(2):112–122.

Rhoton AL, Jr. (1990) Microsurgical anatomy of decompression operations on the trigeminal nerve. In Rovit, Murali and Jannetta (eds.) Trigeminal Nerualgia (pp165–200). Baltimore, MD: Williams and Wilkins.

Rusu MC, Ivaşcu RV, Cergan R, Păduraru D, Podoleanu L. Typical and atypical neurovascular relations of the trigeminal nerve in the cerebellopontine angle: an anatomical study. *Surg Radiol Anat*. 2009;31(7):507–16. *Epub* 2009 Feb 12.

Sade B, Lee JH. Significance of the tentorial alignment in approaching the trigeminal nerve and the ventral petrous region through the suboccipital retrosigmoid technique. *J Neurosurg*. 2007;107(5):932–6.

Saunders RL, Sachs E. Relation of the accessory rootlets of the trigeminal nerve to its motor root: a microsurgical autopsy study. *JNS* 1970;33(3).

Sekula R, Jannetta PJJ. (Isolated V_2 trigeminal neuralgia) Congress of Neurological Surgeons. New Orleans LA, September 2009.

Sjoqvist O. Studies on pain conduction in the trigeminal nerve. A contribution to surgical treatment of facial pain. *Acta Psych Neurol Scand* 1938;17(Suppl):1–139.

Ueyama T, Al-Mefty O, Tamaki N. Bridging veins on the tentorial surface of the cerebellum: a microsurgical anatomic study and operative considerations. *Neurosurg*. 1998 Nov;43(5):1137–45.

Weinberger LM, Grant FC. Experiences with intramedullary tractotomy. III: Studies on sensation. *Arch Neurol Psych* 1942;48:355–381.

3

Typical and Atypical Symptoms

Peter J. Jannetta

Trigeminal neuralgia (TN; "typical" or "classical"), also called *tic douloureux* (painful tic), was traditionally known as an "idiopathic disease." To designate a disorder as *idiopathic* (from the Greek, meaning a problem coming from within itself) indicates that we are ignorant of the root cause of the problem. A certain inertia of thought sometimes attaches itself to such diseases; many clinicians may begin to believe that no "real" cause for an idiopathic illness can ever be found. In this chapter, we will try to clarify the diagnosis of TN in its common presenting form, its permutations, and when it presents in combination with other factors.

Typical TN comes like a bolt out of the blue; the first attack is totally unexpected. It is a terrible facial pain, with most patients describing it as by far the worst pain they have ever suffered. Details of the first attack will be remembered forever. Women who have borne children say unfailingly that childbirth is nothing compared to an attack of TN. The pain is described as lancinating, like electric shocks, like glass grinding into the face, and worse. It is of sudden onset and offset, and we estimate that 5%–8% of TN is precipitated by trauma, most commonly an acute flexion-extension injury, perhaps due to brain and vessels shifting. This may occur immediately or within weeks of the injury. The pain is more commonly located in the lower face. Only a small percentage of people have isolated V_1 pain. (Although I am not as convinced as some that pain is clearly located by divisions, I use them here as descriptive terms.) After the initial attack, which may include the entire side of the face (V_1, V_2, and V_3), the pain usually settles into the lower (V_3), middle (V_2), or upper (V_1) face. Over time, pain may start in one division and spread to the adjacent area, usually V_3 spreading to V_2. This is most likely due to elongation over time of an artery, most commonly the superior cerebellar artery, with advancing compression of the nerve.

Before the onset of TN, some patients have a prodrome of discomfort or moderate pain in the face, jaw, or a tooth. This may precede the actual TN by some time, weeks to months. During this period, or even as the patient is suffering an attack of true TN, he or she usually will go to the dentist. It is very difficult for a dentist, who sees hundreds of patients with common toothaches, to single out the rare case of TN. In many cases, patients may have teeth extracted, root canal procedures done, and be fitted with mouth guards. Not unexpectedly, these patients will "dentist shop" when told that a tooth is normal, until someone is found who will remove it. All to no avail: The pain continues to recur.

On average, over the years, our patients typically have seen more than three dentists and about two physicians before the diagnosis of TN was made. This record is improving as practitioners become more knowledgeable.

ETIOLOGY

Women are more commonly afflicted than men with TN, by a ratio of 3 to 2. In all patients with TN, pain is more commonly located on the right side, again by a ratio of 3 to 2. It is located in the lower face and/or the malar region in 95% of patients. A positive family history of TN exists in about 5% of patients. Bilateral TN occurs sequentially in about 5% of patients. This incidence may be increasing slightly as the patient population ages.

The age of onset of TN, although generally occurring in the sixth, seventh, or eighth decade, follows a Gaussian curve. We have seen and treated many teenagers. Our youngest patient presented at age 7 months, and we operated on him when he was 22 months old. The second youngest, a girl, suffered onset at age 13 months. Her father, a dentist, made the initial diagnosis—just as the parents of the 7-month-old boy did when doctors told them that TN was not the cause of their son's pain, because he was too young to have TN. Rarely do we see a nonagenarian with acute-onset TN, but this is possibly because we see few nonagenarians.

The pain of TN is frequently positional, and the patient often can find a position that mitigates or worsens the pain. Lying on the contralateral side often helps. Some patients are made worse by lying down. We have seen patients who, because of pain exacerbations, have been unable to lie flat in bed for years, forced instead to sleep in a lounge chair with the head elevated. In others, over time, the positional component is lost, implying possibly that the offending blood vessel has become impacted into the nerve.

In addition to the spontaneous onset of pain, attacks are frequently precipitated by various stimuli. These vary from patient to patient but include talking, cold air, cold water on the face, eating, chewing, brushing the teeth, shaving, applying makeup, kissing, air conditioning, and many more. Pain may awake the patient from sleep, usually when lying on the ipsilateral side and not necessarily when the bedclothes have brushed against the face. Trigger points, areas where a minimal stimulus such as a light touch but not pressure, are usually located around the nose and mouth. They are evanescent, not necessarily remaining in one place, as though this sequence is part of a very active process.

Over time, the character of sudden onset and offset lancinating pain of brief duration will alter. The pain will become of longer duration and may become slightly duller. It may become constant. My colleague, R. F. Sekula, Jr., and I have discussed at length what to call this type of modified and altered pain experience, which some have described as a transitional pain period. We finally settled on "mixed TN" to designate this change in pain experience.

With improving understanding of TN, attempts have been made to categorize the pain of this condition into various subdivisions. Burchiel noted seven different varieties of TN, and assigned them numbers. Although a good try and, I think a useful one, Burchiel's categories may be overelaborate. We have tried to classify TN into a simpler classification structure that also takes into account changes with time: (Table 3.1)

- *Typical TN.* Lancinating pain of sudden onset and offset
- *Atypical TN.* Constant pain, usually burning in nature, either from onset or altered from typical TN over time
- *Mixed TN.* Pain with elements of both typical and atypical TN

In addition to the effects of time, which may cause increased compression or distortion of the trigeminal nerve by an elongating artery, medications also may alter tic pain. A moderate dose of carbamazepine may stop the lancinating pain but bring out a more constant, protracted, less severe pain, frequently described as "burning." Increased dosage may cause this pain to disappear.

In some patients, the duration of the typical lancinating pain (typical TN) is brief, and is replaced early on by a constant (burning) pain. Occasionally, in someone with long-duration pain, the lancinating pain period will be recalled by the patient only through specific questioning. Usually, however, the first onset of TN, the true beginning of the real pain, is utterly and totally memorable. A small number of patients have an aura, usually a terrible feeling, as a sense of doom, before the attack. More frequent is a refractory period after an attack, during which the pain cannot be

Table 3.1 Changes in trigeminal neuralgia over time. Symptoms and signs blend into one another depending on several variables including size and location of offending blood vessel(s), duration and degree of stretch of nerve

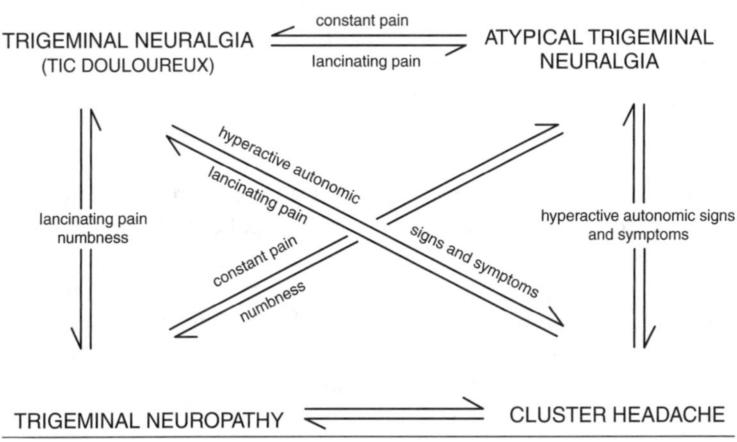

precipitated by the usual inciting measures. The patient will use this brief period to do things which he or she cannot do otherwise, such as eat or brush the teeth.

Atypical TN is a constant focal pain syndrome, usually burning in character. The pain may exacerbate and remit either spontaneously or secondary to the same precipitating factors operant in the typical variety. The pain usually starts out mildly and unobtrusively, gradually worsening over time. It is much more common in women than men.

A patient may come to us years after onset, with her ego destroyed. This occurs in the following sequence: The face pain develops and persists, and the patient goes to her family doctor, who refers her to a neurologist, who sends her to a neurosurgeon, tagging her with the label of "atypical facial pain or neuralgia." Because a firm somatic cause for the disease cannot be found (it is "idiopathic"), she risks being classified as "neurotic," especially if the constant, severe pain of TN has caused a breakdown in the patient's normal coping mechanisms.

It is important, when considering these patients for operation, to clarify with the family the premorbid emotional status of the individual before pain caused ego decompensation. No matter how strong a person's ego, it ultimately crumbles, partly, I fear, because everyone in her environment begins to suspect she is "crazy." The fact that many of these patients have only a modest response to the usual anti-TN drugs but are relieved somewhat by narcotics is only further reason for the failure of emotional well-being.

Atypical TN correlates well pathophysiologically with compression of the distal motor-proprioceptive fascicles of the trigeminal nerve. It is difficult to distinguish it from nervus intermedius neuralgia (NIN), although the latter is more prone to feel as though it is located deeper in the face and not superficially, to have a medial canthus-area component, to be accompanied by deep ear pain (although both trigeminal and glossopharyngeal neuralgia may have a deep ear pain component), and to respond even less well to medications than atypical TN. Both syndromes may end up as cluster headaches, correlating pathophysiologically with stretch of the motor-proprioceptive fascicles of the trigeminal nerve and/or more severe compression of nervus intermedius fascicles. It is not possible to estimate the number of patients with NIN who have been missed over the years because we have concentrated on the trigeminal aspects of this debilitating problem.

A further issue for the treating neurosurgeon to be aware of is the postoperative emotional state of the atypical TN patient after microvascular decompression (MVD). At some time during the hours after the procedure, the patient will say, "The pain was real, wasn't it?" "Of course" is the answer that allays all the patient's self-doubt. Astonishingly, on the afternoon of the second postoperative day, many patients rapidly develop every neurotic symptom in the book with no abnormality on examination, sleep well with sedation, and awaken having returned to their premorbid psychological status. This sequence is currently less common as more physicians recognize and understand the course of TN, and also as patients and their families learn to deal with the symptoms of TN from these knowledgeable physicians and from the Internet.

CONCLUSION

To summarize, the symptoms and signs of TN can present in a variety of ways, dependent upon the location and size of offending blood vessels, duration of the process, severity of nerve compression-distortion, and on the activity engendered by the ongoing process of nerve damage. Trigeminal neuralgia is an active process: The patient's history, changes in physical examination, and even electron microscopic abnormalities all point to this.

4

Medical Therapy: The Dentist's Perspective

Peter J. Jannetta and George J. Hadeed

Because so many patients with severe face and jaw pain think their problem is dental, the dentist is frequently, if not usually, the first contact a person with trigeminal neuralgia (TN) has with the medical profession.

Trigeminal neuralgia is a disorder that affects primarily women in the fourth to seventh decades of life. Often, the dentist sees the patient for what is described as atypical facial pain (AFP). Atypical face pain differs from TN in that it is a broader, more diffuse and poorly localized pain, often described as "burning" by patients. These patients often have had prior magnetic resonance imaging, computed tomography scans, multiple radiographs, and even tooth extractions performed in an attempt to clarify and alleviate the problem.

Nicolas André (André 1756) is the French physician who is generally credited with providing the first full description of the disorder. Of particular interest is his description of a patient who had several teeth extracted in an attempt to alleviate her symptoms, which had been diagnosed then as a "dental infection" of the maxilla. André used the term *tic douloureux* in his description, most likely because this disorder was seen as a form of neurological epilepsy (neuralgia epileptiform). Unfortunately, even today, patients still experience the same treatment—the extraction of teeth—often at their own insistence, at the hands of health care providers before a proper diagnosis is obtained.

When presented with a patient with intractable face or jaw pain who shows no obvious signs of disease, the dentist should take note of the neurological symptoms. Often, the patient will describe trigger points and their resulting symptoms. A diagnostic anesthetic block of the gasserian ganglion can be helpful.

If a tooth is sensitive, it is important to determine the cause. Percussion sensitivity and sensitivity to hot or cold can indicate an acute pulpitis. However, in rare instances, this is not the case. And although good dental and oral health care is important, TN patients should receive the minimal amount of treatment in order to avoid overstimulating their trigger points. These patients are often reluctant to have any dental care because of the severity of pain elicited by treatment. A preemptive measure would be to administer dental anesthesia to have the patient experience relief from trigger point stimulation. This serves to build confidence in having necessary procedures performed at a later date, at the patient's convenience.

If dental procedures are planned in a patient with TN, it is best to increase their dose of TN medication one or two days before the procedure. Analgesics, such as codeine or ibuprofen, should be taken by the patient at least 1–2 hours before the procedure. Long-acting dental anesthetics without epinephrine should be used, and injected as far from the trigger point as possible. Epinephrine can often trigger TN and should be avoided. If all methods of alleviating pain fail, patients should consider dental work done under IV sedation.

At home, the patient should avoid drinking cold or hot liquids, which can stimulate the trigger. If brushing the teeth is difficult, the dentist can prescribe viscous Xylocaine to numb the mouth prior to brushing. If that is not successful, chlorhexidine gluconate (Peridex®) can be prescribed as an anti-plaque mouth rinse, along with fluoride to help sustain the patient's oral health. These patients, especially women, are prone to xerostomia. In addition, TN medications such as phenytoin, carbamazepine, or gabapentin can induce xerostomia in a small percentage of patients. It is for this reason that the dentist must facilitate in any way the patient's oral hygiene and minimize the risk for caries and periodontitis. Finally, it is important to have the patient continue with a periodic dental exams and prophylaxis cleaning to maintain good oral health and minimize any risk of extensive dental work, which would increase the likelihood of trigger point stimulation.

Some patients anecdotally report pain relief with capsaicin, used to relieve trigger point stimulation. If applied intraorally, a plastic dental splint is used to confine the capsaicin.

EVALUATION OF PATIENTS WITH FACE PAIN

In any patient presenting with face pain, it is proper to evaluate the state of the dentition. A few practitioners a number of years ago felt that gingivitis, often subliminal, was causal of TN, but neither conservative nor radical treatments helped very much. The studies were never controlled, nor were they convincing, and this perspective fell into disuse. One wonders, however, if gingival infection might predispose to TN at an earlier state of vascular compression of the trigeminal nerve by altering the baseline that will precipitate pain (resetting the rheostat, so to speak). This is purely speculative, but when dealing with neurogenic pain, it's important to keep an open mind in the discussion of any pathophysiologic concept.

Neurologists and neurosurgeons often have much maligned dentists because they do not recognize nor readily make the diagnosis of TN in their office practice. This is hardly fair: physicians other than neurologists or neurosurgeons do not do much better. In a series of TN patients seen in my office before the diagnosis was made, an average of three dentists saw the patient first. This may sound bad, but the same patients also saw an average of two physicians before the diagnosis.

Its also common to believe that a practitioner cannot be held liable for missing a diagnosis when the disorder is outside his or her area of primary expertise. This may be valid, but in my years as an academic neurosurgeon, I developed my own bias on such a perception—as follows: If a neurosurgery resident does a superb, faultless, and excellent job of evaluating, diagnosing, and treating a patient with a neurosurgical problem, common or rare, that is as it should be. Nothing to brag about. On the other hand, if a neurosurgical resident works at this same level regarding a patient with a non-neurological problem—in a sense, outdoing residents and staff in that particular specialty—then that rates a gold star.

For young medical practitioners today, it is getting harder to have a broader, more global understanding of other areas of medicine and surgery than it was in the past. The wide experience opportunities are limited; the horizons closer; the information more complex and more difficult to find. This may be just a prolonged and apparently degenerative phase of medicine that further technological developments, especially of the computer and the Internet, will alter for the better.

A patient who has had one or more attacks of TN out of the blue is frequently certain that a particular tooth is the culprit. Off to the dentist. The dentist sees and examines the patient, performs plain x-rays, finds no abnormalities, and tells the patient so. Or, the dentist, unaware of TN, atypical TN, or nervus intermedius neuralgia (NIN), may pull the tooth or send the patient for a root canal procedure.

Some patients, upon being told that no pathology has been found, will "dentist shop" until they find someone who will pull the tooth, so it is not always the dentist who is at fault—I have seen many, many patients who have had multiple to total tooth extractions with no help for their TN.

So, what must a dentist do? First, developing an understanding of TN and its variations is essential and easy to do. This diagnostic acumen is perhaps truly the most important skill, even before ruling out the common cause of dental and jaw region pain, which most dentists can do so easily and so well. (Chapter 3 in this volume covers the spectrum of TN diagnosis nicely.)

In screening for TN, listen for the patient who tells you that he had the sudden onset of severe unilateral facial pain: "By far the worst pain I have ever had. It is unbearable." The pain of TN is of sudden onset and offset; it is described as lancinating, "like an electric shock, like someone boring into my face with a drill." It consists most commonly of repetitive shocks but may be more constant. Each attack may consist of a brief single shock or multiple shocks lasting a few seconds to many minutes. The pain rarely exceeds 30 minutes, and usually lasts a much shorter time. The first attack is so severe that it is almost always memorable in great detail to the patient, even many years later. Further attacks may occur spontaneously or be precipitated variously by talking, chewing, brushing the teeth, applying makeup, shaving, cold air or water on the face, air conditioning, and other triggers. In the early years, the pain is frequently precipitated by changes in position and may be eased by returning to the former position. This pain infrequently awakens the patient from a sleep, and when it does, he usually has been sleeping with the impaired side down. (I have had patients who could not lie down at all, but slept in lounge chairs with the head up and the feet elevated.)

Middle-aged and older women most commonly develop TN, and women with TN outnumber men with TN by 3 to 2. The pain occurs on the right side over the left side also by a ratio of 3 to 2. It is of sequentially bilateral onset in 5%, and there is a positive family history of TN in 5% of patients.

The age distribution is a Gaussian curve. Children do develop TN, although it may not be recognized for a long time. My youngest patient developed TN at 7 months of age, and we operated at 22 months. The next youngest was 13 months old at onset. She had a knowledgeable and very bright dentist father who clarified the diagnosis and brought her to us at age 5. Children frequently have multiple veins as the cause of their TN; we had to operate upon the 5-year-old a second time because veins recollateralized. She has now been free of pain for over 20 years.

PHYSICAL EXAMINATION

The physical examination between acute attacks of pain may be completely normal. Trigeminal neuralgia was originally called *tic douloureux* (painful tic) because the patient, when seized by the pain, grimaces, especially on the ipsilateral side. When describing the pain, the patient will not touch the area of involvement but rather keep the indicating fingers away from the skin. He may shake the fingers in a charade of the electric shock-like pain. Sensory changes, which may be very mild but reproducible, are found in about one-third of patients, usually centered over the area of pain. This is more common when the patient is in the midst of a severe attack and when the pain has been present for many years. V_1 pain may present, with a decreased corneal reflex, both subjective and objective, in the upper half of the cornea only; V_2 pain may be present with a lower-half decrease. The cornea, not the sclera must be touched lightly with one small tapered wisp of cotton to test reflexes. V_2 or V_3 pain may present with mild hypalgesia and/or hypoesthesia centered low in the nasolabial fold area. The neurologic convention of going from the area of atypical sensation to the region of typical sensation must be observed to evaluate these sensory changes.

Atypical TN is focal in location, prolonged, has little or no shock-like pain at any time, and is reproducible. Typical TN may change to the more prolonged non–shock-like pain of atypical TN over time. This form of modified or mixed TN is treatable by drugs and operation. Some of these differentiating points are covered in a recent article in the dental literature (Horowitz et al. 2004), which, using our series of patients, made a good attempt to clarify the symptoms of TN, primarily of typical TN.

Medical treatment is covered in Chapters 4, 6, and 14 but will be briefly described here. Gabapentin (Neurontin), starting in small doses of 100 mg bid and increasing every 48–72 hours by 100 mg/day may suffice. Except for drowsiness, there are no serious side effects. Carbamazepine is a better drug, but has some potential side effects. The treating medical person must understand these risks and be able to prevent them if he is to treat TN medically. The drowsiness from gabapentin usually lessens with time. Carbamazepine, early on, can cause drowsiness, memory disturbance, blood dyscrasias, severe and dangerous dermatitis (Stevens-Johnson syndrome) and, with prolonged use, liver damage. These drugs *must* be monitored or should not be given.

Dental manipulations have no place in the treatment of TN pain, and may be responsible for protracted periods of pain.

Barring contraindications, the first treatment offered should be carbamazepine, or other medical therapy. A response to pain medication (especially carbamazepine) not only makes the patient feel better but also helps to solidify the diagnosis of TN.

Nervus intermedius neuralgia (geniculate neuralgia) may be compared to and confused with TN. In NIN, the pain is deeper in location, does not respond well (if at all) to medication, and is often accompanied by deep ear pain. Cluster headache and its variations are the endpoint of NIN. Cluster headache is more common in men than in women, and the patient typically has attacks of ipsilateral face pain/temporal headache accompanied by ipsilateral scleral redness, tearing, and runny nose. Analgesics, including opiates, may help alleviate the pain of NIN and cluster headaches.

REFERENCES

André N. *Traite sur les maladies de l'urethre*. Paris: Delaguette, 1756.

Horowitz M, Horowitz M, Ochs M, et al. Trigeminal neuralgia and glossopharyngeal neuralgia: Two orofacial pain syndromes encountered by dentists. *J Am Dent Assoc* 2004;135:1427–1433.

5

Face Pain in the Front Lines

David Halpert

I was called to the hospital to consult on a 47-year-old woman who was hospitalized for a 1 week history of severe intractable bitemporal headache. Upon close questioning, I identified two separate problems. She did indeed have a one1-week history of bitemporal occipital viselike headache (without any prior history for this) and without a trigger. However, she was driven to the hospital by the symptoms that developed on day 5: shooting or stabbing incapacitating pain in the right temporal area lasting 30 seconds and recurring repetitively for 5 minutes with bouts occurring throughout the day. These shooting pains were associated with slight numbness in a V1 distribution (which resolved). Imaging studies were normal.

My initial treatment of increasing doses of gabapentin (Neurontin) stepping up to 300/300/500 mg/day was directed at the neuralgic pain with some good but not complete improvement over the first days and weeks, allowing the patient to return to work. After 6 weeks, I added 10 mg of amitriptyline (Elavil) because of persisting, frequent, and severe (but no longer daily) viselike headaches with occasional visual blurring. The patient became pain-free at this point, although she had symptoms of mild fatigue and sedation from both the gabapentin and the amitriptyline. A slow gabapentin wean was undertaken over months. After the dose had been reduced to just 300 mg daily at bedtime for a month, we discontinued the drug.

Within 4 or 5 weeks, both the daily vise-like headaches and intermittent daily bouts of right temporal shooting pain had returned. The patient described feeling as if her "nerve was prodded by the dentist during drilling without novocaine." I immediately reinstituted the gabapentin, increasing stepwise back to 300/300/500 mg/day when lower doses did not stop the pain. Once again, both her headache and neuralgia resolved on this regimen, and we were able to decrease her dose of gabapentin to 300/500 mg/day. On this current regimen of amitriptyline and gabapentin, the patient has now been pain-free for 6 months, has no side effects, and is content. This case illustrates that, while the presentation of trigeminal neuralgia (TN) can be quite varied in clinical practice, even in the presence of complicating non-typical features such as associated primarily muscular headache, a detailed history will readily identify the characteristic features of trigeminal neuralgia TN and allow for directed treatment.

THE VARIED PRESENTATION OF TRIGEMINAL NEURALGIA

The spectrum of TN as described by tertiary referral centers is different from what I have seen practicing front-line neurology for 20 years. Academic centers focus on more severe, unremitting, or escalating cases of neuralgia. In an unfiltered general neurology setting, on the other hand, a practitioner encounters not only classic, severe TN, but also many simple variations that would not find their way to a tertiary care setting, either because the symptoms are not severe or because the symptoms resolve within a relatively short time frame, either by themselves or following successful early medical intervention. It is worth looking at the spectrum of facial neuralgic pain that presents in a general neurology setting to develop a strategy for identifying and treating neuralgia.

In my practice, neuralgic pain is a relatively common complaint. Frequently, patients describe typical TN: brief, sharp, shooting pain in the distribution of the trigeminal nerve, often with an escalating pattern. Other patients describe infrequent neuralgia occurring on a weekly or monthly basis. Some describe frequent severe pain that lasts days to weeks but does not persist.

Emergency room physicians, primary care doctors, and dentists often fail to diagnose trigeminal neuralgia TN because patients will report that their severe head pain lasts for hours or days, but they will not specify that their individual unit of pain is brief (lasting seconds) but occurs repetitively over the duration of the attack. In addition to the lancinating pain, there is sometimes a persistent dull ache in the temporal area that persists between the sharp pains. The caregiver needs to ask specific questions about the details of the time course, whether the severe pain is lancinating, and what triggers the pain. Neuralgia is usually readily identified by such careful history taking.

Sometimes the trigger for trigeminal neuralgia TN can obscure the diagnosis. I have seen many patients who have had multiple dental procedures performed, including dental extractions, as treatment for facial pain that is triggered by chewing or by dental manipulation, and that eventually gets diagnosed solely as neuralgia. In these cases, the procedures not only were unnecessary and delayed the diagnosis but seemed to exacerbate the neuralgic pain. On the other hand, clear-cut dental problems, such as abcesses or cavities, can serve as the trigger for neuralgia and need to be identified and treated. As a neurologist, I advise doing dental procedures in patients who have neuralgic pain only when there is a clear-cut indication for the procedure on medical grounds. The consideration of pain relief should not be the sole criterion for performing such a procedure.

In other cases, the diagnosis of TN can be confused by a concomitant diagnosis. I have seen a couple of cases in which a patient with Bells palsy had TN at the same time. More commonly, as in the earlier-described case, I have seen many people who have migrainous (or less commonly muscular) headaches occurring in conjunction with TN. In my experience, such neuralgias tend to occur in middle-aged and younger people and are usually amenable to medical treatment, although at times they can recur.

Although I commonly see patients present in their 50's and 60's, the syndrome presents in childhood as well. I have seen rare cases under age 10; it is not infrequently a complaint in teenagers. These pediatric cases are often benign and resolving, but I have had a handful of young patients who have had severe and persistent neuralgia. Age should not be a criterion for ruling out TN as a potential diagnosis.

In my practice, I will obtain an MRI scan to look for vascular compression of the trigeminal nerve; it is rare to find a specific underlying disease on MRI. I have had only a couple of patients who had multiple sclerosis and trigeminal neuralgia TN, but the trigeminal neuralgia TN presented after the diagnosis of MS had been made already. I had one patient who had a thalamic vascular malformation who presented with burning pain in the face. Although this patient had been referred to me for neuralgia, I thought he had atypical facial pain instead because the pain was constant and burning.

MANAGING TRIGEMINAL NEURALGIA

The most important decision in managing TN is to clinically assess the severity and malignancy of each individual case. Some patients have frequent, severe, escalating pain that needs aggressive medical treatment, and these patients are more likely to need operative intervention. Other patients have a pattern of TN that appears more indolent and is more likely to resolve. Since neuralgic pain is severe and can become so frequent as to incapacitate a person, it is important to treat the pain aggressively. Once the pain is unremitting and incapacitating, there may be no good cure.

In my experience, TN can perpetuate itself. In other words, the TN pain is the most important trigger for more TN pain. A patient's pain may initially result from an external trigger such as trauma, but once the nerve is irritated ongoing volleys of pain can occur. Within a patient's flare of TN, one series of volleys makes it more likely that there will be another series of volleys. I think these are clinical correlations of what likely is happening pathophysiologically at the trigeminal ganglion: axonal and demyelinating loss sets up ephatic discharges of the sensitized ganglion, sometimes occurring circularly and perhaps causing further damage.

A patient who is having sporadic neuralgia occurring as one or two electric jolts every few weeks does not need to be treated with medication. However, it is important to educate the patient to avoid triggers and to return to neurologic care quickly if the pattern of disease intensifies. On the other hand, the person who is having daily bouts of repetitive pain clearly needs medication. In my experience, a bout in which the patient has delayed treatment until the symptoms become more severe is more difficult to treat than a bout in the same person when caught earlier. Such a severe bout often requires higher doses of medications for longer periods of time to quiet the TN. For some patients with a history of recurrent TN, it is prudent to prescribe a continuing low dose of anticonvulsant to keep flares less frequent, escalating the dose if a flare should recur.

The details of specific treatment are left to other chapters of this book. However, my approach in a nutshell is to load with intravenous phenytoin (Dilantin) if the patient is presenting with incapacitating pain. This will achieve therapeutic levels of anticonvulsant drug quickly, often with quick relief of pain. For more chronic management, I usually use other anticonvulsants. I like to use gabapentin since it works about as well as other anticonvulsants and it has a wide therapeutic window, so that it can be titrated up quickly with minimal side effects.

Other treatment considerations include the treatment of associated conditions. Sometimes having a medication that treats both the TN and the comorbid condition, simultaneously treating each separately, is necessary for optimum results; at other times, it might be best to prescribe separately for each condition. For example, if the patient is having insomnia with the pain, a low dose of amitriptyline can be useful for both pain and insomnia. I have had several patients without a prior history of anxiety become quite anxious worrying about their neuralgic pain and when it would strike. Sometimes this anxiety needs to be treated. Migraine and other headache disorders may need to be treated in addition to the TN. Finally, like other patients with chronic pain, there is a risk for addiction and drug- seeking behavior. This vulnerability needs to be discussed with the patient early in the course of medical treatment and dealt with as needed.

The response of my patients with TN to medication follows a certain pattern that has practical implications. The treatment course of the 47-year-old patient described earlier falls within this overall pattern. My observations suggest to me that, in the face of acute neuralgic pain, one needs to reach a certain (relatively high) therapeutic threshold to suppress the active firing of the trigeminal nerve. Once suppression is achieved, the nerve will be quiet at a lower therapeutic range of medication, and sometimes with no medication. However, either with external trigger or with too low a dose of medication, the vulnerable trigeminal nerve "escapes," neuralgia resumes, and higher doses of medication are again needed, which may or may not suppress the neuralgia.

Invasive procedures should be considered when medical treatment fails. However, in patients who have incapacitating pain, it is important to have an aggressively quick medical trial. Within a few weeks of beginning treatment for new TN, one has a good sense of whether medical treatment will likely be successful. While continuing to try other medications if the first or second medication fails to control the neuralgia, one should simultaneously refer the patient to a tertiary center for invasive treatment. It usually takes several weeks for a patient to be seen at a tertiary center and optimally, the patient will be evaluated in the center toward the end of their third medication trial.

CONCLUSION

The natural history of trigeminal neuralgia TN is not clearly understood. However, some individuals may be predisposed to self-perpetuating cycles of worsening, sometimes intractable, neuralgic pain. A careful history of the components of a patient's facial pain can lead to a rapid and accurate diagnosis of TN. Prompt, aggressive medical treatment will best limit the patient's acute pain syndrome and may, in my opinion, decrease the frequency and severity of future bouts of pain. The trigeminal nerve in the neuralgic patient acts as if it has "memory" for synchronized painful discharges; it is the job of the treating physician to make the nerve forgetful.

6

Current Medical Therapy

Jeffrey Cohen

Medication is the first-line treatment for the management of newly diagnosed trigeminal neuralgia (TN). For many patients with chronic or recurrent TN, medication is also the mainstay for management of the pain. Medications are also used if pain returns after a surgical intervention.

MEDICATIONS FOR TRIGEMINAL NEURALGIA

Medications for TN can be divided into antiepileptic medications (AEDs) and non-AEDs. The use of AEDs for TN arose from the observation by Trouseau (1853) that paroxysmal pain might be related to paroxysmal discharges in the trigeminal nerve system. It was further hypothesized that this type of abnormal electrical activity might be similar to what occurs in the production of epileptic seizures. Since this initial observation, many AEDs, as well as non-AED, but central nervous system (CNS)–acting drugs, have been tried to eliminate TN pain. For a choice of drugs, clinicians have had to rely mostly on clinical experience as there are relatively few randomized controlled clinical trials for these medications. The literature contains several small clinical trials, case series, or single case reports. For several drugs that have been used, there are no reports in the literature. The relative rareness of TN, the lack of agreement of definition and trial design, and the presence of older treatments that became available before the current era of randomized clinical trials account for this situation. This makes objective evaluation and comparison of medical therapies difficult.

Antiepileptic Medications

First-generation Antiepileptic Drugs

A distinction is made between those AEDs marketed in the United States before and after 1993. In general, first-generation AEDs have a more complicated metabolism, and are often potent P450 enzyme stimulators or inhibitors. They have relatively narrow therapeutic indices, and many have a history of ill-desired chronic adverse events. Nonetheless, they are still used for the management of TN.

Phenytoin Introduced to market in 1938, phenytoin (5,5-diphenylhydantoin) is an AED first reported as useful for TN in the French literature in 1942 (Bergouignan 1942). A small case series reported in 1958 (Iannone, Baker, & Morrell 1958) seemed to solidify its use. There are no clinical trials for phenytoin in TN, but estimates of its initial effectiveness are 70%, with only about 25% having sustained relief (Braham & Saia 1960). Phenytoin is a voltage-dependent sodium channel blocker with zero-order pharmacokinetics throughout its therapeutic range, and with numerous drug–drug interactions (as a P450 enzyme inducer), making dosing somewhat troublesome. It has well-known dose-dependent adverse events (sedation, ataxia, diplopia, liver function abnormalities), as well as long-term consequences (gingival hyperplasia, bone loss, increased skull thickness, peripheral neuropathy). It is probably not a first-line therapy at present, with some exceptions (see below).

Carbamazepine Carbamazepine (5H-debenz(*b,f*)azepin-5-carboxamide) was approved by the U.S. Food and Drug Administration (FDA) in 1974, for the treatment of TN, and remains the only such approved medication. It is still considered to be a first-line drug by many practitioners. Its presumed mechanism of action is as a voltage-dependent sodium channel blocker. Four randomized clinical trials (RCTs) suggest good efficacy (over 70% initial response rate), with evidence of reduction of severity of pain and reduction of number of attacks (Campbell, Graham, & Zilkha 1966; Killian & Fromm 1968; Nicol 1969; Rockliff & Davis 1966;). It is a P450 enzyme inducer, exhibits autoinduction (of enzymes responsible for its own metabolism), and has significant drug–drug interactions. It may cause hyponatremia, via SIADH, and has black-box warnings for aplastic anemia/agranulocytosis and, more recently, for serious dermatologic reactions, especially in Asians with the HLA-B*1502 allele. Carbamazepine remains the only FDA-approved medical treatment for TN.

Valproate In an open-label comparator study of valproate versus phenytoin for an assortment of pain patients with "shooting pain," which included a small number of TN patients, valproate was found to be useful (Swerdlow 1980). An uncontrolled study of 20 TN patients (new-onset and refractory) treated with valproate, up to 1200 mg/day, suggested that 9 of 20 had either no pain attacks, or a 50% reduction in frequency/severity, for up to 6 months (Peiris, Perera, Devendra, & Lionel 1980).

Next-generation Antiepileptic Drugs

This category refers to AEDs marketed in the United States after 1993. Some of these drugs represent "improved" versions (such as oxcarbazepine) of previously existing AEDs, and others are truly new and novel (such as topiramate). The main advantages of the next-generation AEDs are primarily in their less-complicated pharmacokinetics and better safety and tolerability profiles. There is little information to suggest superior efficacy in reducing pain.

Oxcarbazepine Oxcarbazepine (10,11-dihydro-10-oxo-carbamazepine) is a keto analog of carbamazepine. It is an inhibitor of sustained, high-frequency, repetitive firing of voltage-dependent sodium action potentials. An unblinded study of 13 patients with typical TN treated with oxcarbazepine, and who had been previously refractory to carbamazepine, resulted in a 73% response rate (Farago 1987). An additional six patients refractory to carbamazepine were treated with oxcarbazepine, with good response, in an open-label trial (Zakrzewska & Patsalos 1989). Eleven patients refractory to other medications had a 91% response rate to oxcarbazepine (median dose = 1,650 mg/day) in an open-label trial, with an 11-month follow-up (Cohen 2002). Another prospective open-label trial of 36 TN patients refractory to gabapentin resulted in 60% of the patients reporting a good to excellent pain relief response (Royal et al. 2001). Three randomized, double-blind studies comparing oxcarbazepine to carbamazepine in both newly diagnosed and refractory TN patients (total of 132 patients), with a 24-week maintenance period, revealed no difference in percent of responders (about 70%) or in percent of subjects becoming pain free (about 38%) (Beydoun, Schmidt, & D'Souza 2002). However, fewer oxcarbazepine versus carbamazepine subjects reported adverse effects. The most common adverse effects of oxcarbazepine are dose-dependent and affect the central nervous and gastrointestinal systems. Hyponatremia is also characteristic of oxcarbazepine, although the mechanism may be through impaired renal water excretion (Sachdeo et al. 2002). There are fewer drug–drug interactions versus carbamazepine, in part because a major part of oxcarbazepine metabolism is through reduction, not P450 oxidation.

Gabapentin Gabapentin is structurally related to the major CNS inhibitory neurotransmitter γ-aminobutyric acid (GABA). Although it was designed to enhance GABA activity, there is no clear evidence that its mechanism of action works that way at clinically effective doses. Instead, gabapentin may work via the $\alpha_2\delta$ subunit of calcium ion (Ca^{+2}) channels. Gabapentin has been reported useful in the treatment of refractory TN in multiple sclerosis (MS) patients (Khan 1998). Two additional open-label studies of gabapentin for TN in MS have confirmed this observation (Solaro et al. 1998, 2000). A retrospective analysis of 92 TN patients treated with gabapentin found that 43 (47%) reported a reduction in pain (Cheshire 2002). The mean effective dose was 930 mg/day. In most, gabapentin was fairly well tolerated, although common adverse effects included sedation, nausea, peripheral edema, and weight gain. Gabapentin does not have active metabolites, does not affect the P450 system, and is not highly protein bound. It does not have any significant known drug–drug interactions.

Lamotrigine Lamotrigine (3,5-diamino-6-(2,3-dichlorophenyl)-1,2,4-triazine) is also a voltage-dependent sodium channel blocker, but appears to act on the slow inactivated state. A study of lamotrigine as adjunctive therapy in refractory TN (14 subjects; 2-week evaluation period) suggested efficacy in pain reduction as measured by a composite index (Zakrzewska et al. 1997). An open-label prospective trial of 20 subjects with either refractory idiopathic or symptomatic TN reported that 15 of 20 subjects had complete pain relief with lamotrigine monotherapy (100–400 mg/day) (Lunardi et al. 1997). Lamotrigine is generally well tolerated. However, there is a black-box warning for serious rash (e.g., Stevens Johnson syndrome). The possibility of rash decreases greatly when the titration rate is very slow (4–6 weeks), but slow titration rate limits its clinical effectiveness. Lamotrigine undergoes glucuronidation, has relatively low (55%) protein binding, and relatively few drug–drug interactions. One clinically significant drug interaction is with oral contraceptives: oral contraceptives reduce lamotrigine levels, but lamotrigine does not seem to affect hormone levels.

Topiramate Topiramate (2,3:4,5-Bis-O-(1-methylethylidene)-B-D-fructopyranose sulfamate) has several presumed mechanisms of action: voltage-dependent sodium channel blockade, augmentation of GABA activity at some subtypes of the $GABA_A$ receptor, antagonization of the L-alpha-amino-3-hydroxy-5-methyl-4-isoxazolepropionic acid (AMPA)/kainate subtype of the glutamate receptor, and inhibition of the carbonic anhydrase enzyme. A small (n = 3) randomized, placebo-controlled, multiple-crossover pilot study of topiramate in TN showed a significant reduction of pain in all three subjects (doses 75–600 mg/day), although a confirmatory study failed to show a positive effect (Gilron, Booher, Rowan, & Max 2001). Another small trial also suggested efficacy (Solaro et al. 2001). Siniscalchi et al. (2006) reported a case of MS–associated TN that was refractory to carbamazepine and gabapentin, but responded to topiramate monotherapy (200 mg/day) with a 14-month follow-up with no recurrence.

Felbamate Felbamate (2-phenyl-1,3-propanediol dicarbamate) appears to work by blocking currents evoked by N-methyl-D-aspartic acid (NMDA), and also by facilitating GABAergic responses. Efficacy of pain relief in three patients with TN who were refractory to other medical treatments was reported (Cheshire 1995). However, clinical use of felbamate remains limited due to the possibility of aplastic anemia and fatal hepatotoxicity. An improved version of felbamate, without these presumed risks, is in development.

Levetiracetam Levetiracetam ((–)-(S)-α-ethyl-2-oxo-1-pyrrolidine acetamide) has a unique mechanism of action: it binds to the presynaptic synaptic vesicle protein SV2A and presumably modulates calcium-dependent exocytosis of synaptic vesicles. How it may reduce neuropathic pain is not known. In a single-site, open-label, prospective pilot study of ten patients with TN, 40% of levetiracetam-treated subjects (monotherapy) were considered responders (Jorns, Johnston, & Zakrewska 2009). The average dose for the responders was 60.25 mg/kg/day in twice-daily dosing. Levetiracetam was generally well tolerated.

Pregabalin Pregabalin ((3S)-3-(aminomethyl)-5-methylhexanoic acid) binds with high affinity to the $\alpha_2\delta$ site (an auxiliary subunit of voltage-gated calcium channels) in CNS tissues. In vitro, pregabalin reduces the calcium-dependent release of several neurotransmitters, perhaps contributing to its antinociceptive properties. In an open-label, multicenter, prospective observational study of 12 weeks, with 65 subjects, pregabalin treatment was associated with a reduction in pain and was cost effective in a family medicine setting (Perez et al. 2009a, 2009b). Pregabalin monotherapy was used in 55%. The dosing was controlled by the treating physician, and was 196 + 105 mg in monotherapy and 234 mg + 107 mg in polytherapy. A previous open-label prospective study with a mixed population of TN patients suggested that pregabalin was useful in reducing pain in 74% of patients at a mean dose of 269.8 mg/day when evaluated after 8 weeks (Obermann et al. 2008). Neither study was blinded, and further data are needed to confirm these results.

Other Next-generation Antiepileptic Drugs

Data for tiagabine, lacosamide, rufinamide, vigabatrin, and zonisamide is either scarce or nonexistent. Nonetheless, practitioners have sometimes tried them for TN pain, with mixed results.

OTHER MEDICATIONS

Baclofen

Baclofen (4-amino-3(4-chlorophenyl)-butanoic acid) is a CNS muscle relaxant that possibly decreases excitatory synaptic transmission in the spinal trigeminal nucleus (Fromm, Terrence, Chattha, & Glass 1980). A small, double-blind crossover study showed that baclofen reduced the number of TN painful paroxysms in 7 of 10 versus 1 of 10 on placebo (Fromm, Terrence, & Chattha 1984). In a follow-up crossover, double-blind study of a mixed group of refractory TN patients, L-baclofen was more effective than racemic baclofen in 9 of 15 patients, using a measurement of number of paroxysms. Some of these patients were also taking AEDs (Fromm & Terrence 1987). It was felt that the D-baclofen in the racemic drug was antagonizing the effect of L-baclofen. Although efficacious for pain relief, the often-observed dose-dependent sedation may limit its effectiveness. Other common adverse events include gastrointestinal discomfort. Baclofen has a short half-life and is usually dosed at least three times per day. It is excreted via the kidneys.

Clonazepam

Clonazepam (6-(2-chlorophenyl)-9-nitro-2,5-diazabicyclo(5.4.0)undeca-5, 8,10,12-tetraen-3-one) binds to benzodiazepine receptors, which results in inhibitory effects on the CNS. Two small open-label studies have suggested partial benefit in TN (partial response rates of about 64% in each study), although sedation was a limiting factor (Court & Kase 1976; Smirne & Scarlato 1977).

Clomipramine

Clomipramine (3-(9-chloro-5,6-dihydrobenzo(b)(1)benzazepin-11-yl)-N,N-dimethylpropan) was compared to amitriptyline (3-(10,11-dihydro-5H-dibenzo((a,d)) cycloheptene-5-ylidene)-N,N-dimethyl-1-propanamine) in an older trial for neuropathic pain that included 17 patients with TN (Carasso, Yehuda, & Streifler 1979). Using a single-blind method, 20–75 mg/day of clomipramine was compared to 30–110 mg/day of amitriptyline. Significantly more subjects reported a moderate to marked improvement of TN pain when treated with clomipramine. Predominant adverse events included agitation and dry mouth.

Sumatriptan

Sumatriptan (3-(2-(dimethylamino)ethyl)-N-methyl-indole-5-methanesulforanide succinate) is an agonist for a vascular 5-hydroxytryptamine$_1$ receptor subtype (probably 5-HT$_{1D}$). It has been approved for the treatment of migraine headaches. The rationale for its use in TN has been hypothesized to be related to its agonistic effect on the 1D receptor subtype, which is present in high concentrations in the trigeminal system (Kanai, Suzuki, Kobayashi, & Hoka 2006b). Its potential effectiveness for use in TN pain was assessed in two small clinical trials. In a preliminary trial of 15 subjects with idiopathic TN, some of whom continued to take their carbamazepine, 3 mg of subcutaneous sumatriptan was administered after a placebo injection of saline. This was followed by oral sumatriptan, 50 mg, twice a day for 1 week (Kanai, Suzuki, Osawa, & Hoka 2006b). Using a visual analogue scale (VAS), pain was assessed at rest, during touching, and while eating. There was a significant reduction in VAS in the sumatriptan-treated group, lasting up to 2 weeks. Assessments were done by a blinded investigator. The second study randomized subjects with idiopathic TN to either 3 mg of subcutaneous sumatriptan, or placebo, in a crossover design (Kanai, Saito, & Hoka 2006a). Subjects discontinued other TN medications prior to receiving study drug. Investigators were blinded. Pain was assessed via

VAS scores 30 minutes after injection. Fifty percent of the subjects who received sumatriptan became pain free. A statistically significant effect was noted in number of subjects responding to sumatriptan versus placebo. The duration of effect was 7.9 hours. Adverse events in the two studies included a mild increase in blood pressure, nausea, and rare chest discomfort. While promising, this side-effect profile is likely to limit its use in the usual TN population, which tends to be older and have comorbidities that would make sumatriptan relatively contraindicated. Long-term effectiveness has not been evaluated. More recently, a report using nasal sumatriptan as adjunctive therapy for refractory TN in three cases suggested utility of this form as well (Shimohata et al. 2009).

Intranasal Lidocaine

Lidocaine (2-(diethylamino)-N-(2,6-dimethylphenyl) is a common local anesthetic that stabilizes neuronal membranes by inhibiting the ionic flux required for the initiation and conduction of impulses. Lidocaine has been used for many types of nerve blocks. Intranasal lidocaine (IL) was studied in patients with TN in the V_2 distribution (Kanai et al. 2006c) because the second division of the trigeminal nerve passes through the sphenopalatine ganglion, which is accessible via the nasal passages. Twenty-five subjects with typical TN were randomized to either 8% IL or placebo in a crossover design. Stimulus-evoked paroxysmal pain was assessed with the VAS before and after 15 and 30 minutes of treatment. Other TN medications were discontinued prior to the first study drug dose. There was a significant reduction in VAS after IL, but not after placebo. Forty percent of subjects given IL were pain free. Duration of pain relief averaged 4.3 hours. Adverse events included local irritation, bitter taste, and throat numbness.

Capsaicin

Capsaicin (8-methyl-N-vanillyl-trans-6-nonenamide) selectively blocks primary sensory neurons with possible nociceptive functions. In the first open-label study of 12 patients, 1 gm of capsaicin (0.05%) was applied topically to the area of pain three times daily for 1 year (Fusco & Alessandri 1992). Ten of twelve patients had partial or complete relief, although four of the responders had recurrences (Epstein & Marco 1994).

Tocainide

Tocainide (2-amino-N-(2,6-(dimethylphenyl)-propanamide) is a class I antiarrhythmic and sodium channel blocker that was studied in 12 patients in a double-blind, crossover study with carbamazepine (Lindstrom & Lindblom 1987). Duration of treatment for each drug was 2 weeks. Pain scores improved in both groups; no difference was noted between the two drugs. Nonetheless, the drug is not a practical treatment option at this time as it is no longer marketed in the United States because of unacceptable side effects, including serious hematological problems.

Pimozide

Pimozide (1-(1-(4,4-bis(4-flourophenyl)butyl)-4-piperidinyl)-1,3-dihydro-2H-benzimidazole-2-one) is an antipsychotic that was evaluated in a multicenter, double-blind, crossover trial when compared to carbamazepine in monotherapy (Lechin et al. 1989). Each treatment period was 8 weeks, and consisted of 48 patients having TN in the V_1 or V_2 distributions. Patients were refractory to a number of TN drugs at the outset. One-hundred percent of pimozide versus only 58% of carbamazepine patients exhibited reduced pain. Pimozide pain scores were reduced by 78% versus only 50% of carbamazepine-treated subjects ($p < 0.01$). Adverse effects were present in 83% of pimozide-treated patients, although none chose to drop out. Nonetheless, pimozide is not a viable option for TN pain due to its unacceptable side-effect profile, including extrapyramidal adverse effects and potentially fatal long Q-T syndrome.

Botulinum Toxin

Botulinum toxin-A (BTX-A) has gained widespread use for a number of medical and cosmetic conditions. It is thought to work by blocking the release of acetylcholine from the neuromuscular junction. It has been studied in two open-label trials for TN pain. In the first, eight patients with idiopathic TN were injected with 100 U of BTX-A: 50 U above and 50 U below the zygomatic arch on the affected side (Turk, Ilhan, Alp, & Sur 2005). Other medications were discontinued after receiving the injection. Both VAS scores and frequency of pain analyses showed statistically significant decreases after BTX-A at 1 week, 2 months, and 6 months post treatment. In the second study, 13 patients with idiopathic TN were injected with BTX-A subcutaneously in the area of facial pain (Piovesan et al. 2005). The range of BTX-A used was 6.45 to 9.11 U. Patients were on their concomitant TN meds, but could decrease or eliminate them if their pain improved. The area of pain was statistically significantly reduced at 10, 20, 30 and 60 days post injection. A reduction VAS scores correlated with the reduction of area of pain. Duration of pain relief did not end at 60 days, but there was no additional follow-up. Several of the patients were able to eliminate or reduce their concomitant medications. Although the mechanism of pain relief is unknown, it has been hypothesized to involve the inhibition of release of glutamate and substance P. Although positive, both of these studies should be considered preliminary. A randomized double-blind clinical trial is in progress to assess the potential efficacy of BTX-A in TN.

Homeopathic Agents

A single, noncontrolled observational study of 15 patients with TN was performed to assess the potential of individualized homeopathy to reduce pain (Mojaver et al. 2007). Two medical homeopaths interviewed each patient, and had to agree on the specific individualized homeopathy remedy to control TN pain. For women, *Pulsatilla*, and for men, *Aconite* was most commonly prescribed, although others were used and could be changed at the discretion of the practitioners during the course of the study. Traditional allopathic medication for TN was tapered before the start of the homeopathic treatment. A VAS was used to assess pain intensity. The results indicated a statistically significant reduction in pain intensity over the 4-month observational period. Methodological concerns included the definition of TN, individualization and altered treatments during the course of the study, lack of control or comparison group, and unblinded observations. Although of interest, this observation requires replication with more patients and improved design.

NEGATIVE CLINICAL TRIALS IN TRIGEMINAL NEURALGIA

Topical Proparacaine

Proparacaine (2-(diethylamino)ethyl 2-amino-4propoxybenzoate) was suggested as a treatment for TN based upon a serendipitous observation of pain improvement in a TN patient undergoing ophthalmological examination. A randomized double-blind trial of single-application topical proparacaine 0.5% (vs. placebo) administration to patients with TN was performed in 47 subjects (Kondziolka et al. 1994). Patients remained on previous drug therapy. No improvement was noted in the treatment group over placebo, using several measures on days 3, 10, or 30 after administration. Of interest, no data were reported regarding potential short-term (<1 day) or stimulus-evoked pain relief.

Tizanidine

Tizanidine(4-chloro-N-(4,5-dihydro-1H-imidazol-2yl)-8thia-7,9-diazabicyclo-(4,4,0) nona-2,4,6 9-tetraen-5-amine) is a centrally acting α_2 adrenergic agonist. It was evaluated in a small (n = 12) randomized, double-blind parallel group design with a maximum dose of 18 mg/day versus carbamazepine (900 mg/day, maximum) (Vilming, Lyberg, & Lataste 1986). No significant reduction in pain was noted. In a single crossover double-blind study of 11 patients with TN, some continuing other pain medications, tizanidine (4 mg tid) as adjunctive therapy was compared to placebo over an 8-day treatment period, followed by an open-label extension (Fromm, Aumentado, & Terrence 1993). At best, a modest response was noted, and there were tolerability issues.

Mexiletine

Mexiletine (1-(2,6-dimethylphenoxy)propan-2-amine) is a class 1B antiarrhythmic. It decreases action potentials by shortening the repolarization phase. It was studied in four patients with idiopathic TN at a dose of 10 mg/kg/day for at least a week, without improvement of pain (Pascual & Berciano 1989).

Dextromethorphan

Dextromethorphan ((+)-3-methoxy-17-methyl-(9a, 13a, 14a)-morphinan) is an NMDA glutamate receptor antagonist. A randomized, double-blind, crossover controlled trial of dextromethorphan was performed in patients with facial pain that included three people with TN (Gilron et al. 2000). The study did not reveal a benefit of dextromethorphan in any facial pain patients. It was inconclusive with respect to the three subjects with TN.

MISCELLANEOUS MEDICATIONS

Several case reports or small series have reported positive results with the following agents, although none of these may be taken as proof that these drugs are of true benefit in TN. A single patient with TN who developed hepatotoxicity to carbamazepine was treated with *milnacipran* ((1R,2R)-2-(aminomethyl)-N,N-diethyl-1-phenyl-cyclopropane-1-carboxamide), a serotonin-norepinephrine reuptake inhibitor (50 mg/day) for 2 months and had improvement in TN pain (Ito 2007). *Misoprostol* (methyl 7-(3-hydroxy-(E)-4-mehtyloct-1-enyl)-5-oxycyclopentyl)heptanoate) is a long-acting prostaglandin E1 analogue. It was studied in an open-label design of refractory TN patients with MS, and was suggested to be effective in six of seven research participants (Reder & Arnason 1995).

SPECIAL ISSUES IN CURRENT MEDICAL THERAPY

Acute Exacerbations of Trigeminal Neuralgia Pain

A significant minority of TN patients experience a crisis severe enough so that oral medications do not provide sufficient relief of pain to allow basic functioning. At the same time, high doses of their baseline medications produce significant adverse events. There is little guidance as to how to approach these situations. These patients may resort emergency room (ER) visits, especially in the evenings or on weekends. Often, local ER personnel are unfamiliar with TN, or may actually doubt the diagnosis. ER personnel may not know how to treat TN, and may sometimes give morphine or its equivalents; this may or may not result in pain relief, and may contribute to drug toxicity.

One option may be for the patient to have a separate, predetermined treatment plan for crises, with the notion that this may keep them from

ER visits. Such a plan may include treatments that may not be useful for everyday use, but are helpful for an occasional exacerbation, such as subcutaneous sumatriptan, intranasal lidocaine, or a previously physician-approved titration schedule to increase maintenance medication.

If this is not practical or fails to control pain, the patient may be treated in the ER. Providing the patient with a doctor's note stating the diagnosis and preferred acute treatment often ensures better and quicker pain relief. Intravenous (IV) phenytoin (3–5 mg/kg) given via normal saline, no faster (and preferably slower) than 50 mg/min, with the aid of a cardiac monitor and blood pressure checks, has been reported to be effective in several small case series (Albert 1978; Jensen 1954; Kugelberg & Lindblom 1959). The pain relief is rapid and may last up to 4 days. Common dose-limiting side effects include sedation, ataxia, bradycardia, and hypotension.

The relative negatives of IV phenytoin suspension formulated with 40% propylene glycol and 10% ethanol, adjusted to a pH of 12 with sodium hydroxide (thus leading to the adverse effects mentioned earlier), as well as the possibility of severe skin irritation with extravasation from the IV, has led to the development of the prodrug fosphenytoin. Fosphenytoin is a prodrug of phenytoin, with a pH of 8 in tris buffer. Although its administration also requires cardiac monitoring, it may be given at a faster rate (up to 150 mgPE/min) with less toxicity. Cleavage of the phosphates may lead to pruritus, often in the genital region. In a small case series of TN patients in acute pain crises, a loading dose of 14 mg/kg was needed to provide pain relief for up to 2 days (Cheshire 2001).

Other AEDs with IV formulations, such as valproate and levetiracetam, have not been assessed in the treatment of acute TN crises.

MANAGEMENT OF PREGNANT WOMEN AND WOMEN OF CHILDBEARING AGE

Although TN tends to affect women who are past their childbearing years, a significant minority of TN patients are women of childbearing age. All of the medications discussed above are at least pregnancy category class C; none are classified as class B. Therefore, their use for TN during pregnancy requires a risk–benefit analysis for each individual patient.

Data are emerging regarding the use of AEDs during pregnancy, via reports from various AED pregnancy registries. The North American Antiepileptic Drug Pregnancy Registry has reported an increased incidence of major congenital malformations (MCMs) for valproate (10.7%; Wyszynski et al. 2005), compared to that observed in the general population (roughly 2%). Lamotrigine has been associated with an elevated risk of nonsyndromic oral clefts (8.9/1000), although the overall rate of MCM was only 2.7% (Holmes et al. 2006). Using a different methodology, the

International Lamotrigine Pregnancy Registry reported a rate of 2.6% of MCMs to first-trimester lamotrigine monotherapy exposures (LTG pregnancy interim report, July, 2007).

For carbamazepine monotherapy, other pregnancy registries have reported a range of MCM rates from 2.2% to 8.2% (Meador et al. 2006; Morrow et al. 2006; Vajda et al. 2006).

Pregnancy data for the more commonly used AEDs during TN are either too small to be significant or are lacking. All women with TN who are of childbearing age should take folic acid, to help reduce the possibility of neural tube defects should they become pregnant. Although no drug of choice can be recommended for TN during pregnancy, the available data suggest that lamotrigine may be preferable from a safety point of view.

TREATMENT OF TRIGEMINAL NEURALGIA IN PATIENTS WITH MULTIPLE SCLEROSIS

The incidence of TN in MS patients is estimated to be 1.9% (Hooge & Redekop 1995), higher than in the general population. It is of interest to understand similarities and differences about the medical treatment of these patients. In MS patients, TN is often bilateral (14%) and occurs at a younger age than typical TN patients ($x = 38$ yrs). The etiology of TN in MS patients has traditionally been attributed to MS plaques present at the root entry zone of fifth-nerve fibers, or in the pons involving trigeminal fascicular fibers and nuclear areas (Gass et al. 1997).

There are no formal studies of the use of carbamazepine or oxcarbazepine in the management of TN in MS, although anecdotally it is of value in some patients. Gabapentin has been reported to effective in MS patients with refractory TN, in small open-label series, in mono- or polytherapy, at doses up to 1,200 mg/day (Khan 1998; Solaro et al. 1998, 2000, 2001). There is a report of two cases of refractory TN in MS patients successfully treated with topiramate at 200 mg/day (Solaro et al. 2001).

Misoprostol has been studied in two open-label trials in MS patients with refractory TN and has been reported to be effective (Reder et al. 1995; Evers et al. 2003).

PATIENTS WHO ARE SENSITIVE TO MEDICATIONS

A difficult management issue is the TN patient who is unable to tolerate oral medication. Sometimes patients are truly unable to take adequate doses of medications that are required to reduce pain (pharmacogenomics, hepatic or renal comorbidities). Others become paralyzed by fear of potential adverse effects. Frequently, additional education about medications may be helpful. Other approaches include the use of other than oral medications (commercial or compounded patches, creams, nasal or subcutaneous products). This group may seek procedures earlier than those able to tolerate medications.

COMPARATOR STUDIES: WHICH DRUG IS BETTER?

A meta-analysis of oxcarbazine versus carbamazepine revealed no difference (Beydoun et al. 2002). Carbamazepine was more effective than tizanidine (Vilming et al. 1986). Although baclofen was somewhat more effective than carbamazepine, the side-effect profile favored carbamazepine (Parekh, Shah, Kotdawalla, & Gandhi 1986). Clomipramine was more effective than amitriptyline (Carasso et al. 1979). Pimozide was more efficacious than carbamazepine, although not practical (Lechin et al. 1989).

BRAND VERSUS GENERIC MEDICATIONS

Many of the drugs used for TN have been available as generics for a number of years. Over the last few years, and continuing in the near future, a number of newer TN medications will become available as generics. Although considered to be therapeutically equivalent by the FDA, generics may introduce treatment issues for particular patients. For generics to be considered equivalent, there must be a 90% confidence interval for the mean area under the curve and a C_{max} between 80% and 125% (Lu & Davit 2007). It is conceivable that either loss of pain relief or development of adverse events could occur when patients switch between brand and generics, or among generics. In Canada, it was found that the switch-back rate from generic to brand medications was higher for AEDs than for several other drug classes (Andermann, Duh, Gosselin, & Paradis 2007).

MONO VERSUS POLYTHERAPY

Single drugs are often preferred since they may be effective, tend to produce fewer adverse events, and may be less expensive. However, although polytherapy is often tried in refractory TN patients, no studies suggest which combinations are best. Many of the open-label studies add the new drug to the primary drug and report a benefit. One study has suggested that adding baclofen to carbamazepine is synergistic (Parekh et al. 1986).

HOW MANY MEDICATIONS BEFORE A PROCEDURE?

Unfortunately, the literature does not allow us to directly answer the question of how many medications should be tried before a surgical procedure is recommended. On the one hand, a significant number of newly diagnosed patients with TN respond to the first medical therapy, at least for the short term. One subset of newly diagnosed TN patients gets partial relief from initial medical therapy, then develops unacceptable side effects as the dose is raised to provide complete pain relief. Another group of newly diagnosed TN patients never truly go into remission. These patients often go from one drug to another, sometimes in polytherapy, achieving partial relief, but still with side effects and occasional flare-ups. After several months, and a number of failed or partially effective drug trials, they opt for a surgical procedure.

There is a suggestion that some surgical procedures, such as microvascular decompression (MVD) is more effective if performed within the first 7 years of TN diagnosis. Thus, waiting to try multiple drugs may not be the most effective strategy. A small study of 15 patients with refractory TN were treated with oxcarbazepine and had long-term follow-up. Twelve of these patients required surgery, and most reported better improvement versus oxcarbazepine (Zakrzewska & Patsalos 2002). Using a decision analysis/time trade-off technique of 156 patients with TN, surgical treatments were somewhat preferable to medical treatments in terms of providing improved quality of life (Spatz, Zakrezewska, & Kay 2007).

WHEN TO TAPER MEDS?

There is little formal guidance as to when to taper medications for TN. For patients who truly go into remission, medications may be tapered slowly over 1 month. However, in those in whom the major pain is alleviated, but there are still mild twinges (reminders of pain), maintenance of a low dose of an effective drug is preferable.

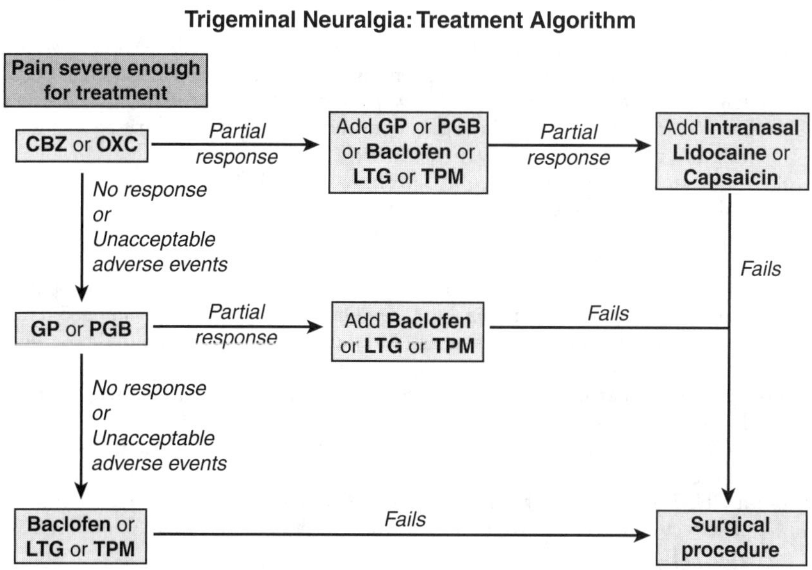

Figure 6.1 Enhanced Enriched Randomised Withdrawal (EERW) design.

ALGORITHM FOR MEDICAL MANAGEMENT

One suggestion for medical management is outline in Figure 6.1. In most patients, the initial choice of oxcarbazine or carbamazepine seems reasonable, given their high rate of initial success. Gabapentin is a reasonable second-line option, although it may be used initially in some cases. After this, further choices are often made depending upon whether the reason for drug failure is due to poor pain control or adverse effects. Drugs with different mechanisms of action may be combined. Other options include combined oral and nonoral adjunctive medications (intranasal lidocaine, subcutaneous sumatriptan).

REFERENCES

Albert HH. Infusionsbehandlung der akuten trigeminusneuralgie mit phenytoin i.v. *Munchener Medizinische Wochenschrift* 1978;120:529–530.

Andermann F, Duh MS, Gosselin A, Paradis PE. Compulsory generic switching of antiepileptic drugs: high switchback rates to branded compounds compared with other drug classes. *Epilepsia* 2007;48:464–469.

Bergouignan M. Cures hereuses de nevralgies faciales essentielles par le diphenyl–hydantoinate de soude. *Rev Laryng Otol Rhinol* 1942;63:34.

Beydoun A, Schmidt D, D'Souza J. Oxcarbazepine versus carbamazepine in trigeminal neuralgia: a meta-analysis of three double blind comparative trials. *Neurology* 2002;58(Suppl 2).

Braham J, Saia A. Phenytoin in the treatment of trigeminal and other neuralgias. *Lancet* 1960;2:893–893.

Campbell FG, Graham JG, Zilkha KJ. Clinical trial of carbamazepine (Tegretol) in trigeminal neuralgia. *J Neurol Neurosurg Psych* 1966;29:265–267.

Carasso RL, Yehuda S, Streifler M. Clomipramine and amitriptyline in the treatment of severe pain. *Int J Neurosci* 1979;9:191–194.

Cheshire WP, Jr. Felbamate relieved trigeminal neuralgia. *Clin J Pain* 1995;11:139–142.

Cheshire WP, Jr. Fosphenytoin: an intravenous option for the management of acute trigeminal neuralgia crisis. *J Pain Sympt Mgmt* 2001;21:506–510.

Cheshire WP, Jr. Defining the role of gabapentin in the treatment of trigeminal neuralgia: a retrospective study. *J Pain* 2002;3:137–142.

Cohen J. Postmarketing experience with oxcarbazepine in the treatment of trigeminal neuralgia, 2002 (abst).

Court JE, Kase CS. Treatment of tic douloureux with a new anticonvulsant (clonazepam). *J Neurol Neurosurg Psych* 1976;39:297–299.

Epstein JB, Marco JH. Topical application of capsaicin for treatment of oral neuropathic pain and trigeminal neuralgia. *Oral Surg Oral Med Oral Pathol* 1994;77:135–140.

Evers S, DMKG Study Group. Misoprostol in the treatment of trigeminal neuralgia associated with multiple sclerosis. *J Neurol* 2003;250:542–545.

Farago F. Trigeminal neuralgia: its treatment with two new carbamazepine analogues. *Eur Neurol* 1987;26:73–83.

Fromm GH, Aumentado D, Terrence CF. A clinical and experimental investigation of the effects of tizanidine in trigeminal neuralgia. *Pain* 1993;53:265–271.

Fromm GH, Terrence CF, Chattha AS, Glass JD. Baclofen in trigeminal neuralgia: its effect on the spinal trigeminal nucleus: a pilot study. *Arch Neurol* 1980;37: 768–771.

Fromm GH, Terrence CF, Chattha AS. Baclofen in the treatment of trigeminal neuralgia: double blind study and long-term follow up. *Ann Neurol* 1984;15:240–244.

Fromm GH, Terrence CF. Comparison of L-baclofen and racemic baclofen in trigeminal neuralgia. *Neurology* 1987;37:1725–1728.

Fusco BM, Alessandri M. Analgesic effect of capsaicin in idiopathic trigeminal neuralgia. *Anesth Analg* 1992;74:375–377.

Galleli L, Scornaienghi D, Mancuso F, De Sarro G. Topiramate therapy for symptomatic trigeminal neuralgia. *Clin Drug Invest* 2006;26:113–115.

Gass A, Kitchen N, MacManus DCR, et al. Trigeminal neuralgia in patients with multiple sclerosis: lesion localization with magnetic resonance imaging. *Neurology* 1997;49:1142–1144.

Gilron I, Booher SL, Rowan JS, et al. A randomized, controlled trial of high-dose dextromethorphan in facial neuralgias. *Neurology* 2000;55:964–971.

Gilron I, Booher SL, Rowan JS, Max MB. Topiramate in trigeminal neuralgia: a randomized placebo-controlled multiple crossover pilot study. *Clin Pharmacol* 2001;24:109–112.

Holmes LB, Wyszynski DF, Baldwin EJ, et al. Increased risk for non-syndromic cleft palate among infants exposed to lamotrigine during pregnancy. *Birth Defects Res (Part A)* 2006;76:5.

Hooge JP, Redekop WK. Trigeminal neuralgia in multiple sclerosis. *Neurology* 1995;45:1294–1296.

Iannone A, Baker AB, Morrell F. Dilantin in the treatment of trigeminal neuralgia. *Neurology* 1958;8:126–128.

International Lamotrigine Pregnancy Registry, interim report, issued July 2007.

Ito M, Yoshida K, Kimura H, et al. Successful treatment of trigeminal neuralgia with milnacipran. *Clin Neuropharm* 2007;30:183–185.

Jensen H. Die Behandlung der trigeminusneuralgie mit diphenylhydantoin. *Arztliche Wochenschrift* 1954;9:105–108.

Jorns TP, Johnston A, Zakrewska JM. Pilot study to evaluate the efficacy and tolerability of levetiracetam (Keppra[R]) in treatment of patients with trigeminal neuralgia. *Eur J Neurol* 2009;16:740–744.

Kanai A, Saito M, Hoka S. Subcutaneous sumatriptan for refractory trigeminal neuralgia. *Headache* 2006a;46:577–582.

Kanai A, Suzuki A, Kobayashi M, Hoka S. Intranasal lidocaine 8% spray for second-division trigeminal neuralgia. *Brit J Anesth* 2006c;97:559–563.

Kanai A, Suzuki A, Osawa S, Hoka S. Sumatriptan alleviates pain in patients with trigeminal neuralgia. *Clin J Pain* 2006b;22:677–680.

Khan OA. Gabapentin relieves trigeminal neuralgia in multiple sclerosis patients. *Neurology* 1998;51:611–614.

Killian JM, Fromm GH. Carbamazepine in the treatment of neuralgia. *Arch Neurol* 1968;19:129–136.

Kondziolka D, Lemley T, Kestle JR, et al. The effect of single-application topical ophthalmic anesthesia in patients with trigeminal neuralgia. *J Neurosurg* 1994;80:993–997.

Kugelberg E, Lindblom U. The mechanism of the pain in trigeminal neuralgia. *J Neurol Neurosurg Psychiat* 1959;22:36–43.

Lechin F, van der Dijs B, Lechin ME, et al. Pimozide therapy for trigeminal neuralgia. *Arch Neurol* 1989;46:960–963.

Lindstrom P, Lindblom U. The analgesic effect of tocainide in trigeminal neuralgia. *Pain* 1987;28:45–50.

Lu SK, Davit BM. Bioequivalence testing in the US for generic drug products, 2007. Accessed March 17, 2008. Available at http://www.fda.gov/cder/audiences/iact/forum/200704_lu.pdf.

Lunardi G, Leandri M, Albano C, et al. Clinical effectiveness of lamotrigine and plasma levels in essential and symptomatic trigeminal neuralgia. *Neurology* 1997;48:1714–1717.

Meador KJ, Baker GA, Finnell RH, et al. In utero antiepileptic drug exposure. *Neurology* 2006;67:407–412.
Mojaver YN, Mosavi F, Mazaherinezhad A, et al. Individualized homeopathic treatment of trigeminal neuralgia. *Homeopathy* 2007;96: 82–86.
Morrow J, Russell A, Guthrie E, et al. Malformation risks of antiepileptic drugs in pregnancy: a prospective study from the UK epilepsy and pregnancy registry. *J Neurol Neurosurg Psychiatry* 2006;77:193–198.
Nicol CF. A four year double-blind study of Tegretol in facial pain. *Headache* 1969;9:54–57.
Obermann M, Yoon MS, Sensen K, et al. Efficacy of pregabalin in the treatment of trigeminal neuralgia. *Cephalgia* 2008;28:174–181.
Parekh S, Shah K, Kotdawalla H, Gandhi I. Baclofen in carbamazepine resistant trigeminal neuralgia: a double blind clinical trial. *Cephalgia* 1989;9:392–393.
Pascual J, Berciano J. Failure of mexiletine to control trigeminal neuralgia. *Headache* 1989;29:517–518.
Peiris JB, Perera GLS, Devendra SV, Lionel NDW. Sodium valproate in trigeminal neuralgia. *Med J Australia* 1980;2:278.
Perez C, Navarro A, Saldana MT, et al. Patient-reported outcomes in subjects with painful trigeminal neuralgia receiving pregabalin: evidence from medical practice in primary care settings. *Cephaligia* 2009a;29:781–790.
Perez C, Saldana MT, Navarro A, et al. Trigeminal neuralgia treated with pregabalin in family medicine settings: its effet on pain alleviation and cost reduction. *J Clin Pharmacol* 2009b;49:582–590.
Piovesan EJ, Teive HG, Kowacs PA, et al. An open study of botulinum-A toxin treatment of trigeminal neuralgia. *Neurology* 2005;65:1306–1308.
Reder AT, Arnason BG. Trigeminal neuralgia in multiple sclerosis relieved by a prostaglandin E analogue. *Neurology* 1995;45:1097–1100.
Rockliff BW, Davis EH. Controlled sequential trials of carbamazepine in trigeminal neuralgia. *Arch Neurol* 1966;15:129–136.
Royal M, Wienecke G, Movva V, et al. Open label trial of oxcarbazepine in neuropathic pain. *Pain Medicine* 2001;2:250–251.
Sachdeo RC, Rajesh C, Wasserstein A, et al. Effects of oxcarbazepine on sodium concentration and water handling. *Ann Neurol* 2002;51:613–620.
Shimohata K, Shimohata T, Motegi R, et al. Nasal sumatriptan as adjunctive therapy for idiopathic trigeminal neuralgia: report of three cases. *Headache* 2009;49: 768–770.
Siniscalchi A, Gallelli L, Scornaienghi D, et al. Topiramate therapy for symptomatic trigeminal neuralgia. *Clinical Drug Investigation* 2006;26(2):113–5, 2006.
Smirne S, Scarlato G. Clonazepam in cranial neuralgias. *Med J Australia* 1977;1:93–94.
Solaro C, Lunardi GL, Capello E, et al. An open-label trial of gabapentin treatment of paroxysmal symptoms in multiple sclerosis patients. *Neurology* 1998;51: 609–611.
Solaro C, Messmen Uccelli M, Ucelli A, et al. Low dose gabapentin combined with either lamotrigine or carbamazepine can be useful therapies for trigeminal neuralgia in multiple sclerosis. *Eur Neurol* 2000;44:45–48.
Solaro C, Uccelli MM, Brichetto G, et al. Topiramate relieves idiopathic and symptomatic trigeminal neuralgia. *J Pain Sympt Mgmt* 2001;21:367–368.
Spatz AL, Zakrzewska JM, Kay EJ. Decision analysis of medical and surgical treatments for trigeminal neuralgia: How patient evaluations of benefits and risks affect the utility of treatment decisions. *Pain* 2007;131:302–310.
Swerdlow M. The treatment of "shooting" pain. *Postgrad Med J* 1980;56:159–161.
Trouseau A. De la neuralgie epileptiforme. *Arch Gen Med* 1853;1:33.
Turk U, Ilhan S, Alp R, Sur H. Botulinum toxin and intractable trigeminal neuralgia. *Clin Neuropharmacol* 2005;28:161–162.

Vajda FJE, Hitchcock A, Graham J, et al. Foetal malformations and seizure control: 52 months data of the Australian pregnancy registry. *Eur J Neurol* 2006;13:645–654.

Vilming ST, Lyberg T, Lataste X. Tizanidine in the management of trigeminal neuralgia. *Cephalgia* 1986;6:181–182.

Wyszynski DF, Nambisan M, Surve T, et al. Increased rate of major malformations in offspring exposed to valproate during pregnancy. *Neurology* 2005;64:961–965.

Zakrzewska JM, Chaudry Z, Nurmikko TJ, et al. Lamotrigine (Lamictal) in refractory trigeminal neuralgia: results from a double-blind placebo controlled crossover trial. *Pain* 1997;73:223–230.

Zakrzewska JM, Patsalos PN. Long-term cohort study comparing medical (oxcarbazepine) and surgical management of intractable trigeminal neuralgia. *Pain* 2002;95:259–266.

Zakrzewska JM, Patsalos PT. Oxcarbazepine: a new drug in the management of intractable trigeminal neuralgia. *JNNP* 1989;52:472–476.

7

Differential Diagnosis, Look–alike Diseases, Atypical Trigeminal Neuralgia

Mark E. Linskey and Peter J. Jannetta

Sensation to the face is governed by the fifth cranial, or trigeminal, nerve. Pain of nerve origin is often termed *neuralgia*. It is thus very common for any pain involving the face to be considered "trigeminal neuralgia"; neglecting the fact that true trigeminal neuralgia (TN) is a distinct and well-defined syndrome. Indeed, TN also represents a subset of facial pain syndromes that include many other conditions that often do not respond to TN medical or surgical therapies in predictable or successful ways. The confusion between true TN and other facial pain syndromes is common among physicians and dentists, and is even more common among patients. This confusion has recently become compounded by the ready exchange of information through the Internet, where patients seeking information and help often compare their symptoms to personal posted anecdotes or testimonials, which may lead patients toward misdiagnosis through apparent similarities in symptoms and experience. Interestingly, the Internet also holds the best promise for dispelling confusion and focusing the search for relief in positive directions, through the development of scientifically advised and well-maintained websites for patient support groups, such as the TNA–The Facial Pain Association website (http://www.endthepain.org).

Two equally important problems exist. The first is avoiding the tragedy of misclassifying a TN patient as not having TN, and thus missing the opportunity to successfully intervene surgically if medical treatment fails. The second is in mislabeling a facial pain patient as having TN and then pursuing TN treatments that carry some risks, without a high likelihood of therapeutic success. The first step in trying to help a patient with facial pain or even one referred for "trigeminal neuralgia" is to carefully determine whether the patient has TN or another "look-alike" syndrome. This chapter is focused on this very issue.

MISSING THE DIAGNOSIS OF TRIGEMINAL NEURALGIA

In our experience, at least three persisting myths are circulating among health practitioners that can mislead well-intentioned practitioners into failing to recognize that their patient actually has TN, rather than one of the other facial pain syndromes to be discussed in this chapter. Missing the diagnosis of TN can have significant negative impact on patients through prolonging their suffering, failing to apply optimal medical TN treatments, or even failing to refer medically refractory patients for potentially beneficial operative intervention. Each of these myths will be addressed in turn.

Myth 1: A Patient with a Detectable Trigeminal Sensory Deficit Does Not Have Trigeminal Neuralgia

It is very unfortunate that the International Headache Society (IHS) in their publication *International Classification of Headache and Related Disorders* (ICHD-II) defined TN as having no detectable sensory deficit on examination (Table 7.1) (Olesen et al. 2004). They thus, by definition, excluded a subset of true TN patients from correct diagnosis and referral for potentially beneficial therapy. It should be obvious that many patients who have undergone trigeminal destructive procedures for TN, such as radiofrequency thermoablation, glycerol rhizotomy, percutaneous balloon compression, or stereotactic radiosurgery, will have sensory loss related to their destructive procedure, even if the procedure fails and their TN persists or recurs. However, this assertion is problematic even for a subset of patients who have never undergone a palliative destructive procedure.

Abundant evidence suggests that a subset of TN patients have subtle sensory deficits that can be picked up by either careful and thorough neurological examination (Bowsher et al. 1997; Nurmikko 1991; Sinay, Bonamico, & Dubrovsky 2003), or by trigeminal sensory-evoked potential study (Bennett & Jannetta 1983; Mursch et al. 2002). In our experience, we find subtle sensory deficits, usually detectable in the medial aspect of the V_2, or less commonly V_3 divisions, in up to 30% of TN cases. Similarly, a carefully performed corneal reflex examination will show a decrease in the upper half of the cornea in V_1 TN and a decrease in the lower half in V_2 TN.

Table 7.1 Diagnostic criteria for classic trigeminal neuralgia

- Paroxysms lasting fraction of a second to 2 minutes, affecting one or more divisions of the trigeminal nerve
- Pain has at least one of these characteristics:
  - Intense, sharp, superficial, or stabbing
  - Precipitated from trigger zones or by a trigger factor
- Attacks are stereotyped in the individual patient
- No evident neurological deficit
- Not attributable to another disorder

From the International Headache Society (IHS). *International Classification of Headache and Related Disorders*, 2nd edition (ICHD-II) (Olesen 2004).

Interestingly, these findings appear to be more common in patients with a longer history of TN, lending support to hypotheses suggesting an ongoing nerve damage process at the root of TN. We also find subtle sensory deficits more commonly in patients who remain predominantly typical in their pain features (>70% of their syndrome), but who are starting to develop minor background (<30% of their syndrome) atypical pain features, such as persisting dull or burning pain between neuralgic episodes. This observation would seem to support the hypothesis first noted by Jannetta and put forward by Burchiel, that TN type 1 (TN1) patients can evolve into TN type 2 (TN2) patients over time (Burchiel & Slavin 2000).

Myth 2: Patients Who Do Not Initially Respond to a Trial of an Appropriate Antiepileptic Drug for Trigeminal Neuralgia Do Not Have Trigeminal Neuralgia

It is very true that most true TN patients will at least initially show improvement with a therapeutic trial of the one of the common and proven antiepileptic drugs (AEDs) used to treat TN (carbamazepine, oxcarbazepine, gabapentin, phenytoin, etc.). Unfortunately, the impression persists that this therapeutic trial is diagnostic for TN and, if the patient does not improve at all with the trial of one or two agents, then the diagnosis of TN is incorrect. The finding of a response to AED treatment is overwhelmingly common, and this should certainly reassure the practitioner that his diagnosis is correct. The absence of response, however, should also lead to very careful reconsideration of the other syndromes to be discussed in this chapter. This finding of nonresponse is not pathognomonic: If the patient has purely typical TN pain features (brief, sharp, electric, stabbing pain; tactile triggers; no pain between episodes), then he or she still likely has TN. In our experience, up to 5% of TN patients who go on to respond to surgical TN interventions never responded to AED therapy.

Myth 3: A Patient with Bilateral Symptoms Does Not Have Trigeminal Neuralgia

Bilateral TN symptoms are much more common in the setting of multiple sclerosis (MS)-related TN. While less common in the setting of non-MS TN, in our own experience approximately 2%–4% of TN patients have bilateral symptoms. Nevertheless, bilateral symptoms should lead to a thorough evaluation to rule out MS. In our practices, this involves not just magnetic resonance (MR) scanning to identify and rule out demyelination plaques, it also includes cerebrospinal fluid (CSF) examination to assess myelin basic protein and rule out oligoclonal bands. When typical TN is bilateral, it almost always begins sequentially and not simultaneously on both sides, with often years between developing symptoms on the other side.

CONSIDERING THE ALTERNATIVES

When interviewing, examining, and evaluating a patient with possible TN, it is important not to confuse typical TN with "look-alike" or overlap conditions and syndromes. When trying to sort this out, we have found it useful to consider alternative facial pain syndromes in two separate categories: Those in which the symptoms are exactly the same as typical TN, and those in which there may only be certain features or characteristics in common.

Conditions with Complete Symptom Overlap

The basic clinical features of typical TN are outline schematically in Figure 7.1 (Zakrzewska & Linskey 2009). The most important features are pain severity (patients stop whatever they are doing and are often frightened), pain character (sharp, electric, shock-like), time course (pain lasts seconds to minutes, unless coming in repetitive clusters), pain-free status between episodes, and the presence of tactile triggers in the trigeminal distribution (Mathews, et al., Youmans, in press; Zakrzewska & Linskey 2008, 2009). Although more than 95% of patients with these features have idiopathic TN, the remainder will be found to have either intraparenchymal or extraparenchymal structural lesions accounting for their syndrome, as outlined in Table 7.2.

The IHS ICHD-II defines this subset as "symptomatic TN" (Olesen et al. 2004). This label is unfortunate and misleading, since all patients with TN are symptomatic. Identifying this subset of patients is usually possible with dedicated neuroimaging, usually in the form of fine-cut, multiplanar, with- and without-contrast MR imaging (MRI). For MS, this may also require CSF examination via lumbar puncture.

Distinguishing this subset from those with classic or typical (sometimes termed *idiopathic*) TN is extremely important for two reasons. First, for

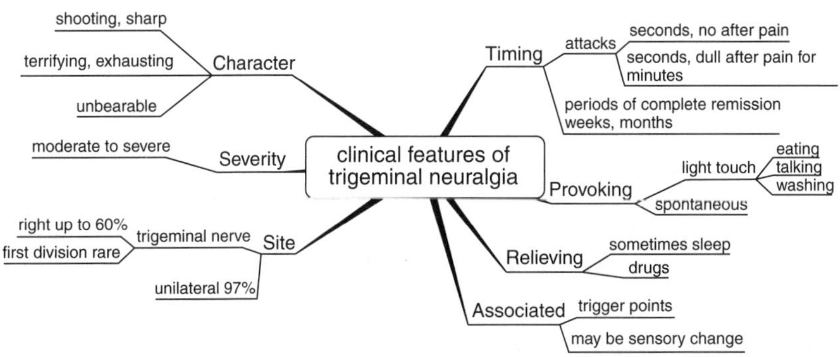

Figure 7.1 Major clinical features of trigeminal neuralgia.

Reprinted with permission from Zakrzewska & Linskey 2009.

Table 7.2 Sorting out Patients with Complete Symptom Overlap: symptomatic versus idiopathic trigeminal neuralgia

Idiopathic TN
Suspected to be caused by nerve root entry zone vascular compression
Symptomatic TN
Intraparenchymal Lesions
Multiple sclerosis*
Lacunar infarction
Trigeminal schwannoma
Extraparenchymal Lesions
Cerebellopontine-angle and/or petrous apex cyst (epidermoid, dermoid)†
Cerebellopontine-angle arachnoid cyst†
Cerebellopontine-angle tumor (meningiomas, other cranial nerve schwannomas, etc.)†
Aneurysm†
Arteriovenous malformation†

*Often associated with vascular compression
†Almost always associated with vascular compression.

those with extraparenchymal lesions, addressing the causative lesion will often eliminate the TN symptoms. Second, for those with intraparenchymal lesions, operative procedures with proven efficacy for idiopathic TN often do not work as well. In this clinical setting, surgical TN procedures can be recommended only with caution and careful preoperative qualification and perspective.

Conditions with Some Symptom Overlap

Conditions with only some symptom overlap are much more difficult to sort through and, at times, can be both frustrating and problematic for both patients and health care providers. We have found it useful to operationally classify these conditions into atypical TN and "look-alike" syndromes. The key point is that there remains significant Venn diagram overlap between the pain characteristics of atypical TN and typical TN, whereas "look-alike syndromes" often have significant differences in presentation and symptoms. The latter group of conditions often do not have a good surgical option for treatment, thus underscoring the need and desirability to evaluate and manage facial pain patients in coordinated multidisciplinary teams, in order to achieve optimal patient outcomes.

Atypical Trigeminal Neuralgia

Atypical TN is a syndrome in which the patient has persisting pain in the trigeminal distribution between neuralgic episodes. The neuralgic episodes are usually typical in character with sharp, electric, or shock-like pains superimposed upon the constant background pain component. The neuralgic episodes may be characteristically brief, as in typical TN, but atypical TN patients are more likely to report longer-duration, superimposed pain episodes lasting minutes to hours. While they may occasionally mean a clustering of brief episodes in a tetanic chain, the longer a single sharp pain episode lasts, the more the patient differs from typical TN. The background constant chronic pain is often described as dull, aching, or burning, implying a certain degree of deafferentation origin. There may be spread of the constant background pain outside of the trigeminal distribution to involve the head, ear, or retroauricular region.

In evaluating patients with atypical TN components, it is important to try to get them to distinguish the episodic, brief, neuralgic pain components from the constant background components. Burchiel does so with a classification system that classifies patients with less than 50% atypical features as TN1 and with more than 50% atypical features as TN2 (Burchiel 2003; Eller, Raslan, & Burchiel 2005; Limonadi, McCartney, & Burchiel 2006). This system is easy for patients to use to self-assess and self-classify. However, under this system, the TN1 classification includes typical TN patients (pure classic syndrome), those with minor atypical components (<30% atypical features), as well as those with significant atypical features (30%–50% atypical features). Such heterogeneity may not recognize the likely disparity in natural history, as well as likelihood of response to TN interventions among these three groups within the TN1 classification. Indeed, 100% of typical TN through 99% of atypical TN may represent a spectrum of nerve pathology, natural history, and prognosis with TN interventions. The TN1 versus TN2 classification may thus represent an arbitrary cut point in this assessment and analysis.

The main reason for distinguishing typical TN from atypical TN, and the gradations in between, is that it has become increasingly apparent that the closer to 100% typical TN a patient's syndrome is, the more likely he is to have a good outcome from operative interventions (Miller, Acar, & Burchiel 2009; Miller, Magill, Acar, & Burchiel 2009). Conversely, the more atypical features are present, the less likely the patient is to benefit from operative interventions. This appears to be true not only for the overall pain syndrome, but for the components as well. Indeed, in our practice, we usually do not recommend microvascular decompression (MVD) as a front-line therapy for patients with more than 50% atypical features, and for those with 1%–50% atypical features, we carefully counsel them preoperatively that the procedure is more likely to completely relieve the typical component, but may leave them with some or all of their background persistent pain. This has been our standard practice; however, as we have learned more about nervus intermedius (geniculate) neuralgia (NIN) and how to treat it, and have had better results, we have lowered the bar. Patients must understand what the surgeon can and cannot do, and the surgeon must go beyond the standard TN MVD procedure.

Other "Look-alike" Syndromes:

The remaining differential diagnosis for overlapping syndromes that are not TN are listed in Table 7.3. Although patients and referring practitioners may believe a patient to have TN, it is very important to recognize these "look-alike" syndromes, since the natural history, treatments, and prognoses differ a good deal. The list should not be considered definitive or complete,

Table 7.3 Sorting out "look-alike" syndromes: The differential diagnosis of trigeminal neuralgia

Other cranial nerve or peripheral nerve neuralgias
Glossopharyngeal neuralgia
Geniculate neuralgia/nervus intermedius neuralgia
Hemifacial spasm
Occipital neuralgia
Trigeminal autonomic cephalgias (TACs)
Episodic cluster headache
Chronic cluster headache
Short-lasting unilateral neuralgiform headaches with conjunctival injection and tearing (SUNCT)
Sporadic paroxysmal hemicrania
Chronic paroxysmal hemicrania
Other headache syndromes
Ocular migraine
Muscular tension headache
Dental/oral-maxillofacial disorders
Atypical odontalgia
Temporal mandibular joint (TMJ) syndrome
Neuralgia-inducing cavitational osteonecrosis (NICO)
Burning mouth syndrome
ENT disorders
Sinusitis
Peripheral trigeminal branch entrapment
Peripheral trigeminal branch neuroma
Infectious or inflammatory disorders
Herpes zoster infection
Temporal arteritis
Musculoskeletal disorders
Facial tendonitis
Myofascial pain syndrome
Fibromyalgia
Trigeminal deafferentation/neuropathic pain syndromes
Postherpetic neuralgia
Anesthesia dolorosa
Persistent idiopathic facial pain (PIFP; atypical facial pain syndrome)

as new syndromes are described on a regular basis, and it would appear that reorganization and renaming of existing syndromes continues to occur on a regular basis among the many disciplines and associations involved with pain management.

Other Cranial Neuralgias

The trigeminal nerve is not the only sensory cranial nerve serving the head and neck region. On occasion, there can be perceived overlap in the areas of the head and neck involved in the pain syndrome, prolonged or severe facial muscular spasms can become painful, and multiple cranial nerve syndromes can be involved at once. Glossopharyngeal neuralgia has very similar pain severity, characteristics, time course, and tactile trigger tendency as typical TN, but instead involves the back of the throat and frequently the ear. The same can be said for geniculate neuralgia, which frequently leads to pain deep within the ear. Confusion between these two syndromes and TN comes into play when patients are not precise about localizing their pain and when trigeminal pain is also associated with ear pain. The latter confusion results from the complexity of the sensory innervation of the ear that develops from contributions from several branchial arches. Different parts of the ear have sensory representation in the trigeminal system, the sensory component of the facial nerve (nervus intermedius), as well as the glossopharyngeal and vagus systems.

Similar ear pain overlap, as well as head pain overlap, is operative in distinguishing occipital neuralgia. In this case, the head and ear pain is retroauricular, involving the neck and posterior cranial vertex. Severe or prolonged muscle contractions (tonus phenomenon) of hemifacial spasm (HFS) can lead to pain of muscular origin within the facial muscles. This type of pain is not likely to be confused with TN, however. Trigeminal neuralgia can rarely be associated with HFS in a combined syndrome known as *tic convulsif* (Cook & Jannetta 1984; Cushing 1920), or with HFS and glossopharyngeal neuralgia in a triple combination (Kempe & Smith 1969, Kobata, Kondo, Iwaski, & Nishioka 1998).

Trigeminal Autonomic Cephalgias

The International Headache Society has classified trigeminal autonomic cephalgias into episodic and chronic cluster headache and paroxysmal hemicrania (Radford & Kitimolmard 2009). Cluster headache is an ipsilateral episodic and paroxysmal hemicranial pain syndrome that tends to center in the upper trigeminal sensory distribution, particularly in and around the orbit. It is often associated with facial flushing, vasomotor rhinitis, ipsilateral lacrimation, meiotic pupil, and conjunctival injection suggesting ipsilateral parasympathetic discharge. It has overlap with the rare case of isolated V_1 division TN, but the other parasympathetic features usually distinguish it. Hemicranial migraine is also episodic, but it involves the hemicranium posterior to the V_1–C2 dermatomal border and is distinguished by additional features characteristic of migraine (photophobia, nausea, prolonged throbbing pain, response to migraine treatments, potential dietary associations, +/– an aura).

Dental/Oromaxillofacial Disorders

Given that TN most often affects the second and third divisions of the trigeminal nerve (either singly or in combination), which also innervate the teeth, it is not surprising that a dentist is often the first health care provider sought out by a new TN patient. The evaluating dentist is in the position of trying to distinguish TN from dental and oromaxillofacial conditions such as odontalgia from local dental conditions (e.g., cracked tooth, caries, pulpitis, neuritis, abscess, periodontitis, dry socket, etc.) and other less-common dental conditions (Vickers & Zakrzewska 2009). The standard odontalgias and their proximate cause are usually apparent by dental examination and x-ray. Difficulty can arise when the proximate cause is not immediately apparent. With temporomandibular joint syndrome (TMJ), pain is localized to the face and temple. There is often pain with TMJ palpation or motion, restricted TMJ motion, palpable crepitus or catching with attempted motion, and often abnormal TMJ x-rays (Forsell & Ohrbach 2009). Neuralgia-inducing cavitational osteonecrosis (NICO) is a very serious, painful disorder with mandibular or maxillary osteonecrosis usually visible by x-ray. *Burning mouth syndrome* is an enigmatic condition characterized by a burning sensation in the oral mucosal associated with taste disturbance and xerostomia (Woda & Grushka 2009). It is usually readily distinguishable from TN by these symptoms, as well as by bilateral oral involvement limited to the mouth.

Ear, Nose, and Throat Disorders

Sinusitis can be associated with significant pain. While most often confused with headache, maxillary sinus or frontal sinus pain can lead to localized V_1 or V_2 pain. Fortunately, the pain is usually localized and is often a pressure pain worsened by palpation or percussion of the involved area. Somatic and/or laboratory signs of infection or inflammation are often present, there may be nasal discharge, and transillumination and x-ray imaging are usually diagnostic. Less common and more problematic ENT causes include trigeminal peripheral branch entrapment or neuroma formation. Patients should be carefully queried for a history of head or facial trauma that might have led to an undiagnosed facial fracture near an exiting foramen, as well as a history of facial or sinus surgery (including face lift), which could have placed traction or tension on the peripheral nerve at the point of anchorage in a facial foramen. These situations characteristically involve one distal branch of the peripheral trigeminal nerve rather than a whole division, often include sensory loss in the specific distribution of the peripheral branch, and may include palpation or percussion tenderness at the involved area. A fine-cut computed tomography (CT) scan coupled with MRI with fat suppression can be useful in the posttraumatic or postsurgical setting to visualize the facial foramen, assess for old fractures, and occasionally visualize neuromas.

Infectious or Inflammatory Disorders

Herpes zoster commonly affects the trigeminal nerve. Most of us are exposed to a subclinical infection early in life and carry the latent virus in the trigeminal ganglion. If the virus reactivates or if a primary infection occurs as an adult, the resultant infectious neuritis can be very painful. This is especially true if it involves the V_1 distribution, which can lead to corneal de-epithelialization and additional corneal pain as a result. Pain is usually severe, often episodic, and limited to the trigeminal distribution. The source of the syndrome is usually readily apparent within days, as the onset of pain is shortly followed by the appearance of the characteristic vesicles. The pain usually resolves with resolution of the infection, but occasionally enough nerve damage is caused by the infection to create a chronic deafferentation pain syndrome known as *postherpetic neuralgia.*

Temporal arteritis can lead to V_1 distribution pain. However, it is associated with polymyalgia rheumatic, pain over the temples manifest when palpating the artery or doing activities such as combing the hair, as well as from laboratory indications of inflammation, such as an elevated erythrocyte sedimentation rate (ESR). Diagnosis is made by temporal artery biopsy.

Musculoskeletal Disorders

Musculoskeletal disorders include facial tendinitis, myofascial pain syndrome, and fibromyalgia. The former is limited to the face, can be bilateral, and has associated tenderness with tendon movement and palpation. Spontaneous neuralgic pain is not common. The latter two syndromes are distinguished by common spread outside of the trigeminal distribution to involve the neck, tenderness to muscle movement and palpation, and frequent identification of myofascial "trigger points."

Trigeminal De-Afferentation/Neuropathic Pain Syndromes

Any form of nerve damage can lead to deafferentation pain. This damage can take the form of complete or partial nerve section, nerve damage from trauma or infection (as in postherpetic neuralgia), or even iatrogenic nerve damage from destructive therapeutic procedures such as radiofrequency thermoablation, glycerol rhizotomy, percutaneous balloon compression, or stereotactic radiosurgery.

It is an unfortunate truth that, deprived of sensory input from the periphery, the primary sensory reception areas in the brain sometimes do not remain inactive. Instead, in the absence of input they substitute spontaneous noxious activity. The classic example of this phenomenon is phantom limb pain experienced by some amputees despite the absence of the portion of the body perceived to be in pain. *Anesthesia dolorosa* of the face is a similar situation effecting the trigeminal nerve distribution.

Trigeminal deafferentation pain syndromes are always associated with severe sensory loss (often anesthesia) in the region of the trigeminal distribution experiencing the pain. Unlike TN, the pain is constant, burning, boring, and unremitting. It abates very little in response to any medication tried. The character of this pain is not likely to be confused with TN. However, its distribution is trigeminal and, unfortunately, several syndromes can occur in combination, especially in circumstances where the original syndrome was TN, but a component anesthesia dolorosa has developed from repeated trigeminal palliative destructive procedures that may have only temporarily worked, thus requiring multiple repeat procedures.

Postherpetic neuralgia can also exist as a combination of background constant deafferentation pain with superimposed neuralgic pains. Gabapentin, pregabalin, and lidocaine topical patch 5% are all U.S. Food and Drug Administration (FDA)-approved for use in postherpetic neuralgia. Unfortunately, these interventions are more likely to help the episodic neuralgic pain component, rather than the constant deafferentation pain component.

Atypical Facial Pain Syndrome

What has traditionally been referred to as "atypical facial pain syndrome" has been redefined by the IHS as persistent idiopathic facial pain (PIFP). Persistent idiopathic facial pain presents solely with the background constant features of atypical TN, without any episodic neuralgic component. The pain is constant, ipsilateral trigeminal in distribution, usually dull, aching, throbbing, or even burning, but is not associated with any sensory loss (List & Feinmann 2009). The exact cause and pathophysiology of this syndrome is not known, and the syndrome may be a collection of different conditions. In oral cases, there appears to be a large overlap with atypical odontalgia, and in other cases, with more diffuse musculoskeletal conditions such as fibromyalgia, myofascial pain syndrome, and chronic fatigue syndrome. Antidepressant medications and cognitive behavioral therapy may play a beneficial role in treating PIFP (List & Feinmann 2009).

CONCLUSION

Getting the diagnosis right is the first step toward reassuring patients with TN that their condition is understood and that there is hope for success through directed therapy, whether that therapy is medical or surgical. A correct diagnosis gives patients an important feeling of control over their condition and their future, and allows them the freedom and confidence to research and explore their therapeutic options. Getting the diagnosis right as soon as possible limits their period of suffering during the evaluation phase and brings relief at the soonest possible moment. Getting the diagnosis right allows patients the freedom to explore and understand surgical options well before they might need to be considered, and avoids the need to consider the pros and cons of surgical options under conditions of pain duress, time urgency, and maximal cognitive side effects of high-doses AEDs.

For patients without TN, or with overlap variants, getting the diagnosis right prevents false starts and avoids false hopes. It will hopefully lessen the likelihood of exposure to treatment risks for medical or surgical treatments that only have reasonable success rates for typical TN. It will hopefully allow for direction to the proper health practitioner and/or intervention targeted for their actual condition. As with medicine in general, everything begins with the correct diagnosis.

REFERENCES

Bennett MH, Jannetta PJ. Evoked potentials in trigeminal neuralgia. *Neurosurgery* 1983;13(3):242–247.

Bowsher D, Miles JB, Haggett CE, et al. Trigeminal neuralgia: a quantitative sensory perception threshold study in patients who had not undergone previous invasive procedures. *J Neurosurg* 1997;86(2):190–192.

Burchiel KJ. A new classification for facial pain. *Neurosurgery* 2003;53(5):1164–1166.

Burchiel KJ, Slavin KV. On the natural history of trigeminal neuralgia. *Neurosurgery* 2000;46(1):152–154;discussion 154–155.

Cook BR, Jannetta PJ. Tic convulsif: Results in 11 cases treated with microvascular decompression of the fifth and seventh cranial nerves. *J Neurosurg* 1984;61: 949–951.

Cushing H. The major trigeminal neuralgias and their surgical treatment based on experiences with 332 gasserian operations. *Am J Med Sci* 1920;160:157–184.

Eller JL, Raslan AM, Burchiel KJ. Trigeminal neuralgia: definition and classification. *Neurosurg Focus* 2005;18(5):E3.

Forsell H, Ohrbach R. Temporomandibular disorders (TMD). In Zakrzewska JM, ed. *Orofacial pain*. New York: Oxford University Press, 2009;105–118.

Kempe LG, Smith DR. Trigeminal neuralgia, facial spasm, intermedius and glossopharyngeal neuralgia with persistent carotid basilar anastomosis. *J Neurosurg* 1969;31:445–451.

Kobata H, Kondo A, Iwaski K, Nishioka T. Combined hyperactivity dysfunction syndrome of the cranial nerves: trigeminal neuralgia, hemifacial spasm, and glossopharyngeal neuralgia: 11-year experience and review. *Neurosurgery* 1998;43:1351–1561.

Limonadi FM, McCartney S, Burchiel KJ. Design of an artificial neural network for diagnosis of facial pain syndromes. *Stereotact Funct Neurosurg* 2006;84(5–6):212–220.

List T, Feinmann C. Persistent idiopathic facial pain (atypical facial pain). In Zakrzewska JM, ed. *Orofacial pain*. New York: Oxford University Press, 2009;93–104.

Mathews MS, Binder DK, Linskey ME. Trigeminal neuralgia: Diagnosis and non-operative management. In Winn HR, ed. *Youmans textbook of neurological surgery*, 6th ed. Philadelphia: Saunders (In Press).

Miller JP, Acar F, Burchiel KJ. Classification of trigeminal neuralgia: clinical, therapeutic, and prognostic implications in a series of 144 patients undergoing microvascular decompression. *J Neurosurg* 2009 Apr 24. [Epub ahead of print.]

Miller JP, Magill ST, Acar F, Burchiel KJ. Predictors of long-term success after microvascular decompression for trigeminal neuralgia. *J Neurosurg* 2009;110(4):620–626.

Mursch K, Schafer M, Steinhoff BJ, et al. Trigeminal evoked potentials and sensory deficits in atypical facial pain–a comparison with results in trigeminal neuralgia. *Funct Neurol* 2002;17:133–136.

Nurmikko TJ. Altered cutaneous sensation in trigeminal neuralgia. *Arch Neurol* 1991;48(5):523–527.

Olesen J, Bousser MG, Diener HC, et al. The international classification of headache disorders, 2nd edition. *Cephalalgia* 2004;24(Suppl 1):24–150.

Radford SG, Kitimolmard S. Trigeminal autonomic cephalgias. In Zakrzewska JM, ed. *Orofacial pain*. New York: Oxford University Press, 2009;157–172.

Sinay VJ, Bonamico LH, Dubrovsky A. Subclinical sensory abnormalities in trigeminal neuralgia. *Cephalalgia* 2003;23(7):541–544.

TNA–Facial Pain Association website. Accessed 6/26/09. Available at http://www.endthepain.org.

Vickers ER, Zakrzewska JM. Dental causes of orofacial pain. In Zakrzewska JM, ed. *Orofacial pain*. New York: Oxford University Press, 2009;69–82.

Weigel G, Casey KF. *Striking back. The trigeminal neuralgia and face pain handbook.* Gainesville FL: The Trigeminal Neuralgia Association, 2004.

Woda A, Grushka M. Burning mouth syndrome (BMS). In Zakrzewska JM, ed. *Orofacial pain.* New York: Oxford University Press, 2009;83–92.

Zakrzewska JM. Insight: facts and stories behind trigeminal neuralgia. Gainesville FL: The Trigeminal Neuralgia Association, 2006;1–403.

Zakrzewska JM, Linskey M. Trigeminal neuralgia. *BMJ Clin Evid* 2008;2(1207):1–9.

Zakrzewska JM, Linskey M. Trigeminal neuralgia. In Zakrzewska JM, ed. *Orofacial pain*. New York: Oxford University Press, 2009;119–134.

8

The Evaluation of the Preoperative Patient

Raymond F. Sekula, Jr. and Peter J. Jannetta

In our center, following medication failure or debilitating side effects as a result of medications, we perform microvascular decompression (MVD) as the first-line procedure for trigeminal neuralgia (TN) in patients able to undergo MVD, regardless of age or subtype of TN because MVD provides the highest likelihood of success (i.e., pain-free without medication), the best quality of life (no numbness), and the lowest long-term recurrence rate. Evaluation of the risk–benefit ratio for each patient before operation, however, is essential in optimizing care. With this in mind, this chapter is dedicated to the preoperative evaluation of the patient with TN, including appropriate supplemental testing in anticipation of MVD.

The diagnosis of TN is based on the history. In most instances, the diagnosis can be made over the telephone. Trigeminal neuralgia, or *tic douloureux*, is a syndrome characterized by paroxysmal attacks of facial pain. Thinking their pain is of a dental origin, patients often present to the dentist first for evaluation, and, thus, the dentist is often afforded the first opportunity to make a correct diagnosis of TN. Although the diagnosis of TN should be easily made by the history, misdiagnosis occurs not infrequently throughout the medical community. Eighty percent of the patients, in our series of over 3,000 patients who have undergone MVD for TN, were initially evaluated by their dentists. Tooth extractions and, now more commonly, root canal procedures are commonly performed. Further dental treatments, all ineffective, include jaw equalization, implants, and periodontal treatments. Although many dentists have learned to diagnose TN, the high rate of unnecessary dental procedures persists, partly because patients may "dentist shop" until a procedure is performed. Here, we will attempt to clarify the signs and symptoms of TN and its variations, to help with decision-making regarding medical and surgical therapy.

CLINICAL CHARACTERISTICS

Epidemiology

The incidence of TN increases with age, ranging from 4 in 100,000 to greater than 20 in 100,000 (Katusic, Beard, Bergstralh, & Kurland 1990; Katusic et al.

1991), and occurs more frequently in women than in men (3:2). Trigeminal neuralgia occurs in more than one person in a family in slightly over 5% of patients. Although the pain more commonly occurs in middle aged and older patients, small children and teenagers are also affected. Our youngest patient was 7 months of age at onset and was operated upon when he was 22 months old.

History

In the great majority of patients, the onset of TN is sudden, acute, and highly memorable: "The worst pain I have ever had in my life." The pain is described in many ways ("electrical shocks," "a lightning bolt," "an ice pick jabbing me over and over," etc.). Physicians describe this kind of pain as lancinating. We have seen patients who, many years later (i.e., 30 or 40 years), could recall the precise details of their first attack of TN pain. In a small minority, patients with TN may have a prodromal state with the insidious onset of mild pain or paresthesias in the face, in the area where TN will eventuate. This may persist for many months. The pain may be limited to the area of a tooth or to the skin over the mandible or cheek. In these patients, it is imperative that other causes of face pain (e.g., dental caries, myofascial pain, temporomandibular joint dysfunction, or neoplasm) are excluded by history, physical examination, and radiography.

Typical attacks are of sudden onset and offset, "Like turning a switch on and off." The pain may last a fraction of a second or longer, and rarely more than 30 minutes. Attacks of pain most often occur spontaneously. A small majority of patients experience a very brief aura before an episode of pain. This aura may consist of a sense of foreboding, a dire moment, or a feeling of doom. The pain may be brought on or exacerbated by stimuli or "triggers" in the area of the face and mouth. These triggers include a gust of cold air on the face, cold water, washing the face, brushing the teeth, chewing food, showering or applying makeup, kissing, or lightly touching the face. Trigger points are usually, but not always, located in the distribution of the pain. They are most frequently located in the area of the nose and mouth, which has a rich supply of nerve endings and is innervated solely by the trigeminal nerve, without overlap by the upper cranial segments. Trigger points are frequently evanescent and variable in location and distribution. Rubbing the face or applying deep pressure is not likely to precipitate an attack, whereas a light touch will do so.

Trigeminal neuralgia occurs on the right side more often than on the left side (3:2), and in the lower and central face (V_3, V_2, V_{2-3}) more often than in the upper face (V_1) distribution (Barker et al. 1996). Trigeminal neuralgia occurs bilaterally in just over 5% of patients, almost always with sequential asymmetrical onset. The first side usually precedes the other by some time. Positional changes of the head, neck, or body may exacerbate or ease the pain. The offending or easing position may consist of the head turning in a certain way, or of leaning forward or lying down (left, supine, or right side).

Patients may infrequently experience a short time of relief from their pain after an attack, a refractory period, when the usual inciting causes of pain will not precipitate it. They will use this period to do what they cannot usually do because of the pain—eat rapidly, talk, brush their teeth, and the like.

Over a prolonged period of time, prolonged burning or even constant, nonlancinating pain may precede the sudden onset and offset of TN pain. Carbamazepine of less than optimal dose may have the same effect, with an increase in the doses causing the pain to be relieved. Apfelbaum has shown that prolonged duration of TN over 10 or more years is associated with a decrease in efficiency of MVD, suggesting that the trigeminal nerve might be injured by repetitive vascular pulsations and has less capacity for recovery (Apfelbaum 1977).

Classification

Despite well-intentioned attempts at classifying the various forms of facial pain, no classification scheme has been uniformly accepted. The majority of practitioners continue to divide TN into "typical" (i.e., *tic douloureux*) and "atypical" forms, or use the Burchiel classification scheme (Burchiel 2003; Sweet 1969). Recently, some authors have proposed the term *transitional TN* (Tyler-Kabara et al. 2002). Although many cases of TN do transition from strictly typical TN to atypical TN (Burchiel 2003), others begin with constant background pain (usually "burning"), with crescendos or paroxysms of lancinating pain throughout the day, and these patients do not fit into this proposed transitional subgroup. Most recently, in response to Heros, Burchiel wrote "Type 2 TN may well be a composite category, containing one or more other diagnoses. The results of our studies would tend to support this thesis. Perhaps, it would make more sense to divide Type 2 TN into two subdivisions: cases in which there is some history of lancinating pain (Type 2a), and those in which there is no such history (Type 2b)" (Miller, Magill, Acar, & Burchiel 2009b). For similar reasons, our group has previously referred to all TN comprised of considerable components of both typical and atypical TN as "mixed." In the future, despite additional complexity, we may need to further classify multiple subgroups within type 2 TN (TN2).

We now administer a detailed questionnaire (modified from Miller et al. 2009b) to all patients presenting with face pain, in order to classify their TN pain according to the Burchiel scheme. Patients who experience paroxysmal or lancinating pain greater than 50% of the time and who had a memorable onset of facial pain, trigger points, periods of remission, and response to antiepileptic drugs (AEDs) are considered to have type 1 TN (TN1). Patients who experience dull constant pain greater than 50% of the time and who had an insidious onset of facial pain, no trigger points, no periods of remission, and no response to AEDs are considered to have TN2. Patients with TN2 are further divided into two groups. Patients with TN2a had a history of at least some paroxysmal pain at some time. Patients with TN2b have strictly constant pain, with no history of paroxysmal or lancinating pain (Heros 2009; Miller, Acar, & Burchiel 2009a).

Physical Examination

On physical examination, jaw movements may not be smooth and symmetrical. Sensory changes are common and easily missed. We have noted mild hypalgesia and/or hypesthesia in one-third of our patients. This is not a new finding. In 1938, Lewy and Grant (Lewy & Grant 1938) found that 25% of their TN patients had mild sensory loss as tested by von Frei hairs. The sensory loss is more prone to occur in two situations: first, prolonged TN (over 5 years) and second, during an exacerbation of pain.

Sensory loss follows a rather standard pattern (Fig. 8.1). It almost invariably occurs in the area of pain. The loss in V_2 and V_3 pain occurs around the

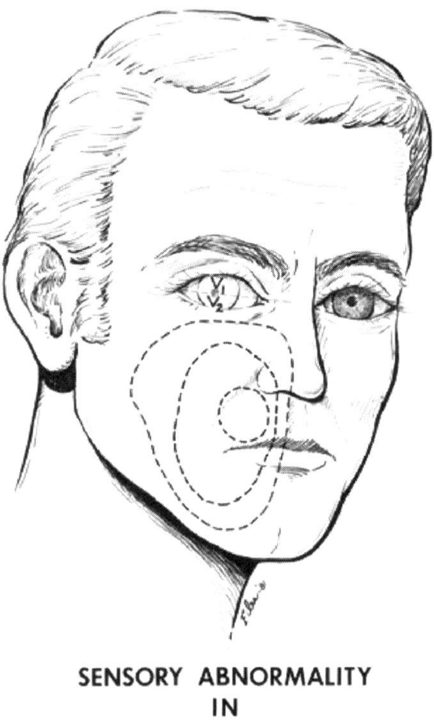

SENSORY ABNORMALITY
IN
TRIGEMINAL NEURALGIA

Figure 8.1 V_2 and/or V_3 pain may have mild hypalgesia and hypesthesia centered at the nasolabial fold. One must touch the skin lightly with a single strand of cotton and with a pin, and use the neurological convention of proceeding from the abnormal to the normal to trace out these abnormalities. V_2 pain may have a decreased corneal reflex in the lower half of the corneal; V_1 pain may have decreased corneal reflex in the upper half of the cornea. The corneal reflex is tested with a wisp of cotton, just touching (not dragging across) the cornea.

nasolabial fold. V_2 pain may be accompanied by a decrease in the lower half of the corneal reflex; V_1 pain by a decrease in the upper half of the corneal reflex (Vonderahe 1928, *courtesy of J. Keller*). Careful technique is necessary to find these changes. First, one must use the neurological convention of proceeding from the abnormal to the normal. One strand of cotton, touched not dragged, and a pin, again touched not dragged across the skin is necessary. The corneal reflex is tested with one strand of cotton, comparing sensation and response in the upper compared with lower cornea, ipsilateral versus contralateral, subjectively and objectively. Bennett and colleagues showed abnormality in trigeminal evoked potentials in 86% of trigeminal patients, with 83% returning to normal after MVD (Bennett & Jannetta 1980).

SUPPLEMENTAL TESTING

Diagnostic Imaging

Some confusion exists amongst clinicians regarding the utility of magnetic resonance imaging (MRI) in predicting which patients may benefit from proposed MVD. This confusion occurs, in part, because of conflicting reports regarding the ability to detect vascular compression of the trigeminal nerve with MRI and the significance of any vascular compression detected by MRI. Occasionally, patients are not referred for MVD because the interpreting radiologist, neurologist, or neurosurgeon does not note neurovascular compression of the trigeminal nerve. Lack of visible neurovascular compression, however, can be attributed to technical inadequacies of MR sequencing or simply the inability of even the most advanced MR sequencing to detect certain neurovascular conflicts (i.e., many compressing vessels are small and venous). We frequently note apparent compression of a nerve on MRI and subsequently find another vessel causing the problem and/or multiple vessels in contact with the nerve.

As MR technology has evolved, various authors have demonstrated that neurovascular conflict of the trigeminal nerve (i.e., the putative cause of TN) [Jannetta 1967] can be visualized with MR imaging. Naidich et al. (Yousry et al. 2004) were the first to reliably identify vascular contacts with the motor and sensory roots of the trigeminal nerve using three-dimensional (3D) Fourier transform constructive interference in steady state (CISS) imaging and time-of-flight (TOF) sequences. In their study, 33 patients and seven cadaveric specimens (80 sides) were studied. All study patients were known to be free of TN. At least one motor root was identified in all sides examined: in 51% of the sides a single motor root, in 37% of the sides two motor roots, and in 11% of the sides three motor roots were identified. The sensory roots of the trigeminal nerve were identified on all 66 sides in the patients and on all 14 sides of the specimens. In their study, the sensory root of the trigeminal nerve was contacted by the anterior inferior cerebellar artery (4.5% of sides), the superior cerebellar artery (45.5% of sides), and diverse veins (54.5% of sides). The authors emphasized, however, that the root was not distorted or grooved in any instance. More recently, however, radiographic atrophy of the trigeminal nerve, measured by MRI during gamma-knife surgery (GKS) planning, was seen 24%–96% of patients with TN prior to MVD or ablative procedures (Devor, Govrin-Lippmann, & Rappaport 2002; Erbay et al. 2006; Lorenzoni et al. 2008; Park et al. 2009). Despite these results, one cannot know whether certain arteries or veins are "missed" by MRI, or whether patient positioning during MRI (i.e., lying supine versus lateral decubitus vs. upright) influences the results of neurovascular conflict as detected by MRI. In 20 cadavers free of facial pain, Haines et al. (1980) noted that 35% of trigeminal nerves had a proximate artery, but only 10% showed evidence of "compression or distortion" of the nerve. This study provided evidence that the majority of individuals without facial pain were free of vascular compression of the trigeminal nerve. In another study of 18 patients undergoing preoperative MRI for MVD, Miller et al. (2008) reported the results of 18 patients with the "classic" signs and symptoms of TN undergoing 3D reconstructed high-resolution balanced fast-field echo (BFFE) imaging fused with 3D TOF MR angiography and gadolinium (Gd)-enhanced 3D spoiled-gradient recalled sequence. Fifteen patients were predicted to have neurovascular compression on the symptomatic side (nine arterial and six venous compressions). At operation, all patients had a vascular structure that was identical in location and configuration to that predicted on preoperative analysis. The three patients without predicted compression underwent operation because they manifested the classic symptoms. While exploration in two of these patients revealed no offending vessel, a third patient was found to have a small vein embedded in the trigeminal nerve that was beyond the resolution of the 3D Gd-enhanced study.

Taken together, these studies would suggest that vascular conflict of the trigeminal nerve can frequently be detected with appropriate MR sequencing, but certain vessels, veins in particular, will be missed by even the most sophisticated MR sequencing. In our experience, MRI is necessary in the preoperative evaluation of the patient with TN for exclusion of structural lesions (i.e., tumors, arteriovenous malformations [AVMs], aneurysms, Chiari I malformation) or demyelinating disease (i.e., multiple sclerosis), but convincing evidence for its use in preoperative planning or in predicting which vessels will require decompression is not yet possible with contemporary technology.

Electrophysiological and Other Testing

Preoperative testing for every patient involves audiometry (pure tone and speech), acoustic middle ear reflexes, and brainstem auditory evoked potentials (BAEPs). The audiometric tests are performed preoperatively to obtain a baseline for quantitatively determining deteriorations or improvement in hearing function. Additionally, preoperative BAEPs provide baseline information for the clinical neurophysiology team, so that they may warn the surgeon of any deviations during monitoring of the intraoperative auditory-evoked potentials.

PATIENT SELECTION

In consideration of MVD for TN, the utility of distinguishing between the various subtypes of TN is becoming more clear. Reviewing Jannetta's results over a 24-year period, Tyler-Kabara et al. (2002) showed that patients with typical TN fare far better than those with atypical TN. Li et al. (2004) suggested that patients with typical TN of a shorter duration fare better following MVD. Sindou et al. (2006), however, reported equivalent rates of success with MVD in a consecutive series of typical and atypical TN patients. A close examination, however, of inclusion and exclusion criteria in Sindou's study may help to clarify their results: Although 2,232 patients were evaluated for surgery for TN, only 362 were randomized to MVD, whereas 1,680 were randomized to thermal rhizolysis. In fact, only those patients with typical TN or atypical TN characterized as "paroxysmal pain (at least at the beginning of the disease) but later accompanied by a constant deep aching or burning pain" were offered MVD. In addition, all patients, at least initially, responded to anticonvulsants (Sindou et al. 2006) In effect, Sindou et al. report on outcomes in a highly selected series of typical and so-called "transitional" TN patients. With this selection in mind, one cannot conclude from Sindou's report that both typical and atypical TN (as classified by most clinicians) respond equally well to MVD. From Sindou's report, however, one may conclude that typical and transitional TN responds equally well to MVD. Sandell and Eide (2008) recently showed that patients with variable degrees of constant pain did as well as those who did not have constant pain. Like Sindou et al., (2006), however, the authors included only those patients with constant pain whose TN started with purely episodic pain (i.e., TN1 or typical and transitional TN). Most recently, Burchiel et al. (2003) provided more evidence that TN1 or typical TN patients fare better with MVD, and acknowledged that further partitioning of TN2 or atypical patients may be useful (Miller et al. 2009b). In most cases, outcomes of MVD for TN appear to be strongly related to exclusion, classification, and outcome criteria.

MEDICAL CLEARANCE PRIOR TO MICROVASCULAR DECOMPRESSION

The ultimate goals of preoperative medical assessment are to reduce the morbidity associated with operation, to increase the quality and decrease the cost of perioperative care, and to restore the patient quickly to the desired level of functioning. Years ago, physicians relied primarily on history taking and physical examination, supplemented with carefully chosen laboratory tests to confirm clinical impressions when making decisions regarding which patients could safely undergo an intended surgical procedure. Today, with an expanding array of diagnostic tests available to the physician, and growing medicolegal and financial pressures, neurosurgeons are more often abrogating the medical clearance of patients for MVD to internists and medical subspecialists, or simply following hospital-based guidelines for general anesthesia (typically based on age). Although this makes sense in some instances, all patients can benefit from a thorough review of their medical systems by their neurosurgeon; in so doing, more patients may be carefully considered for MVD. We routinely operate on patients classified as grades I–IV according to the American Society of Anesthesiologists scale (Dripps 1963).

Stroke, although rare, is one of the most feared complications of MVD surgery and may occur for a variety of reasons. Although risk factors for stroke following MVD are not specifically known, general risk factors for perioperative stroke include advanced age, female sex, hypertension, diabetes mellitus, renal insufficiency, smoking, chronic obstructive pulmonary disease, peripheral vascular disease, cardiac disease, history of prior stroke or transient ischemic attack (TIA), carotid stenosis, and abrupt discontinuation of antithrombotic therapy preoperatively (Selim 2007). Perioperative strokes result in prolonged hospital stays, increased disability rates, and death following operation (McKhann et al. 2006).

Both hemorrhagic and ischemic strokes may occur following MVD. Hemorrhagic strokes may be of venous or, less commonly, arterial origin. One common reason includes hemorrhagic conversion of a venous infarction following intentional sacrifice of veins (i.e., petrosal vein complex) during exposure of the trigeminal nerve. Although most believe the superior petrosal vein complex can be safely sacrificed during exposure of the trigeminal nerve, at least one group has reported the development of a hemorrhagic venous infarction following sacrifice of the superior petrosal vein complex in an elderly patient (Ryu et al. 1999). In addition, excessive mechanical retraction of the cerebellum during exposure of the trigeminal nerve has been associated with hemorrhagic venous infarction. The responsible mechanism for both types of hemorrhagic venous infarcts involves a cascade of events beginning with venous congestion with resultant interstitial edema and cell necrosis, followed by disruption of veins, and finally hemorrhage into areas of infarction (Fujita et al. 1984).

In addition, infarction of the brainstem or cerebellum may occur with prolonged ischemia or emboli. Embolic infarction is a particular concern in the elderly or otherwise predisposed (i.e., tobacco smokers) with atherosclerotic plaques, which may be dislodged and migrate upstream with any manipulation of intracranial blood vessels (Sekula et al. 2008). The utility of aspirin in the perioperative setting of MVD, as it has been used with carotid endarterectomy (Taylor et al. 1999) to reduce embolic complications, is unknown and such a study would be difficult to complete due to the low number of embolic infarcts associated with MVD. In addition, the safety of aspirin in the perioperative setting of MVD has not been established. Anecdotal evidence, however, would suggest that, at least, low-dose aspirin could ameliorate the effect of platelet aggregation in evolving embolic strokes. For the present, however, we discontinue aspirin in our patients for 10 days preoperatively and resume the dose on the fifth post-operative day.

Elderly Patients with Trigeminal Neuralgia

Because TN affects those in the latter half of their life more commonly than those in first half of their life (Amador & Pollock 2008; Katusic et al. 1990, 1991), the development of an algorithm regarding the most appropriate management of TN in the elderly is important. In 2007, 4,215 patients were discharged from hospitals in the United States with the principal diagnosis of TN. Of the 4,215 patients, 46% were age 65 or older (Agency for Healthcare Research and Quality 2003). In the past few decades, the neurosurgical community has begun to ease absolute "age cutoffs" for patients undergoing craniotomy (O'Brien, Nagaria, & Rawluk 1996), and in the past decade, numerous groups have published their experience with MVD in TN patients older than 60 (Ashkan & Marsh 2004), 65 (Ferroli et al. 2009; Gunther et al. 2009; Jodicke et al. 1999; Ogungbo et al. 2000), 70 (Javadpour et al. 2003), and 75 (Ryu et al. 1999; Sekula et al. 2008) years of age. Each group sought to establish the efficacy and safety of MVD in the elderly by comparing the elderly group to a younger group of controls. These studies have demonstrated that comparable results (i.e., pain-free without medication status) can be achieved in appropriately selected elderly patients undergoing MVD for TN. Considerable debate, however, exists regarding the safety of MVD in the elderly with TN. Primarily, critics site inadequacies of study design (e.g., retrospective nature, small sample size, misleading or inappropriate statistical methods, and patient selection bias). Critics argue, perhaps appropriately, that the safety of MVD in the elderly has not been established.

SURGICAL ALGORITHM OF THE MANAGEMENT OF TRIGEMINAL NEURALGIA

Once the diagnosis of TN has been established, a variety of steps can be taken to increase the probability of a pain-free future for the patient. When medications fail, five operative procedures are available to the patient: percutaneous glycerol rhizotomy (PGR), percutaneous radiofrequency rhizotomy (RFR), percutaneous balloon compression (PBC), stereotactic radiosurgery (SRS), and MVD. The first four procedures, although "less invasive," are variably destructive, producing intentional injury to the nerve.

Microvascular decompression is a nondestructive procedure with preservation of the nerve. Although most neurosurgeons experienced with MVD for TN prefer MVD as the first-line treatment for patients with TN, many still apply an "age-cutoff" in recommending MVD (Apfelbaum 1988). Because of presumed increases in morbidity and mortality with general anesthesia and MVD surgery, elderly patients in particular are increasingly offered ablative procedures for TN. In addition, some neurosurgeons, particularly those less experienced with MVD, have been led to believe that some of the ablative procedures, particularly, SRS, represent a good first choice for even younger patients.

Citing a lower incidence of trigeminal sensory dysfunction with radiosurgical rhizolysis of the trigeminal nerve (i.e., using the Leksell Gamma Knife®, GKS) as compared to other ablative techniques, Lunsford et al., in a proposed surgical management algorithm for TN, have recommended GKS, when latency to response is acceptable, in favor of other ablative techniques when MVD is deemed unsafe for the patient (Lunsford, Niranjan, & Kondziolka 2007). The notion, however, that GKS is associated with a lower rate of trigeminal sensory disturbances than other ablative techniques is not supported by the only systematic review of ablative techniques which included GKS (Lopez, Hamlyn, & Zakrzewska 2004). In that report, the authors found that dysesthesias severe enough to interfere with the quality of life were noted with all techniques, although they were twice as common with GKS, glycerol rhizotomy (GR), and balloon compression (BC), as with radiofrequency lesioning (RF) surgery. One can conclude that RF followed by GR/BC provides the highest initial rates of relief from TN (GKS has the lowest initial rate of relief). Radiofrequency ablation appears to provide the highest rate of long-term complete pain relief, with GKS, BC, and GR having very similar long-term rates of complete pain relief at 1 and 3 years follow-up (long-term response of GKS is perhaps slightly superior to GR and BC). Radiofrequency lesioning, however, has the highest overall complication rate (Han et al. 2009; Henson et al. 2005; Kang et al. 2008; Linskey, Ratanatharathorn, & Penagaricano. 2008; Lopez et al. 2004; Pollock 2005; Taha & Tew 1996). Currently, a prescription dose of 80 Gy is considered optimal with GKS for TN, and a review of series involving a maximum prescription dose of 80 Gy or less reveals the risk of numbness following GKS for TN to be 6%–19% (Dhople et al. 2007, 2009; Han et al. 2009; Rogers et al. 2000). Although exceptionally low, MVD comes with certain important risks (i.e., stroke, cerebellar hematoma, deaths) not associated with ablative procedures including GKS (Barker et al. 1996; Linskey et al. 2008; Sindou, Leston, Decullier, & Chapuis 2007). In addition, GKS for TN is often recommended after failed MVD or MVD without lasting benefit. In terms of pain-free status at follow-up, published results would suggest that MVD, rather than GKS, is a superior salvage procedure (Amador & Pollock 2008; Cho et al. 1994; Jannetta & Bissonette 1985; Lee et al. 2000; Little et al. 2009; Longhi et al. 2007; Maesawa et al. 2001). Although the risk of major morbidity is absent with any of the ablative procedures, all ablative procedures have a half-life of between 1 and 3 years, with increasing complications referable to the trigeminal nerve with repeat procedures.

Special Considerations Regarding Atypical or Type 2 Trigeminal Neuralgia

In light of these findings, many patients with atypical TN are denied MVD because of inferior results, as compared to patients with typical TN. This has led some practitioners to offer ablative procedures (i.e., balloon rhizolysis, GR, thermal rhizolysis, radiosurgical rhizolysis) first for those with atypical TN with stereotactic radiosurgical rhizolysis increasingly offered as first-line treatment despite marginal results (Maesawa et al. 2001; Regis et al. 2006; Sheehan, Pan, Stroila, & Steiner 2005). Although patients with typical or TN1 fare better than those with atypical or TN2 generally with any treatment, subgroups of atypical or TN2 patients are more responsive to MVD, such as the subgroup of patients with isolated V_2 TN (Sekula et al. 2009). In addition, no evidence exists to suggest that ablative treatments provide superior pain relief from atypical or TN2 over MVD. Most importantly, the risk of adverse consequences relative to the trigeminal nerve is far higher with ablative procedures (Apfelbaum 1977, 2000).

CONCLUSION

In our center, following medication failure or debilitating side effects as a result of medications, we perform MVD as the first-line procedure for TN in patients able to undergo MVD, regardless of age or TN subtype because MVD provides the highest likelihood of success (i.e., pain-free without medication), the best quality of life (no numbness), and the lowest long-term recurrence rate. Evaluating the risk–benefit ratio for each patient before operation is essential in optimizing care.

REFERENCES

Agency for Healthcare Research and Quality: HCUP Quality Control Procedures. Healthcare Cost and Utilization Project (HCUP). Agency for Healthcare Research and Quality, 2003.

Amador N, Pollock BE. Repeat posterior fossa exploration for patients with persistent or recurrent idiopathic trigeminal neuralgia. *J Neurosurg* 2008;108: 916–920.

Apfelbaum RI. A comparision of percutaneous radiofrequency trigeminal neurolysis and microvascular decompression of the trigeminal nerve for the treatment of tic douloureux. *Neurosurgery* 1977;1(1):16–21.

Apfelbaum RI. Neurovascular decompression, the procedure of Choice. *Clin Neurosurg* 2000;46:473–498.

Apfelbaum R. Comments. *Neurosurgery* 1988;22:352.

Ashkan K, Marsh H. Microvascular decompression for trigeminal neuralgia in the elderly: a review of the safety and efficacy. *Neurosurgery* 2004;55:840–848; discussion 848–850.

Barker FG, 2nd, Jannetta PJ, Bissonette DJ, et al. The long-term outcome of microvascular decompression for trigeminal neuralgia. *N Engl J Med* 1996;334: 1077–1083.

Bennett MH, Jannetta PJ. Trigeminal evoked potentials in humans. *Electroencephalogr Clin Neurophysiol* 1980;48:517–526.

Burchiel KJ. A new classification for facial pain. *Neurosurgery* 2003;53:1164–1167.

Cho DY, Chang CG, Wang YC, et al. Repeat operations in failed microvascular decompression for trigeminal neuralgia. *Neurosurgery* 1994;35:665–669; discussion 669–670.

Devor M, Govrin-Lippmann R, Rappaport ZH. Mechanism of trigeminal neuralgia: an ultrastructural analysis of trigeminal root specimens obtained during microvascular decompression surgery. *J Neurosurg* 2002;96:532–543.

Dhople A, Kwok Y, Chin L, et al. Efficacy and quality of life outcomes in patients with atypical trigeminal neuralgia treated with gamma-knife radiosurgery. *Int J Radiat Oncol Biol Phys* 2007;69:397–403.

Dhople AA, Adams JR, Maggio WW, et al. Long-term outcomes of gamma knife radiosurgery for classic trigeminal neuralgia: implications of treatment and critical review of the literature. *J Neurosurg* 2009;111:351–358.

Dripps R. New classification of physical status. *Anesthesiology* 1963;24:111.

Erbay SH, Bhadelia RA, O'Callaghan M, et al. Nerve atrophy in severe trigeminal neuralgia: noninvasive confirmation at MR imaging: initial experience. *Radiology* 2006;238:689–692.

Ferroli P, Acerbi F, Tomei M, et al. Advanced age as a contraindication to microvascular decompression for drug-resistant trigeminal neuralgia: evidence of prejudice? *Neurol Sci* 2009;31(1):23–28.

Fujita K, Kojima N, Matsumoto S. [Experimental model of venous hemorrhagic infarction by cerebral sinus occlusion]. *No Shinkei Geka* 1984;12:1061–1067.

Gunther T, Gerganov VM, Stieglitz L, et al. Microvascular decompression for trigeminal neuralgia in the elderly: long-term treatment outcome and comparison with younger patients. *Neurosurgery* 2009;65:477–482; discussion 482.

Haines SJ, Jannetta PJ, Zorub DS. Microvascular relations of the trigeminal nerve. An anatomical study with clinical correlation. *J Neurosurg* 1980;52:381–386.

Han JH, Kim DG, Chung HT, et al. Long-term outcome of gamma knife radiosurgery for treatment of typical trigeminal neuralgia. *Int J Radiat Oncol Biol Phys* 2009;75(3):822–827.

Henson CF, Goldman HW, Rosenwasser RH, et al. Glycerol rhizotomy versus gamma knife radiosurgery for the treatment of trigeminal neuralgia: an analysis of patients treated at one institution. *Int J Radiat Oncol Biol Phys* 2005;63:82–90.

Heros RC. Results of microvascular decompression for trigeminal neuralgia. *J Neurosurg* 2009;110:617–618; author reply 618–619.

Jannetta PJ. Arterial compression of the trigeminal nerve at the pons in patients with trigeminal neuralgia. *J Neurosurg* 1967;26(Suppl):159–162.

Jannetta PJ, Bissonette DJ. Management of the failed patient with trigeminal neuralgia. *Clin Neurosurg* 1985;32:334–347.

Javadpour M, Eldridge PR, Varma TR, et al. Microvascular decompression for trigeminal neuralgia in patients over 70 years of age. *Neurology* 2003;60:520.

Jodicke A, Winking M, Deinsberger W, Boker DK. Microvascular decompression as treatment of trigeminal neuralgia in the elderly patient. *Minim Invasive Neurosurg* 1999;42:92–96.

Kang JH, Yoon YS, Kang DW, et al. Gamma knife radiosurgery for medically refractory idiopathic trigeminal neuralgia. *Acta Neurochir Suppl* 2008;101:35–38.

Katusic S, Beard CM, Bergstralh E, Kurland LT. Incidence and clinical features of trigeminal neuralgia, Rochester, Minnesota, 1945–1984. *Ann Neurol* 1990;27: 89–95.

Katusic S, Williams DB, Beard CM, et al. Epidemiology and clinical features of idiopathic trigeminal neuralgia and glossopharyngeal neuralgia: similarities and differences, Rochester, Minnesota, 1945–1984. *Neuroepidemiology* 1991;10: 276–281.

Lee SH, Levy EI, Scarrow AM., et al. Recurrent trigeminal neuralgia attributable to veins after microvascular decompression. *Neurosurgery* 2000;46:356–361; discussion 361–362.

Lewy FH, Grant FC. Physiologic and pathoanatomic aspects of major trigeminal neuralgia. *Arch Neurol & Psychiat* 1938;40:1126.

Li ST, Pan Q, Liu N, et al. Trigeminal neuralgia: what are the important factors for good operative outcomes with microvascular decompression. *Surg Neurol* 2004;62:400–404; discussion 404–405.

Linskey ME, Ratanatharathorn V, Penagaricano J. A prospective cohort study of microvascular decompression and gamma knife surgery in patients with trigeminal neuralgia. *J Neurosurg* 2008;109(Suppl):160–172.

Little AS, Shetter AG, Shetter ME, et al. Salvage gamma knife stereotactic radiosurgery for surgically refractory trigeminal neuralgia. *Int J Radiat Oncol Biol Phys* 2009;74:522–527.

Longhi M, Rizzo P, Nicolato A, et al. Gamma knife radiosurgery for trigeminal neuralgia: results and potentially predictive parameters—part I: Idiopathic trigeminal neuralgia. *Neurosurgery* 2007;61:1254–1260; discussion 1260–1261.

Lopez BC, Hamlyn PJ, Zakrzewska JM. Systematic review of ablative neurosurgical techniques for the treatment of trigeminal neuralgia. *Neurosurgery,* 2004;54:973–982; discussion 982–923.

Lorenzoni JG, Massager N, David P, et al. Neurovascular compression anatomy and pain outcome in patients with classic trigeminal neuralgia treated by radiosurgery. *Neurosurgery* 2008;62:368–375; discussion 375–376.

Lunsford LD, Niranjan A, Kondziolka D. Surgical management options for trigeminal neuralgia. *J Korean Neurosurg Soc,* 2007;41:359–366.

Maesawa S, Salame C, Flickinger JC, et al. Clinical outcomes after stereotactic radiosurgery for idiopathic trigeminal neuralgia. *J Neurosurg* 2001;94:14–20.

McKhann GM, Grega MA, Borowicz LM, Jr., et al. Stroke and encephalopathy after cardiac surgery: an update. *Stroke* 2006;37:562–571.

Miller J, Acar F, Hamilton B, Burchiel K. Preoperative visualization of neurovascular anatomy in trigeminal neuralgia. *J Neurosurg* 2008;108:477–482.

Miller JP, Acar F, Burchiel KJ. Classification of trigeminal neuralgia: clinical, therapeutic, and prognostic implications in a series of 144 patients undergoing microvascular decompression. *J Neurosurg* 2009a;111(6):1231–1234.

Miller JP, Magill ST, Acar F, Burchiel K J. Predictors of long-term success after microvascular decompression for trigeminal neuralgia. *J Neurosurg* 2009b;110:620–626.

O'Brien DP, Nagaria J, Rawluk D. Neurosurgery for the elderly: facts and figures. *Gerontology* 1996;42:1–6.

Ogungbo BI, Kelly P, Kane PJ, Nath FP. Microvascular decompression for trigeminal neuralgia: report of outcome in patients over 65 years of age. *Br J Neurosurg* 2000;14:23–27.

Park SH, Hwang SK, Lee SH, et al. Nerve atrophy and a small cerebellopontine angle cistern in patients with trigeminal neuralgia. *J Neurosurg* 2009;110:633–647.

Pollock BE. Percutaneous retrogasserian glycerol rhizotomy for patients with idiopathic trigeminal neuralgia: a prospective analysis of factors related to pain relief. *J Neurosurg* 2005;102:223–228.

Regis J, Metellus P, Hayashi M, et al. Prospective controlled trial of gamma knife surgery for essential trigeminal neuralgia. *J Neurosurg* 2006;104:913–924.

Rogers CL, Shetter AG, Fiedler JA, et al. Gamma knife radiosurgery for trigeminal neuralgia: the initial experience of The Barrow Neurological Institute. *Int J Radiat Oncol Biol Phys* 2000;47:1013–1019.

Ryu H, Yamamoto S, Sugiyama K, et al. Neurovascular decompression for trigeminal neuralgia in elderly patients. *Neurol Med Chir (Tokyo)* 1999;39:226–229; discussion 229–230.

Sandell T, Eide PK. Effect of microvascular decompression in trigeminal neuralgia patients with or without constant pain. *Neurosurgery* 2008;63:93–99; discussion 99–100.

Sekula RF, Frederickson AM, Jannetta PJ, et al. Microvascular decompression in patients with isolated maxillary division trigeminal neuralgia, with particular attention to venous pathology. *Neurosurg Focus* 2009;27:E10.

Sekula RF, Marchan EM, Fletcher LH, et al. Microvascular decompression for trigeminal neuralgia in elderly patients. *J Neurosurg* 2008;108:689–691.

Selim M. Perioperative stroke. *N Engl J Med* 2007;356:706–713.

Sheehan J, Pan HC, Stroila M, Steiner L. Gamma knife surgery for trigeminal neuralgia: outcomes and prognostic factors. *J Neurosurg* 2005;102:434–441.

Sindou M, Leston J, Decullier E, Chapuis F. Microvascular decompression for primary trigeminal neuralgia: long-term effectiveness and prognostic factors in a series of 362 consecutive patients with clear-cut neurovascular conflicts who underwent pure decompression. *J Neurosurg* 2007;107:1144–1153.

Sindou M, Leston J, Howeidy T, et al. Micro-vascular decompression for primary Trigeminal Neuralgia (typical or atypical). Long-term effectiveness on pain; prospective study with survival analysis in a consecutive series of 362 patients. *Acta Neurochir (Wien)* 2006;148:1235–1245; discussion 1245.

Sweet W. Atypical facial neuralgia. In White J, Sweet W, eds. *Pain and the neurosurgeon.* Springfield, IL: Charles C. Thomas, 1969.

Taha JM, Tew JM, Jr. Comparison of surgical treatments for trigeminal neuralgia: reevaluation of radiofrequency rhizotomy. *Neurosurgery,* 1996;38:865–871.

Taylor DW, Barnett HJ, Haynes RB, et al. Low-dose and high-dose acetylsalicylic acid for patients undergoing carotid endarterectomy: a randomised controlled trial. *ASA and Carotid Endarterectomy (ACE) Trial Collaborators. Lancet* 1999;353:2179–2184.

Tyler-Kabara EC, Kassam AB, Horowitz MH, et al. Predictors of outcome in surgically managed patients with typical and atypical trigeminal neuralgia: comparison of results following microvascular decompression. *J Neurosurg* 2002;96:527–531.

Vonderahe A. Corneal and scleral anesthesia of the lower half of the eye in a case of trauma of the superior maxillary nerve. *Arch Neurol Psychiatry* 1928;20:836–837.

Yousry I, Moriggl B, Holtmannspoetter M, et al. Detailed anatomy of the motor and sensory roots of the trigeminal nerve and their neurovascular relationships: a magnetic resonance imaging study. *J Neurosurg* 2004;101:427–434.

9

Current Operative Procedures: Overview

Toba Niazi, Paul A. House, and Ronald I. Apfelbaum

Treatment of trigeminal neuralgia (TN) is mandated by the severity of the pain produced in this condition. Nontreatment (i.e., "living with it") is not an option. The initial treatment for TN should be medical therapy, which reduces or eliminates pain in approximately 75% of patients (Brown, McDaniel, & Weaver 1993; Pollock & Ecker 2005). Unfortunately, the relief provided by medical therapy may diminish over time, and the condition frequently becomes resistant even to multidrug regimens. Medical therapy can also be associated with intolerable and debilitating side effects such as imbalance, hyponatremia, and cognitive dysfunction, which limit the dosage that can be used and hence its effectiveness (Baker, Taylor, & Lilly 1985; Campbell, Graham, & Zilkha 1966; Rockliff & Davis 1966; Zakrzewska & Patsalos 2002). These side effects tend to occur more commonly in elderly patients than in younger patients. Operation is indicated for patients in whom medical therapy becomes ineffective, leaving the patient with intractable pain, or for those patients in whom the side effects from medical therapy become intolerable.

Surgical treatment options can be divided into procedures that directly decompress the trigeminal nerve, procedures that partially injure the nerve, and palliative procedures separate from the nerve itself. Direct decompression of the nerve is achieved through a posterior fossa craniectomy and translocation of the offending (usually vascular) structure. Destructive procedures include percutaneous thermal radiofrequency ablation, percutaneous glycerol rhizotomy, mechanical balloon compression, trigeminal rhizotomy, and stereotactic radiosurgery (SRS). Palliative procedures that may help with the chronic pain when all other avenues have been exhausted include deep brain stimulation of the periaqueductal and periventricular gray matter and motor cortex stimulation.

Multiple factors must be weighed by the physician in making a decision as to which procedure to recommend. The patient's age, the pain location, and any associated medical comorbidities all need to be considered, as must the patient's preference based on what risks he or she is willing to assume to relieve the tic pain. Destructive lesions placed within the trigeminal system usually provide effective pain relief. However, destructive procedures do not treat the cause of the TN, making it more likely that the pain will recur over a period of time. These procedures are also more likely to produce sensory disturbances involving the trigeminal nerve that can vary from minor dysesthesias to more severe symptoms such as analgesia dolorosa or anesthesia dolorosa, which may be more bothersome than the initial paroxysms of pain (Sweet 1986; Taha & Tew 1996; Tatli, Satici, Kanpolat, & Sindou 2008). The destructive procedures, however, tend to be less invasive than direct nerve decompression. The nerve-sparing microvascular decompression (MVD) procedure is more invasive but treats the apparent cause of the disease process and, as a result, may be curative and usually will not produce sensory disturbances.

DESTRUCTIVE PROCEDURES

Decompressive procedures involve a craniotomy and therefore will always carry more potential morbidity. For this reason, percutaneous trigeminal rhizolysis techniques have been developed and are the appropriate choice for some patients. When used in the treatment of TN, these percutaneous techniques produce a partial destructive lesion in the preganglionic trigeminal rootlets or the ganglion itself to relieve the symptoms, with the hope of sparing some sensory nerve function. Since these procedures destroy some of the nerve, they will produce numbness. This can be minimal or partial numbness limited to certain areas of the face or may be more diffuse and dense. In addition, dysesthesias ranging from mild to quite severe can occur, resulting in analgesia dolorosa or the even more severe anesthesia dolorosa. Corneal hypesthesia can also occur and may result in neuroparalytic keratitis. Because these procedures address the symptoms, rather than the cause of the patient's pain, there is a high probability of future recurrence of symptoms, although many patients may go years without recurrence (Arias 1986; Laghmari et al. 2007; Lopez, Hamlyn, & Zakrzewska 2004; Lunsford 1982; Nugent & Berry 1974; Nugent 1982). The procedures may also be repeated to relieve recurrences, but doing so can increase the numbness and increase the risk of dysesthetic sequelae (Arias 1986; Laghmari et al. 2007; Lopez et al. 2004; Lunsford 1982; Nugent & Berry 1974; Nugent 1982). The percutaneous approach is well tolerated by most patients and, given the minimally invasive nature of the procedures, is especially favored for elderly patients with multiple medical comorbidities. Such patients also have a lower overall life expectancy, and therefore the need for repeated percutaneous procedures will usually be less than in younger patients with TN (Liu & Apfelbaum 2004).

Percutaneous Radiofrequency Thermorhizotomy

Sweet and Wepsic (1974) introduced percutaneous radiofrequency thermorhizotomy in 1974, for the treatment of TN. This was based on earlier work using electrocoagulation with monopolar cautery, which, while effective in relieving pain, produced almost total anesthesia and frequent anesthesia dolorosa and hence had been essentially abandoned (Kirschner 1931). Their modified technique focused on using shorter-acting anesthetic agents to allow for clinical assessment, electrical stimulation for localization of the gasserian ganglion, reliable radiofrequency current for focused lesionectomy, and a temperature probe to monitor the temperature to try to control the degree of damage to the rootlets. The rationale behind this technique, as well as other destructive procedures directed at the preganglionic trigeminal nerve or nerve rootlets, is based on the findings in a cat model of Letcher and Goldring (1968), who noted that compound action potentials of the nociceptive fibers (poorly myelinated and unmyelinated Aδ and C fibers) are blocked at lower temperatures given their architectural make-up than the larger and heavily myelinated (Aα and Aβ) fibers that mediate tactile stimulation. Despite this observation, histological studies examining the injured gasserian ganglion in animal models demonstrated global injury to the nerve rather than differential injury to the nociceptive versus the tactile fibers (Letcher & Goldring 1968). It is thought, however, that this technique helps to reduce the overall sensory input and perhaps aberrant transmission of impulses from the demyelinated fibers to the nociceptive fibers.

Depending on the surgeon's preference and institutional variation, this procedure may be performed in the operating room or a fluoroscopy suite with the assistance of an anesthesiologist. Appropriate monitoring to assess heart rate, blood pressure, and respiratory rate and oxygen saturation should be initiated before the procedure. Short-acting sedatives should be administered intravenously throughout the procedure as needed. In the fluoroscopy suite, the patient is placed supine, with the neck extended and rotated about 15 degrees to the contralateral side. In the operating suite, the desired oblique near-submental view can be obtained with an appropriately positioned C-arm fluoroscope unit. At the beginning of the procedure, 0.4 mg of intramuscular atropine is given to reduce oral secretions and prevent bradycardia (Taha, Tew, & Buncher 1995). Using the Hartel technique (Hartel 1914) and anatomical landmarks, a 100 mm 18-gauge needle containing a stylet is inserted into the cheek approximately 2.5 cm lateral to the oral commissure. Two guide lines from this entry point, one going toward the medial aspect of the pupil and the other to a point approximately one-third of the way along an imaginary line from the external auditory canal to the external canthus of the eye, can be drawn on the patient's face (Fig. 9.1). Keeping the needle close to the pathway defined by the intersection of the two planes perpendicular to the skin through these guidelines will place the needle tip in close proximity to the foramen ovale. The final positioning through the medial end of the foramen ovale is done under direct fluoroscopic guidance. Once the needle is through the foramen ovale, the stylet is withdrawn to assess for flow of cerebrospinal fluid (CSF).

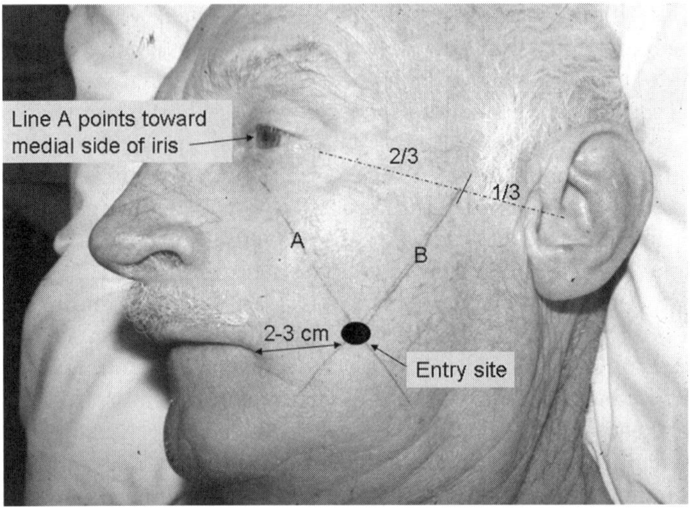

Figure 9.1 Hartel technique for placing a needle into the foramen ovale. The entry site is about 2.5 cm lateral to the mouth. Two lines are drawn through this site. Line A extends from the entry point toward the medial side of the iris with the eyes in a neutral position. Line B goes from the entry point to a point one-third the distance between the external canal of the ear and the lateral canthus of the eye. The needle is placed so that it would pass along the junction of two imaginary planes, one through each line perpendicular to the skin. Final positioning is achieved under fluoroscopy, and a gloved finger in the mouth helps prevent penetration of the oral mucosa as the needle is advanced toward the foramen.

In some patients who have had multiple procedures there may not be egress of CSF because of repeated scarring in that area.

When the needle is in the appropriate location, the electrode is introduced through the needle. There are two different techniques used for the lesioning (Laghmari et al. 2007; Lopez et al. 2004; Taha et al. 1995). In the first technique, an electrode with a flexible curved tip that is capable of both stimulation and temperature sensing is used. The curved tip is used to help localize the area to be lesioned more precisely. Once the electrode is in the region of the gasserian ganglion, stimulation is used to localize the divisions of the trigeminal nerve that are most affected by the tic pain. Patients generally perceive the sensation as a vibration or a paresthetic sensation in the affected division at a threshold between 0.1 and 0.4 V (50 Hz, 2.5-msec continuous pulse train). Prior to lesioning, the depth of the electrode and its orientation are modified to find the location with the lowest threshold of stimulation in the desired division(s). Anesthesia is then induced intravenously, and the radiofrequency current is applied to the electrode, slowly raising the temperature to the desired level for the planned time, to create a lesion in the region of the preganglionic trigeminal rootlets. The patient is then brought out of anesthesia and clinically assessed in regard to residual pain and sensation in the trigeminal nerve.

The alternative technique described by Nugent and Berry (1974) uses a thin wire electrode with about 2.5 mm of the tip exposed, but without temperature monitoring. The needle is placed in the same manner, and the electrode tip location is optimized with stimulation. With this technique, lesioning is done by making small incremental increases in the duration of the radiofreqency current, and if necessary its intensity, with repeated clinical testing of the patient. Initial lesions are made at 50–100 mA for 10 seconds and enlarged in increments of 3–5 seconds. To facilitate repeated testing of the patient, a neuroleptic anesthetic technique is used. Tew (1996) stressed the importance of obtaining a dense hypalgesia rather than analgesia in the affected trigger zone during clinical testing during the procedure. By obtaining hypalgesia, the risk of bothersome dysesthesias is decreased by half, although the long-term pain recurrence rate is similar to that with analgesia (Taha et al. 1995; Taha & Tew 1997; Tew 1996).

Percutaneous radiofrequency thermal rhizotomy is generally well tolerated by the elderly and those with multiple medical comorbidities. In a prospective analysis of 154 patients undergoing percutaneous radiofrequency thermal rhizotomy (Taha et al. 1995), 99% of patients obtained initial pain relief after one procedure. Recurrence of pain over 15 years occurred in 33 patients (21.4 %). Of these 33 patients who had pain recurrence, 10 patients had pain that was well controlled with medication and 23 required additional procedures for pain relief (Taha & Tew 1997).

The price for successful pain relief in the series by Taha et al. (1995) was significant numbness, with 46% of patients having analgesia and 42% having dense hypesthesia. In addition, dysesthesia was reported as mild in 15% of patients, moderate in 5%, and severe in 3%. Although most were affected by dysesthesias less severe than anesthesia dolorosa, those patients affected by the most severe of the postoperative dysesthesias are plagued by frequent or continuous crawling, burning, and itching sensations that for many are very bothersome and for some are almost as intolerable as their initial tic symptoms. Unfortunately, these are usually refractory to treatment. If thermocoagulation of the first division of the trigeminal nerve is performed during the procedure, there is a risk of corneal anesthesia with subsequent development of neurogenic keratitis, which can lead to blindness over time (Taha et al. 1995; Taha & Tew 1997). Thus, clinical examination of the patient during the lesioning is of paramount importance to ensure that facial numbness during the procedure is tolerable and that the corneal reflex is not abolished. Patients must be aware of the inherent risks associated with the procedure and must be willing to cope with and accept permanent alteration in facial sensation. The risk of meningitis, albeit small, must also be discussed with patients and must be considered if there is significant fever, headache, nuchal rigidity, or photophobia in the first several days after the procedure.

Glycerol Chemoneurolysis

Glycerol chemoneurolysis was first introduced by Håkanson (1981). The use of glycerol as the chemoneurolytic agent was discovered serendipitously. During early use of the Leksell gamma knife, Dr. Leksell tried to radiate the gasserian ganglion to treat TN (Leksell 1971). Tantalum powder suspended in glycerol as a vehicle was injected into Meckel's cave to serve as a permanent marker to create a visible target for future treatments (Linderoth & Håkanson 1989); however, many patients in whom this mixture was injected had complete resolution of their paroxysmal pain before any radiosurgery was performed. The exact mechanism behind the action of glycerol is unknown, although its neurolytic properties are thought to be due to its hypertonicity, which may injure thin, unmyelinated and then myelinated fibers in succession (Linderoth & Håkanson 1989). Sweet and colleagues (1981) noted that glycerol injected into the gasserian ganglion in patients plagued with TN caused a decrease in the degree of firing of the nociceptive fiber (Aδ and C) components of trigeminal root potentials recorded during electric stimulation on the surface of the cheek. However, Fruhstorfer and Hensel (1973) used quantitative sensory testing and found that, over time, glycerol acts mainly on the large myelinated or tactile fibers. It is possible therefore that the effect of glycerol may be due to its action on the large myelinated fibers that have been focally demyelinated from arterial or venous compression and thereby prevent aberrant impulses to the nociceptive fibers. The degree of hyperosmolarity appears to be paramount in the mechanism of action of glycerol in the gasserian ganglion region, and it is the rate of change of the osmolarity that is critical for its effect on the nociceptive fibers. For this reason, pure, anhydrous (99.5%) glycerol rather than more dilute glycerol is required (Fruhstorfer & Hensel 1973).

Glycerol chemoneurolysis is generally performed in the radiology suite with the assistance of an anesthesiologist, but can also be done in an operating room. Vital signs monitoring during the procedure and supine patient positioning are as described earlier. The Hartel technique (Hartel 1914) described earlier is used to cannulate the foramen ovale under direct fluoroscopic guidance with a 100-mm 18-gauge spinal needle that has a short beveled tip (Crawford point) and stylet. Short-acting intravenous anesthetic drugs are administered prior to needle placement. Brief, fairly deep anesthesia is used to prevent pain during the initial placement of the needle into the trigeminal cistern. As the needle is inserted through the foramen ovale, the patient positioning allows direct fluoroscopic visualization of the foramen ovale, which must be punctured at its most medial aspect in order to enter the trigeminal cistern. Once the needle is in the appropriate location, the stylet is removed and egress of CSF should be noted (again, patients who have undergone multiple procedures may not have free flow of CSF because of prior scarring). The patient is then allowed to awaken and is placed in a sitting position by securely affixing the table's footboard

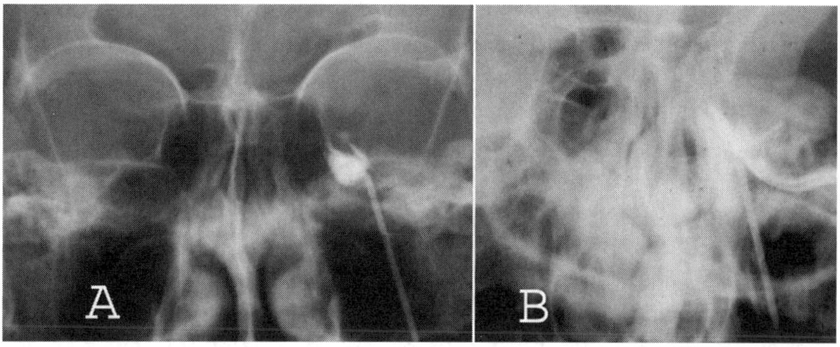

Figure 9.2 Anteroposterior fluoroscopic images of the cisternogram performed to assure correct localization as well as quantify the size of the trigeminal cistern.

(A) The needle is correctly positioned and the dye pools within the cistern. (B) The needle is not in the cistern despite cerebrospinal fluid flow. The dye is outlining the subarachnoid space below the temporal lobe, indicating that the needle has been inserted too deeply or at too steep a trajectory and is above the tentorium.

underneath the patient's buttocks and rotating the fluoroscopy table 90 degrees. A cisternogram is performed by injecting iohexol contrast into the needle; if the needle is placed in the correct location within the foramen, the contrast will be observed fluoroscopically to fill Meckel's cave (Fig. 9.2) and will then start to overflow into the posterior fossa. If the needle is not in the preganglionic trigeminal cistern, it must be repositioned. Using a calibrated syringe, the amount of contrast used to fill the cistern can be measured from the fluoroscopic visualization. The patient is then placed back in the supine position, and the stylet is removed from the needle to allow the contrast to flow out of the cistern. This is confirmed through fluoroscopy. In patients without good CSF flow, sterile saline can be injected to flush out the contrast agent, which could block the glycerol from coming in contact with the trigeminal nerve preganglionic rootlets.

The patient is then transferred onto a hospital bed, positioned into a near 90-degree sitting position, and an amount of glycerol equal to the size of Meckel's cave is slowly instilled. The sitting position helps keep the glycerol within the cistern. The patient is maintained in this position for about 2 hours after the procedure. Patients are generally pretreated with an intravenous analgesic agent during the instillation of glycerol because the procedure may provoke the trigeminal tic pain.

Glycerol injection is well tolerated by the elderly and those patients who have multiple comorbidities. The percentage of patients who have relief of their paroxysmal trigeminal pain within 2 weeks of glycerol neurolysis ranges from 67% to 97% in different series (Arias 1986; Cappabianca et al.

1995; Henson et al. 2005; Laghmari et al. 2007; Liu & Apfelbaum 2004; Lopez et al. 2004; Lunsford 1982; Lunsford & Bennett 1984). In the senior author's experience with 303 patients who underwent this procedure, 90% had relief within 2 weeks (Liu & Apfelbaum 2004). Similarly, Cappabianca and colleagues (1995) presented a series of 191 patients treated with glycerol chemoneurolysis and showed that 93% were pain free immediately after treatment. Long-term follow-up monitoring after 10 years demonstrated that 77% of patients remained pain free. If recurrence of pain does occur, the injection can be repeated. Although the initial success rate for subsequent injections is similar to that of the initial injections, the duration of effectiveness subsides. Of the 303 patients treated by the senior author (Liu & Apfelbaum 2004), 181 underwent one injection, 83 underwent two injections, 19 underwent three injections, and 20 underwent four or more injections. The average time to recurrence of symptoms after one injection was 21 months, whereas the average time to recurrence with more than one injection was 16 months. With each successive injection, however, the patient must be counseled as to the risk of further sensory damage and the risk (albeit small) of development of anesthesia dolorosa. In the series by Cappabianca et al. (1995), no cases of anesthesia dolorosa were observed, but mild hypesthesia was observed in 46% of patients. In the senior author's experience, only one case of anesthesia dolorosa has been observed. Trigeminal glycerol rhizolysis appears to have a lower incidence of postoperative sensory disturbance than thermal radiofrequency ablation (Liu & Apfelbaum 2004). Other complications of glycerol rhizolysis are similar to those of other modalities used to make a lesion. Patients must be counseled as to the signs and symptoms of meningitis after this procedure, as this is a rare but serious complication. Activation of latent herpes simplex virus infections after any manipulation of the trigeminal system is well known. This not infrequent occurrence generally is mild and self-limited (Liu & Apfelbaum 2004).

Percutaneous Balloon Compression

The benefits of compression of the gasserian ganglion were noted by Shelden et al. (1955). They performed subtemporal craniotomies in an effort to decompress the trigeminal ganglion, but instead noted that compression and mechanical injury to the nerve with resultant sensory deficits produced better results. The technique was mostly abandoned over time, however, because of recurrences, which may have been related to the difficulty in standardizing a reproducible degree of mechanical injury. Mullan and Lichtor (1983) reintroduced the technique through a percutaneous approach with the aid of balloon compression. Balloon compression is distinct from the other two percutaneous procedures because it requires a completely anesthetized, intubated patient. An external pacemaker is frequently used to help control the bradyarrhythmias that occur during the procedure.

Compression of the trigeminal ganglion is thought to selectively injure the large myelinated fibers but does not seem to affect the smaller unmyelinated and nociceptive fibers, which are responsible for mediating the corneal reflex. Thus, treatment of first-division pain is reported to be safer because the possibility of injuring this reflex is reduced (Brown & Preul 1988, 1989; Brown et al. 1993).

Percutaneous balloon compression may be performed in the radiology suite or the operating room, depending on the surgeon's preference. As indicated earlier, full general endotracheal anesthesia and an external pacemaker are required for the procedure. As in the other procedures, the patient is placed in the supine neutral position, and the Hartel technique (Hartel 1914) is used to locate the foramen ovale under direct fluoroscopic guidance; however, a larger 14-gauge, 100 mm needle is used. The needle is advanced to the external orifice of the foramen ovale but not passed into the foramen. A balloon catheter is then directed through the foramen and into Meckel's cave, and, depending upon which division is involved, the catheter is directed toward the medial portion for the first division, the lateral portion for the third division, or the midpoint of Meckel's cave for the second division or for multidivision compression. The balloon is then inflated to a pressure of 1.3–1.5 atmospheres (about 1,000 mm Hg), and inflation is confirmed with direct fluoroscopic visualization (Brown & Preul 1988, 1989; Brown et al. 1993). The compression is maintained for no longer than 1.5 minutes, because the risk of dysesthesias increases with increased compression (Brown & Preul 1988, 1989; Brown et al. 1993). Transient bradycardia may occur, with appropriate intervention by the external pacemaker signaling the trigeminal depressor response and confirming trigeminal stimulation. The balloon is then deflated, and the catheter and needle are removed. The patient is monitored overnight after awakening from anesthesia.

Brown and colleagues (1993) found that 93% of patients who underwent balloon compression had pain relief. Of those, 25% had recurrence of pain within 5 years and required an additional procedure. Sixty-eight percent achieved lasting pain relief after a second balloon compression. The occurrence of dysesthesia is slightly decreased compared with the other percutaneous procedures; however, masseter muscle weakness, which is rarely seen with radiofrequency thermocoagulation and virtually never occurs with glycerol injection, occurs not infrequently in these patients. It usually resolves over a 12-month period (Brown & Preul 1989; Brown et al. 1993; Brown 2002). In the series by Brown and colleagues (1993), there was no occurrence of anesthesia dolorosa or corneal anesthesia. Although this is a relatively well-tolerated procedure, it may not be the ideal approach for use in those patients that have multiple comorbidities because general endotracheal anesthesia is required. Special caution should be used in those patients with a history of cardiac arrhythmias, as the trigeminal cardiac reflex response may aggravate them.

Stereotactic Radiosurgery

Stereotactic radiosurgery for treatment of TN was pioneered by Leksell (1971) using a technique in which the gasserian ganglion was exposed to large amounts of ionizing radiation. The initial procedures in two patients who had symptoms of TN were successful, but as more patients had radiation exposure to the gasserian ganglion, there was less consistency of pain relief, so the target evolved to the nerve root entry zone (REZ) of the trigeminal root near the pons. The use of magnetic resonance imaging (MRI) has allowed a third target zone to be identified, the anterior portion of the cisternal nerve just proximal to Meckel's cave (plexus triangularis) (Chavez et al. 2005; Cole, Liu, & Apfelbaum 2005; Haines, Jannetta, & Zorub 1980; Kondziolka et al. 1996a). With the advent of modern technology, including improved neuroimaging targeting techniques and the development of newer stereotactic planning devices, more stereotactic options are available to patients, namely gamma knife radiosurgery (GKRS) and the newer linear accelerator (LINAC)-based systems. The rationale behind the use of radiosurgery for relief of TN pain is that focal radiation targeted at the trigeminal nerve induces injury to the large myelinated fibers and, like the other destructive procedures, may thereby inhibit aberrant nerve transmission to the nociceptive Aδ and C fibers, preventing the "trigger" of paroxysms (Haines et al. 1980; Kondziolka et al. 1996b; Kondziolka et al. 1996a; Kondziolka, Lunsford, Habeck, & Flickinger 1997). The effect of radiosurgery, whether through the GKRS or the LINAC system, is not immediate but instead takes several days to weeks to take effect, so this is not the best intervention for those patients with severe intractable pain. In essence, the high dose of radiation causes a delayed lesion in the nerve. The use of radiosurgery may be especially ideal for those patients who are elderly with multiple comorbidities that preclude them being weaned off anticoagulation for percutaneous procedures or who are high anesthetic risks.

Both GKRS and LINAC require stereotactic high-resolution MRI and stereotactic computed tomography (CT) to be performed with image fusion for optimal targeting. Failure to use high-resolution MRI results in less than ideal visualization of the trigeminal nerve and the REZ, and this compromises the most important part of the radiosurgical procedure, accurately targeting the nerve (Haines et al. 1980; Kondziolka et al. 1996b; Kondziolka et al. 1996a; Kondziolka et al. 1997). A head frame is affixed with percutaneous screws before scanning and then treatment planning is undertaken with the help of a physicist. The ideal target has not yet been determined, but the REZ of the trigeminal nerve and the plexus triangularis are favored over the gasserian ganglion. The degree of radiation exposure to the brainstem is decreased when the plexus triangularis is used, and this site is therefore preferred by some surgeons in consideration of the large doses of radiation that are used (Chavez et al. 2005; Haines et al. 1980; Kondziolka et al. 1996b; Kondziolka et al. 1996a; Kondziolka et al. 1997).

Accuracy is of paramount importance in radiosurgery because of the small target size, as inaccuracy can lead to a failure in treating the target and in radiation being delivered to a different site, such as the prepontine cistern or the brainstem, leading to unwanted side effects and continued trigeminal pain (Chavez et al. 2005).

The ideal radiation dose to treat TN has not yet been clearly defined; however, Kondziolka and colleagues (1996a) have seen success with a dosage between 70 and 90 Gy. Doses greater than 100 Gy in primate models caused axonal necrosis and should be avoided (Kondziolka et al. 2000). Other clinical studies have evaluated the outcomes after varying radiation doses (Goss et al. 2003).

Kondziolka et al. (1996a) reported a nonrandomized multicenter study of 50 patients treated with GKRS to the proximal trigeminal nerve near the pons. The target dose varied between 60 and 90 Gy, and the median time to pain relief was 30 days. A greater proportion of patients gained complete trigeminal pain relief after a maximum dose greater than 70 Gy (range 70–90 Gy) than after a dose less than 70 Gy. Pollock et al. (2001) examined a series of 68 patients treated with GKRS at the REZ and compared outcomes in patients who received doses of 70 Gy or 90 Gy. Initial pain relief was experienced by 86% of the patients who received 70 Gy and 93% of the patients who received 90 Gy. More patients at the lower dose experienced recurrence of pain (26% vs. 15%); however, only 15% of patients at the lower dose had postprocedure trigeminal anesthesia, whereas 54% of patients at the higher dose did. The difference in the rate of pain relief was not statistically significant, but the greater degree of numbness observed was. Goss et al. (2003) reviewed a series of 25 patients treated with GKRS at 90 Gy at the REZ; 76% of patients achieved excellent pain relief and 24% achieved good pain relief. Of these, 32% developed facial paresthesias and numbness, and 12% experienced decreased corneal sensation necessitating treatment with eyedrops daily. Thus, it appears likely the ideal radiation dose is between 70 and 90 Gy, and there is a range in the success rate that must be balanced with the development of possible complications.

Radiosurgery, like the other neurolytic techniques that have been discussed, does not treat the cause of the disease, but acts to produce a delayed lesion and can incur the same side effects as other destructive procedures. The most frequently reported complication of radiosurgery is facial numbness, which is bothersome in a minority of cases (Petit et al. 2003; Pollock et al. 2002; Pollock & Ecker 2005). As with other destructive techniques, cases of anesthesia dolorosa and corneal keratitis have also been reported. No mortality due to SRS has been reported in the literature to date, although very low mortality rates have been described with the other destructive techniques (Kondziolka et al. 1996b; Kondziolka et al. 1996a; Kondziolka et al. 1997; Petit et al. 2003; Pollock et al. 2002; Pollock & Ecker 2005).

Although radiosurgery for TN may be considered a less invasive destructive treatment and offers initial pain relief in greater than 90% of patients, with complete absence of pain in 75% of patients and recurrence of pain in 10%–35%, it remains controversial (Kondziolka et al. 1996b; Kondziolka et al. 1996a; Kondziolka et al. 1997; Petit et al. 2003; Pollock et al. 2002; Pollock & Ecker 2005). This treatment regimen is fairly new, with very few long-term studies with large numbers of patients. Instead, many publications compare competing radiosurgery techniques (GKRS vs. LINAC) using limited numbers of patients with shorter follow-up (Villavicencio et al. 2008). In addition, many studies define "good" and "excellent" results as just a reduction in pain (Rogers et al. 2000; Villavicencio et al. 2008; Young et al. 1997). In studies evaluating other destructive procedures, however, complete pain relief without medication is the standard for "excellent" outcomes, and "good" outcomes are those in which the patient is pain free on tolerable doses of medication (Rogers et al. 2000; Villavicencio et al. 2008; Young et al. 1997). Although reporting the data using less strenuous criteria may make the radiosurgical techniques seem comparable with the other techniques, such results are far from optimal for the patient. With further long-term studies looking at follow-up, safety, efficacy, ideal targeting location, and dose optimization, and using standardized reporting techniques, the true role of SRS may be established. Currently, we reserve this technique for those patients who are unable to undergo other procedures because of underlying medical comorbidities, such as conditions that require anticoagulant therapy, or for those patients who are unwilling to accept the small but real risks associated with the other procedures.

DECOMPRESSIVE PROCEDURES

Microvascular Decompression

In 1934, Dandy described vascular compression of the trigeminal nerve at the REZ and thought this might incite TN (Fig. 9.3), but did not consider decompression. Intracranial surgery was commonly used in the midportion of the 20th century, but primarily consisted of Dandy's nerve section from the posterior fossa approach or the much more commonly used subtemporal middle fossa approach (Gelber, Gogela, & Pierson 1989; Hanraets 1954; Peet & Schneider 1952; Pinkus 1984; Spiller & Frazier 1901). Jannetta (1967) pioneered the use of microsurgical technique to explore the trigeminal nerve, and clearly demonstrated pathological vascular compression of the trigeminal nerve as it was exiting the brainstem. He was the first to advocate moving the vessel away from the trigeminal nerve's REZ rather than sectioning the nerve, and in so doing he revolutionized the approach to the treatment of TN (Jannetta 1967; Cook & Jannetta 1984). His surgical efforts led to the development of an operative technique, MVD via a microsurgical retromastoid craniotomy, in which the offending compressive vessels were displaced from the affected nerve by transposition of the

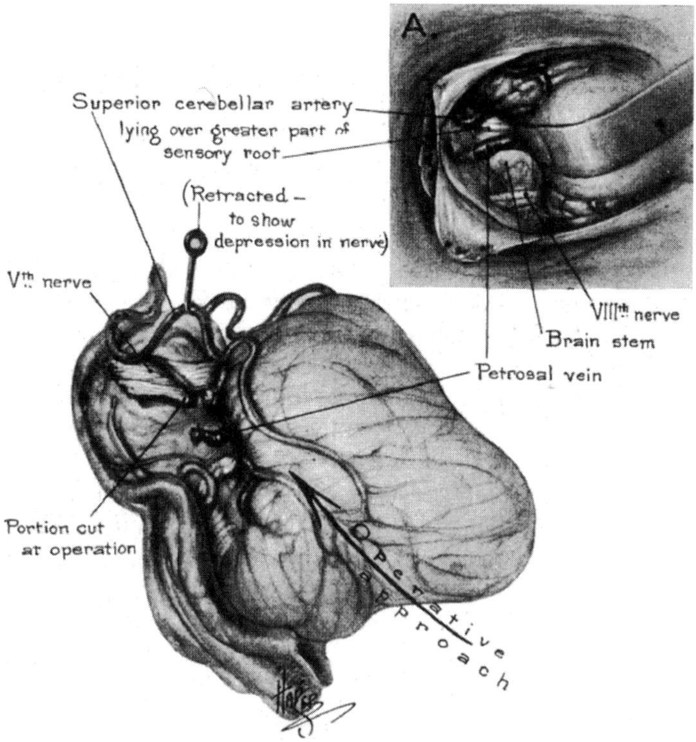

Figure 9.3 Illustration published by Walter Dandy showing his surgical approach.

He commented that "Since the writer has been dividing the sensory root by the cerebellar route, tumors and aneurysms have been found in 10% of cases, over 500. And in almost every additional case, a large arterial branch of the anterior inferior artery lies upon or under the sensory root. In many instances, the nerve is grooved or bent in an angle by the artery. This I believe is the cause of tic douloureux" (Dandy 1932). Although Dandy wrote "anterior inferior artery," his illustration clearly shows the offending vessel to be the superior cerebellar artery. Figure reproduced from Dandy 1932.

vessel and placement of a small implant between the vessels and nerve (Cook & Jannetta 1984; Jannetta 1967). This operation continues to be widely employed, with shredded Teflon felt (PTFE fiber), most commonly used as the implant.

The advantage of MVD compared with the other techniques is that it treats the primary cause of the disease, resulting in complete resolution of symptoms, while preserving neural integrity. Fewer patients experience recurrence of their pain after MVD. Because the nerve is not intentionally damaged, the denervation sequelae seen in destructive procedures, such as facial numbness, dysesthesias, and corneal anesthesia, are avoided.

However, this treatment modality necessitates that the patient tolerate an open surgical procedure under general anesthesia, must take into account any comorbidities that may preclude the safe execution of an open craniotomy, and must address the risks the patient is willing to assume to relieve the pain. The ideal candidate is a younger patient with fewer medical comorbidities, who can tolerate a surgical procedure better than an older patient. There is no exact cut-off age at which patients can no longer undergo this procedure, but we have generally used an age of about 70 years in healthy patients as a guideline. With modern anesthetic techniques, however, the risks of open surgery have clearly decreased, and many surgeons are comfortable recommending MVD even in more elderly patients. A report by Sekula et al. (2008) supports this. These authors reviewed MVD in elderly patients and found that, with proper patient selection, MVD can be performed in physically fit elderly patients without a higher rate of postoperative complications. The generalized atrophy and widened cisterns in these patients allowed ease of access to the cerebellopontine angle. The authors concluded that age alone should not be a contraindication to MVD, but instead the fitness of the patient should be used to identify those who are candidates for neurosurgical intervention.

Positioning of the patient in the sitting position is preferred by the senior author; however, the lateral decubitus position can also be used with similar results. The risk of air embolism is highest in the sitting position but is not negligible in the lateral decubitus position, so monitoring as described here is recommended with both positions. The advantages of the sitting position are that it allows easy access for the anesthesiologist to the patient and it avoids compressing the chest by the patient's weight and the pooling of fluid unilaterally in the dependent lung, which can be an issue with larger patients. It produces a relaxed operative field without venous distension and with the intracranial structures in their normal anatomic relationships. In addition, blood and CSF will flow out of the wound, so that suctioning is not required, thereby possibly reducing the chance of injury to the cranial nerves and or brainstem.

General endotracheal anesthesia using a neuroparalytic technique with controlled mechanical ventilation is required to ensure that the patient does not move while under the operating microscope and obscure the microsurgical field while the surgeon is dissecting around the brainstem. Paralysis also prevents the patient from developing a gasp reflex should a small amount of air embolization occur. The gasp reflex occurs with very small amounts of air and can result in a massive air embolization. Precordial Doppler ultrasound and an end-tidal carbon dioxide monitor are used to detect any air embolization. If embolization is detected, the anesthesiologist raises the venous pressure by increasing positive end-expiratory pressure or by jugular compression, which prevents further entrainment of air and defines its entry site, so that it can be occluded. This technique is so sensitive that even small entrainments are detected, allowing prevention of more massive air embolism, which can be a serious complication. No central lines are required or used, as the amount of entrainment is so small when first detected that they are not useful in treating it.

With either selected position, the patient's head is held with three-point rigid skull fixation and an 8 cm linear paramedian incision is made 3–5 mm medial to the mastoid notch, centered so that two-thirds of the incision is above the notch and one-third lies below the notch. A limited suboccipital retromastoid craniectomy is then performed below the transverse sinus and medial to the sigmoid sinus. By opening the dura close to these dural sinuses, access to the cerebellopontine angle along the superior lateral margin of the cerebellum is obtained. With gentle traction, the petrosal vein is then identified and may be coagulated to allow for better visualization of the trigeminal nerve and access to the arachnoid surrounding the nerve. Whenever possible, however, we try to spare the petrosal vein and work around it. Elongated arterial loops compressing the REZ of the nerve are the most frequently observed phenomenon in patients undergoing this procedure; however, venous channels can also be the cause of compression. The arterial loops are completely dissected off the REZ of the nerve and positioned so that the arterial pulsation is directed away from the nerve. The vessel is secured in this position by interposing a device made of either Ivalon sponge or shredded Teflon felt (PTFE fiber), shaped and positioned in such a manner as to interlock between the vascular structures and nerve to prevent the vessel from coming back in apposition to the nerve (Fig. 9.4). If venous channels are observed to be the offending source of compression of the REZ, they can be carefully dissected off the nerve, cauterized, and sectioned (to prevent them from recanalizing) to decompress the REZ.

Once decompression of the REZ is deemed sufficient, the dura is closed in a watertight fashion, and the wound is closed in sequential layers to prevent any postoperative sequelae of CSF leaks and infection. Postoperatively, patients should be monitored closely overnight in an intensive care setting to ensure that there are no signs of neurological deterioration due to posterior fossa swelling or hematoma. On the first postoperative day, most patients are able to get out of bed and walk. Many patients who undergo the procedure in the sitting position may complain of a postoperative headache. This is not usually a significant problem and is usually managed with oral analgesics. Most patients recover quickly from the procedure and often can be discharged from the hospital by the third postoperative day.

Barker et al. (1996) described the long-term results of MVD in 1,185 patients with a median follow-up period of 6.2 years. They found that the trigeminal root was compressed by the superior cerebellar artery in 75% of cases and that an offending vein was the second most common compressing agent. Immediate postoperative tic relief was seen in 82% of patients, partial relief in 16%, and no relief in 2%. Ten years after MVD, 70% of patients had excellent pain relief, requiring no medications and free from

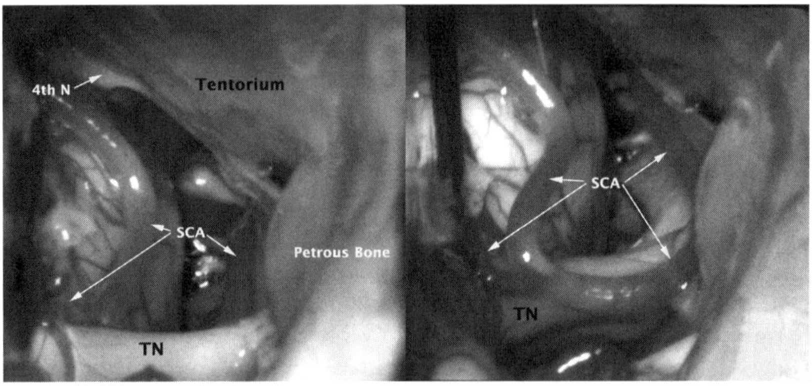

Figure 9.4 Intraoperative photographs of a retromastoid craniectomy performed in the sitting position. In the left panel, a superior cerebellar artery (SCA) loop is seen behind and cross-compressing the root entry zone of the trigeminal nerve. In the right panel, the full extent of the vascular loop is appreciated as it has been dissected free of the nerve and transposed posterior to it. The proximal portion of the vessel is to the left, i.e., more lateral on the image. A shredded Teflon felt prosthesis will be placed above the nerve, extending between the nerve and artery, to elevate the vascular loop from the nerve and redirect the vessel's pulsations into a horizontal plane away from, rather than into, the nerve.

tic pain, and 4% had occasional pain that did not require long-term medication. Ten years after surgery, the annual rate of recurrence of tic pain was less than 1%.

The senior author has had similar results in his series (Apfelbaum 2000) of more than 500 patients with TN treated with MVD. Complete relief of tic pain was seen in 91% of patients who underwent the procedure, and partial relief was seen in another 6% of patients. In 82% of the patients, an artery, most frequently the superior cerebellar artery, was the compressing agent of the trigeminal root. Fourteen years after MVD, 81% of patients had good pain control without the use of medications, and there was a 1% recurrence of pain refractory to treatment per year in the patients who were analyzed. In both series (Apfelbaum 2000; Barker et al. 1996), there was no steady increase in the frequency of recurrences over time, as has been observed with the ablative procedures.

Despite the relative success achieved with MVD, the procedure is not without complications, including but not limited to cerebellar hematomas, transient cranial nerve palsies, unilateral hearing loss, supratentorial and brainstem ischemia and infarction, and death. The incidence of the latter has been less than 1% (Apfelbaum 2000; Barker et al. 1996).

Microvascular decompression has provided patients with the longest optimal long-term pain-free intervals among the procedures discussed, and relieves the apparent cause of the pain without sacrificing the integrity of the trigeminal nerve, thereby preventing the unwanted sequelae of nerve damage, such as dysesthesias. Patient selection is paramount. Motivated patients must be willing to undergo a limited craniotomy and be deemed medically fit so as to minimize the small risk of the serious and possibly potentially lethal complications that can ensue from such a procedure.

Trigeminal Rhizotomy

In 1891, Horsley et al. (1891) first described sectioning of the trigeminal root between the brainstem and the gasserian ganglion through a subtemporal approach. Spiller and Frazier (1901) further popularized trigeminal nerve root sectioning through a middle fossa extradural procedure. In 1925, Dandy advocated a posterior fossa retromastoid intradural approach, with sectioning of the sensory root of the trigeminal nerve at the pons. As his experience increased, he only partially sectioned the nerve, so that only 30%–50% of the lower fascicles of the portio major were sectioned. With the advent of the percutaneous ablative procedures, however, trigeminal rhizotomy fell out of favor with the majority of practitioners because the percutaneous procedures were essentially able to accomplish the similar ablation of the nerve by a less invasive approach to relieve the pain of TN

Partial sectioning of the posterior half of the nerve, the portio major of the trigeminal nerve near the brainstem, however, can provide excellent long-lasting relief of trigeminal pain while preserving the majority of the touch sensation, sparing corneal sensation, and avoiding neuroparalytic keratitis (Bederson & Wilson 1989; Gelber et al. 1989). This procedure is now considered for use in those rare patients who are found during MVD to have no compression on the trigeminal root or in those patients who are afflicted with demyelinating and or neurodegenerative diseases and whose pain has not been relieved by percutaneous procedures (Jensen, Rasmussen, & Reske-Nielsen 1982). This may also serve as the last option for many patients who have had multiple procedures performed and have failed to obtain adequate relief of their tic pain.

The approach is similar to the one used for MVD. Once the trigeminal nerve is identified, and any compression of the nerve is ruled out, the lower 30%–50% of the portio major is sectioned, 2–5 mm lateral to its junction with the brainstem. Despite the destructive nature of this procedure, postoperative facial anesthesia is rare, but facial hypalgesia with relative preservation of light touch perception is common. Impairment of the corneal reflex can be seen with this procedure, although complete loss of the reflex is uncommon (Burchiel & Slavin 2000; Jensen et al. 1982).

Bederson and Wilson (1989) described their experience with partial sensory trigeminal rhizotomy in a series of 86 patients, 56 of whom underwent MVD and trigeminal rhizotomy, and 30 of whom underwent rhizotomy alone. After the median follow-up period of 5 years, no statistical difference in outcome was seen between MVD and partial sensory trigeminal rhizotomy, with 75% of patients obtaining excellent pain relief. Aggressive nerve root sectioning was undertaken in these patients, with greater than 50% of the nerve roots sectioned. Anesthesia dolorosa was seen in two patients, and corneal hypesthesia was seen in four patients.

Young and Wilkins (1993) reported a series of 83 patients who underwent partial sensory trigeminal rhizotomy, with an average follow-up of 72 months. Sixty-four patients had no evidence of microvascular compression of the trigeminal root and partial rhizotomy alone was performed; the remaining 19 patients underwent MVD in conjunction with partial trigeminal rhizotomy because the offending vessel could not be moved adequately or because the vascular contact was deemed insignificant. Only 48% of patients had an "excellent" outcome, defined as pain free without medications, whereas 30% of patients had persistent pain or complete pain recurrence. In this series, fewer than 50% of the roots were sectioned.

In the senior author's experience (Apfelbaum 2002), 40 patients who had a negative exploration during MVD or refractory TN underwent partial sensory trigeminal rhizotomy. Between 30% and 50% of the portio major was sectioned. In this series, 80% of patients achieved complete relief of their tic pain, and an additional 5% achieved adequate pain control in conjunction with medical therapy.

Partial sensory trigeminal rhizotomy is therefore an alternative procedure that can be used in those patients undergoing MVD in whom there is a negative exploration and no compression by a vascular structure is noted, or when the anatomy precludes the safe transposition of the vessels off of the nerve. This allows the surgeon and patient to salvage some benefit from the invasive procedure. This is also an appropriate avenue to pursue in those patients with known demyelinating diseases and neurodegenerative procedures, in whom previous percutaneous procedures have been futile in relieving tic pain. The degree of relief of tic pain is directly proportional to the extent of rhizotomy, with aggressive sectioning leading to a greater relief of tic pain, but also with greater morbidity of dysesthesias and anesthesia dolorosa. This should not be considered first-line treatment for patients with TN but, as previously stated, may be considered after other standard therapies have been exhausted. An informed, motivated, and medically fit patient is the ideal candidate for this technique, as the risks associated with this procedure are the same as for MVD but also include sensory dysfunction because neural integrity is not preserved.

PALLIATIVE PROCEDURES

Deep Brain Stimulation

Deep brain stimulation for the treatment of chronic pain was first introduced by Heath (1954), who implanted temporary electrodes in the septum pellucidum in a region anterior and inferior to the foramen of Monro for the treatment of pain secondary to metastatic carcinoma in schizophrenic patients. Pool and colleagues (1956) reported pain relief after septal stimulation in patients with chronic pain disorders who were not afflicted with any psychiatric ailments. This led to a series of studies (Mazars, Merienne, & Cioloca 1980; Rasche, Rinaldi, Young, & Tronnier 2006) in which different targets were investigated in an effort to relieve chronic pain. Deep brain stimulation for the treatment of TN has been described in the literature (Coffey 2001; Rasche et al. 2006), although no firm conclusions regarding this treatment modality can be made with the sparsity of data that are available. Two large multicentered trials (reviewed by Coffey 2001) demonstrate that deep brain stimulation of well-defined targets in the sensory thalamus and periaqueductal or periventricular gray matter with stereotactic placement have not proven to be efficacious (>50% of patients reporting at least 50% improvement in pain at 1 year) in those patients with chronic pain of various sources. Although these multicenter trials revealed improvement in the severity of neuropathic facial pain, in general, this improvement unfortunately proved not to be robust as indicated by an extremely high rate of patient drop-out in the trials. Further research must be performed before deep brain stimulation is deemed more than an experimental option in those patients who have exhausted all other conventional treatment modalities to alleviate their pain.

Motor Cortex Stimulation

Motor cortex stimulation was first introduced by Tsubokawa and colleagues (1991a, 1991b) in 1991 for the treatment of central and thalamic pain syndromes. Since then, numerous reports have described its use in intractable pain syndromes, but most have focused on post-stroke pain. This technique was then extrapolated for use in patients with facial neuropathic pain in whom traditional treatments were unsuccessful. In several small studies (Tsubokawa et al. 1991a, 1991b; Velasco et al. 2008), good or excellent pain relief was obtained in 75%–100% of patients. Motor cortex stimulation appears to hold promise for these patients who have exhausted the more traditional treatment modalities, but despite the reported success of motor cortex stimulation in several small series, there have been no large, controlled, prospective, randomized trials of this modality.

CONCLUSION

Multiple surgical procedures offer hope for pain relief or control for patients afflicted with TN. Proper patient selection to exclude those with "atypical TN" and other forms of chronic or deafferentation pain should precede any surgical treatment, as results are much inferior in such cases. For patients with typical TN refractory to medication, many good options are available, and the surgeon can advise the patient on the best choice based on risk tolerance and desired benefits.

ACKNOWLEDGMENTS

The authors thank Kristin Kraus, MSc, Medical Editor in the Department of Neurosurgery at the University of Utah, for her excellent editorial assistance in preparing this chapter.

REFERENCES

Apfelbaum RI. Neurovascular decompression: the procedure of choice? *Clin Neurosurg* 2000;46:473–498.

———. Trigeminal rhizotomy. In KJ Burchiel, ed., *Surgical management of pain*. New York: Thieme, 2002;898–902.

Arias MJ. Percutaneous retrogasserian glycerol rhizotomy for trigeminal neuralgia. A prospective study of 100 cases. *J Neurosurg* 1986;65(1):32–36.

Baker KA, Taylor JW, Lilly GE. Treatment of trigeminal neuralgia: use of baclofen in combination with carbamazepine. *Clin Pharm* 1985;4(1):93–96.

Barker FG 2nd, Jannetta PJ, Bissonette DJ, et al. The long-term outcome of microvascular decompression for trigeminal neuralgia. *N Engl J Med* 1996;334(17): 1077–1083.

Bederson JB, Wilson CB. Evaluation of microvascular decompression and partial sensory rhizotomy in 252 cases of trigeminal neuralgia. *J Neurosurg* 1989;71(3): 359–367.

Brown JA. Trigeminal neuralgia: treatment by percutaneous balloon compression. In KJ Burchiel, ed., *Surgical management of pain*. New York: Thieme, 2002;874–877.

Brown JA, McDaniel MD, Weaver MT. Percutaneous trigeminal nerve compression for treatment of trigeminal neuralgia: results in 50 patients. *Neurosurgery* 1993;32(4):570–573.

Brown JA, Preul MC. Trigeminal depressor response during percutaneous microcompression of the trigeminal ganglion for trigeminal neuralgia. *Neurosurgery* 1988;23(6):745–748.

———. Percutaneous trigeminal ganglion compression for trigeminal neuralgia. Experience in 22 patients and review of the literature. *J Neurosurg* 1989;70(6): 900–904.

Burchiel KJ, Slavin KV. On the natural history of trigeminal neuralgia. *Neurosurgery* 2000;46(1):152–154; discussion 54–55.

Campbell FG, Graham JG, Zilkha KJ. Clinical trial of carbamazepine (Tegretol) in trigeminal neuralgia. *J Neurol Neurosurg Psychiatry* 1966;29(3):265–267.

Cappabianca P, Spaziante R, Graziussi G, et al. (1995) Percutaneous retrogasserian glycerol rhizolysis for treatment of trigeminal neuralgia. Technique and results in 191 patients. *J Neurosurg Sci* 1995;39(1):37–45.

Chavez GD, De Salles AA, Solberg TD, et al. Three-dimensional fast imaging employing steady-state acquisition magnetic resonance imaging for stereotactic radiosurgery of trigeminal neuralgia. *Neurosurgery* 2005;56(3):E628; discussion E28.

Coffey RJ. Deep brain stimulation for chronic pain: results of two multicenter trials and a structured review. *Pain Med* 2001;2(3):183–192.

Cole CD, Liu JK, Apfelbaum RI. Historical perspectives on the diagnosis and treatment of trigeminal neuralgia. *Neurosurg Focus* 2005;18(5):E4.

Cook BR, Jannetta PJ. Tic convulsif: results in 11 cases treated with microvascular decompression of the fifth and seventh cranial nerves. *J Neurosurg* 1984;61(5): 949–951.

Dandy W. Section of the sensory root of the trigeminal nerve at the pons: preliminary report of the operative procedure. *Bull Johns Hopkins Hosp* 1925;36:105–106.

———. Surgery of the brain. In *Lewis' practice of surgery*, vol. 12. Hagerstown, MD: W.F. Prior Co., 1932;1–671.

———. Concerning the cause of trigeminal neuralgia. *Am J Surg* 1934;24:447–455.

Fruhstorfer H, Hensel H. Thermal cutaneous afferents in the trigeminal nucleus of the cat. *Naturwissenschaften* 1973;60(4):209.

Gelber BR, Gogela LJ, Pierson EW. Posterior fossa partial trigeminal rhizotomy: an alternative to microvascular decompression. *Nebr Med J* 1989;74(5):105–108.

Goss BW, Frighetto L, DeSalles AA, et al. Linear accelerator radiosurgery using 90 gray for essential trigeminal neuralgia: results and dose volume histogram analysis. *Neurosurgery* 2003;53(4):823–828; discussion 28–30.

Haines SJ, Jannetta PJ, Zorub DS. Microvascular relations of the trigeminal nerve. An anatomical study with clinical correlation. *J Neurosurg* 1980;52(3):381–386.

Håkanson S. Trigeminal neuralgia treated by the injection of glycerol into the trigeminal cistern. *Neurosurgery*. 1981;9(6):638–646.

Hanraets PR. Trigeminal neuralgia; comparison of the various surgical methods to combat trigeminal neuralgia, especially, the Spiller Frazier and the Dandy method. *Folia Psychiatr Neurol Neurochir Neerl* 1954;57(4–5):382–404.

Hartel F. Uber die intracranialle injektions behandlung der trigeminus neuralgie. *Med Klin* 1914;10:582.

Heath R. Studies in schizophrenia: A multidisciplinary approach to mind-brain relationships. Cambridge, MA: Harvard University Press, 1954.

Henson CF, Goldman HW, Rosenwasser RH, et al. Glycerol rhizotomy versus gamma knife radiosurgery for the treatment of trigeminal neuralgia: an analysis of patients treated at one institution. *Int J Radiat Oncol Biol Phys* 2005;63(1):82–90.

Horsley V, TJ, Colman WS. Remarks on the various surgical procedures devised for the relief or cure of trigeminal neuralgia (tic douloureux). *BMJ* 1891;2:1139–1143, 91–93, 249–252.

Jannetta PJ. Arterial compression of the trigeminal nerve at the pons in patients with trigeminal neuralgia. *J Neurosurg* 1967;26(1 Suppl):159–162.

Jensen TS, Rasmussen P, Reske-Nielsen E. Association of trigeminal neuralgia with multiple sclerosis: clinical and pathological features. *Acta Neurol Scand* 1982;65(3):182–189.

Kirschner M. Zur Elektrichirurgie. *Arch Klin Chir* 1931;167:761–768.

Kondziolka D, Lacomis D, Niranjan A, et al. Histological effects of trigeminal nerve radiosurgery in a primate model: implications for trigeminal neuralgia radiosurgery. *Neurosurgery* 2000;46(4):971–976; discussion 76–77.

Kondziolka D, Lunsford LD, Flickinger JC, et al. Stereotactic radiosurgery for trigeminal neuralgia: a multiinstitutional study using the gamma unit. *J Neurosurg* 1996a;84(6):940–945.

Kondziolka D, Lunsford LD, Habeck M, Flickinger JC. Gamma knife radiosurgery for trigeminal neuralgia. *Neurosurg Clin N Am* 1997;8(1):79–85.

Kondziolka D, Somaza S, Comey C, et al. Radiosurgery and fractionated radiation therapy: comparison of different techniques in an in vivo rat glioma model. *J Neurosurg* 1996b;84(6):1033–1038.

Laghmari M, El Ouahabi A, Arkha Y, et al. Are the destructive neurosurgical techniques as effective as microvascular decompression in the management of trigeminal neuralgia? *Surg Neurol* 2007;68(5):505–512.

Leksell L. Stereotaxic radiosurgery in trigeminal neuralgia. *Acta Chir Scand* 1971; 137(4):311–314.
Letcher FS, Goldring S. The effect of radiofrequency current and heat on peripheral nerve action potential in the cat. *J Neurosurg* 1968;29(1):42–47.
Linderoth B, Håkanson S. Paroxysmal facial pain in disseminated sclerosis treated by retrogasserian glycerol injection. *Acta Neurol Scand* 1989;80(4):341–346.
Liu JK, Apfelbaum RI. Treatment of trigeminal neuralgia. *Neurosurg Clin N Am* 2004;15(3):319–334.
Lopez BC, Hamlyn PJ, Zakrzewska JM. Systematic review of ablative neurosurgical techniques for the treatment of trigeminal neuralgia. *Neurosurgery* 2004;54(4): 973–982;discussion 82–83.
Lunsford LD. Treatment of tic douloureux by percutaneous retrogasserian glycerol injection. *JAMA* 1982;248(4):449–453.
Lunsford LD, Bennett MH. Percutaneous retrogasserian glycerol rhizotomy for tic douloureux: Part 1. Technique and results in 112 patients. *Neurosurgery* 1984;14(4):424–430.
Mazars G, Merienne L, Cioloca C. Control of dyskinesias due to sensory deafferentation by means of thalamic stimulation. *Acta Neurochir Suppl (Wien)* 1980; 30:239–243.
Mullan S, Lichtor T. Percutaneous microcompression of the trigeminal ganglion for trigeminal neuralgia. *J Neurosurg* 1983;59(6):1007–1012.
Nugent GR. Technique and results of 800 percutaneous radiofrequency thermocoagulations for trigeminal neuralgia. *Appl Neurophysiol* 1982;45(4–5):504–507.
Nugent GR, Berry B. Trigeminal neuralgia treated by differential percutaneous radiofrequency coagulation of the Gasserian ganglion. *J Neurosurg* 1974;40(4): 517–523.
Peet MM, Schneider RC. Trigeminal neuralgia; a review of six hundred and eighty-nine cases with a follow-up study of sixty five per cent of the group. *J Neurosurg* 1952;9(4):367–377.
Petit JH, Herman JM, Nagda S, et al. Radiosurgical treatment of trigeminal neuralgia: evaluating quality of life and treatment outcomes. *Int J Radiat Oncol Biol Phys* 2003;56(4):1147–1153.
Pinkus RL. Innovation in neurosurgery: Walter Dandy in his day. *Neurosurgery* 1984;14(5):623–631.
Pollock BE, Ecker RD. A prospective cost-effectiveness study of trigeminal neuralgia surgery. *Clin J Pain* 2005;21(4):317–322.
Pollock BE, Phuong LK, Foote RL, et al. High-dose trigeminal neuralgia radiosurgery associated with increased risk of trigeminal nerve dysfunction. *Neurosurgery* 2001;49(1):58–62; discussion 62–64.
Pollock BE, Phuong LK, Gorman DA, et al. Stereotactic radiosurgery for idiopathic trigeminal neuralgia. *J Neurosurg* 2002;97(2):347–353.
Pool J, Clark W, Hudson P, Lombardo M. *Hypothalamus-hypophyseal Interrelationships*, ed. Springfield, IL: Charles C. Thomas, 1956.
Rasche D, Rinaldi PC, Young RF, Tronnier VM. Deep brain stimulation for the treatment of various chronic pain syndromes. *Neurosurg Focus* 2006;21(6):E8.
Rockliff BW, Davis EH. Controlled sequential trials of carbamazepine in trigeminal neuralgia. *Arch Neurol* 1966;15(2):129–136.
Rogers CL, Shetter AG, Fiedler JA, et al. Gamma knife radiosurgery for trigeminal neuralgia: the initial experience of The Barrow Neurological Institute. *Int J Radiat Oncol Biol Phys* 2000;47(4):1013–1019.
Sekula RF, Marchan EM, Fletcher LH, et al. Microvascular decompression for trigeminal neuralgia in elderly patients. *J Neurosurg* 2008;108(4):689–691.
Shelden CH, Pudenz RH, Freshwater DB, Crue BL. Compression rather than decompression for trigeminal neuralgia. *J Neurosurg* 1955;12(2):123–126.

Spiller W, Frazier C. The division of the sensory root of the trigeminus for relief of tic douloureux: an experimental pathological and clinical study with a preliminary report of one surgical successful case. *Phila Med J* 1901;8:1039–1049.

Sweet WH. The treatment of trigeminal neuralgia (tic douloureux). *N Engl J Med* 1986;315(3):174–177.

Sweet WH, Poletti CE, Macon JB. Treatment of trigeminal neuralgia and other facial pains by retrogasserian injection of glycerol. *Neurosurgery* 1981;9(6):647–653.

Sweet WH, Wepsic JG. Controlled thermocoagulation of trigeminal ganglion and rootlets for differential destruction of pain fibers. 1. Trigeminal neuralgia. *J Neurosurg* 1974;40(2):143–156.

Taha JM, Tew JM, Jr. Comparison of surgical treatments for trigeminal neuralgia: reevaluation of radiofrequency rhizotomy. *Neurosurgery* 1996;38(5):865–871.

———. Treatment of trigeminal neuralgia by percutaneous radiofrequency rhizotomy. *Neurosurg Clin N Am* 1997;8(1):31–39.

Taha JM, Tew JM, Jr., Buncher CR. A prospective 15-year follow up of 154 consecutive patients with trigeminal neuralgia treated by percutaneous stereotactic radiofrequency thermal rhizotomy. *J Neurosurg* 1995;83(6):989–993.

Tatli M, Satici O, Kanpolat Y, Sindou M. Various surgical modalities for trigeminal neuralgia: literature study of respective long-term outcomes. *Acta Neurochir (Wien)* 2008;150(3):243–255.

Tew JM, Jr. Percutaneous rhizotomy in the treatment of intractable facial pain (trigeminal, glossopharyngeal and vagal nerves). In H Schmidek, W Sweet, eds., *Operative neurosurgical techniques: Indications, methods and results*. Philadelphia: WB Saunders, 1996.

Tsubokawa T, Katayama Y, Yamamoto T, et al. Chronic motor cortex stimulation for the treatment of central pain. *Acta Neurochir Suppl (Wien)* 1991a;52:137–139.

———. Treatment of thalamic pain by chronic motor cortex stimulation. *Pacing Clin Electrophysiol* 1991b;14(1):131–134.

Velasco F, Arguelles C, Carrillo-Ruiz JD, et al. Efficacy of motor cortex stimulation in the treatment of neuropathic pain: a randomized double-blind trial. *J Neurosurg* 2008;108(4):698–706.

Villavicencio AT, Lim M, Burneikiene S, et al. Cyberknife radiosurgery for trigeminal neuralgia treatment: a preliminary multicenter experience. *Neurosurgery* 2008;62(3):647–655; discussion 47–55.

Young JN, Wilkins RH. Partial sensory trigeminal rhizotomy at the pons for trigeminal neuralgia. *J Neurosurg* 1993;79(5):680–687.

Young RF, Vermeulen SS, Grimm P, et al. Gamma Knife radiosurgery for treatment of trigeminal neuralgia: idiopathic and tumor related. *Neurology* 1997;48(3): 608–614.

Zakrzewska JM, Patsalos PN. Long-term cohort study comparing medical (oxcarbazepine) and surgical management of intractable trigeminal neuralgia. *Pain* 2002;95(3):259–266.

10

Percutaneous Stereotactic Rhizotomy

Andrew Grande, Chad Morgan, and John M. Tew, Jr.

The treatment of trigeminal neuralgia (TN) represents one of the most gratifying aspects of the practice of neurosurgery, as patients, originally transfixed by pain, can achieve substantial relief with little therapeutic sequelae. Of the three primary therapeutic options of microvascular decompression (MVD), percutaneous stereotactic rhizotomy (PSR), and radiosurgery, we focus on PSR of the gasserian ganglion and sensory root. In the treatment of our patients with TN, we strive to integrate the newest techniques, therapies, and devices with the historically successful neurosurgical options. Thus, we approach the treatment paradigm with a full complement of modalities that can best address the pathophysiological nuances, preferences, medical history, and needs of each patient.

Challenged to meet the rapid growth in the field, neurosurgeons face an ever-increasing push toward subspecialization. With this specialization, many young surgeons favor a particular modality in treating TN; for example, MVD may be preferred for its efficacy, or radiosurgery as a single-point treatment for many conditions. However, our experience dictates that inclusion of PSR in the neurosurgeon's armament of skills can better ensure effective treatment for all TN patients. To address its importance and how PSR fits into our practice, here we describe its crucial role in the comprehensive treatment paradigm. Finally, we provide case histories that highlight the importance of a tailored approach for patients with facial pain. For the most challenging cases, we discuss the surgeon's notes that lead to a specific treatment decisions.

PERCUTANEOUS STEREOTACTIC RHIZOTOMY TECHNIQUE

Preparation

One hour before the procedure, 0.4 mg of atropine is administered intramuscularly to reduce oral secretions and prevent bradycardia. In preparation for PSR, the patient lies supine on the radiographic table (Fig. 10.1).

Blood pressure and oxygen (O_2) saturation are monitored often during the procedure; we favor an external cuff rather than an arterial line. Several studies have reported paroxysmal hypertension during lesion generation (Kanpolat et al. 2001; Sweet, Poletti, & Roberts 1985) that in rare instances may be associated with intracerebral or subarachnoid hemorrhage (Sweet

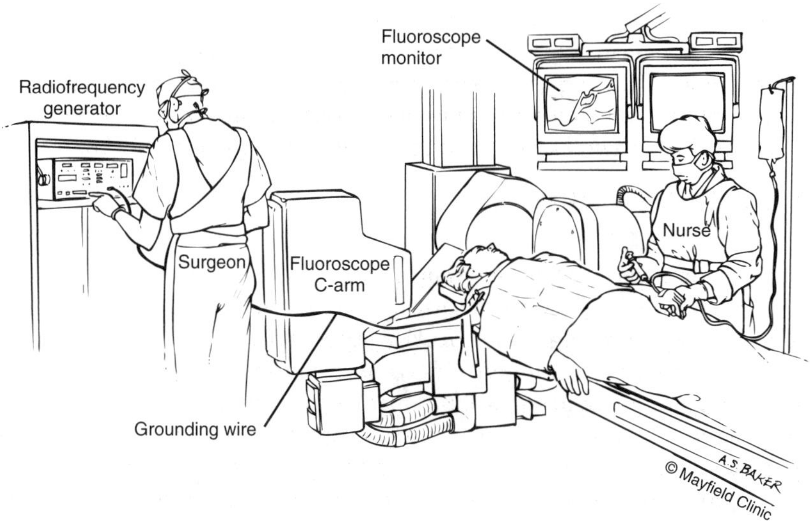

Figure 10.1 Equipment, personnel, and patient positioning for PSR in a fluoroscopic suite.

The surgeon stands on the patient's right side, regardless of pain location. Equipment positioning allows the surgeon to control the radiofrequency generator, view the fluoroscopy screen, and see the patient's face during stimulation. Opposite the surgeon, on the patient's left side, stands a well-trained nurse or anesthesiologist, who can administer anesthetic when needed, monitor blood pressure, and take notes on the lesion parameters. Reprinted with permission Mayfield Clinic.

et al. 1985). Appropriate levels of anesthetic prevent an unwanted rise in blood pressure. However, intravenous antihypertensive agents may occasionally be needed to control elevated pressures.

With the patient lying supine and the head positioned midline, three anatomical marks are made on the face to guide the cannula placement in the foramen ovale (Hartel 1914) (Fig. 10.2). The patient's face is prepped with ChloraPrep while avoiding contact with the eyes. Sterile towels cover the remainder of the neck and chest (Fig. 10.3). The ground pad is placed on the patient's right shoulder or arm.

Before beginning the procedure, a fluoroscopic x-ray should confirm the proper positioning of the patient. A *true lateral* image will clearly show the sella turcica, clivus, and petrous apex, and is confirmed by overlap of the orbital roofs and petrous bone.

Insertion of Cannula and Electrode

A 9-mm airway turned sideways or a bite block inserted into the patient's mouth on the opposite side, protects the surgeon's finger. Anesthesia includes a rapid intravenous injection of 30–50 mg of methohexital (Brevital)

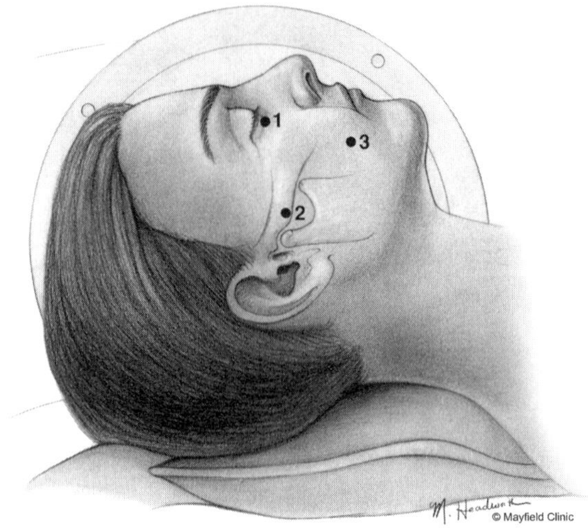

Figure 10.2 To guide the needle into the foramen ovale, the surgeon marks three points on the patient's face as follows: (1) beneath the medial aspect of the pupil on the lower lid, (2) 3 cm anterior to external auditory meatus, and (3) 2.5 cm lateral to the oral commissure.

Reprinted with permission Mayfield Clinic.

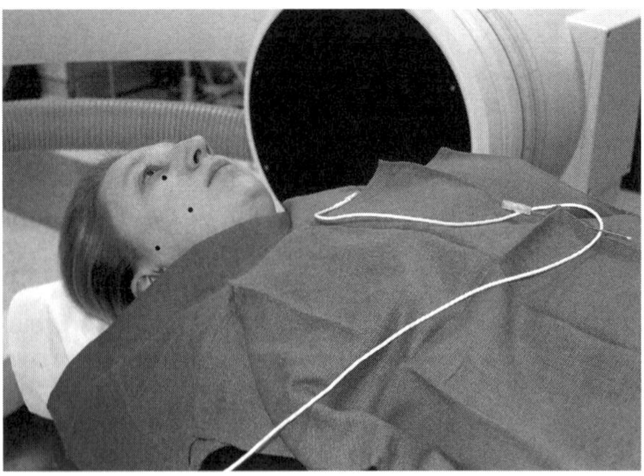

Figure 10.3 Photograph of the sterile field and correct head alignment for true lateral fluoroscopy.

A 20-gauge needle is threaded through the drape and holds the cable in place. Reprinted with permission Mayfield Clinic.

followed by a 10-cc saline flush. Nasal oxygen is administered if the patient's O_2 saturation decreases during sedation. The risk of airway obstruction can be overcome by manually elevating the chin. Preoperative steroids may be advisable for patients with asthma or emphysema, to reduce the risk of bronchial irritation and spasm, which may be aggravated by Brevital.

Understanding the importance of a patient being calm and able to give feedback on stimulus location, the surgeon carefully does not reveal the needle. Once the patient is fully asleep, the surgeon guides the cannula, avoiding mucosal penetration (Fig. 10.4A). The radiofrequency (RF) cannula, with its stylet in place, is inserted into the cheek 2.5 cm lateral to the oral commissure. The cannula is aimed toward the intersection of an axial plane, passing 3 cm anterior to the external auditory meatus, and a sagittal plane passing through the medial aspect of the pupil (Fig. 10.4B).

Intermittent lateral fluoroscopy tracks the advancement of the cannula toward the foramen ovale, which is located at the intersection of the petrous ridge and clivus below the sella turcica (Fig. 10.5). Positioning of the cannula is done with expectation that the RF electrode, when inserted into the cannula, will extend 5–10 mm beyond the cannula's tip. When cannulating the foramen ovale, we advocate either direct continuous or sequential palpation. In the latter case, the surgeon processes the cannula down

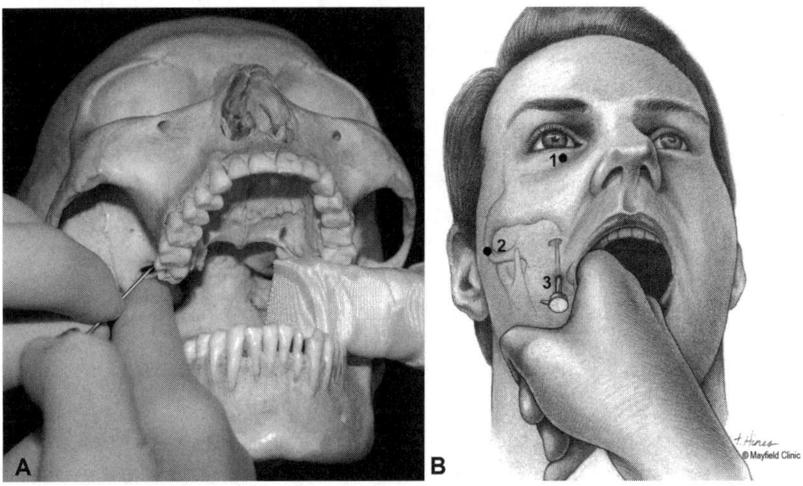

Figure 10.4 (A) Surgeon's gloved index finger resting along the side of the molars, against the lateral pterygoid, guides the cannula toward the foramen ovale, preventing penetration of the oral mucosa. (B) Cannula is inserted 2.5 cm lateral to the oral commissure (*point* 3), aimed at a point along the mid-papillary line (*point 1*) and at 3 cm anterior to the exterior auditory canal (*point* 2).

Reprinted with permission Mayfield Clinic.

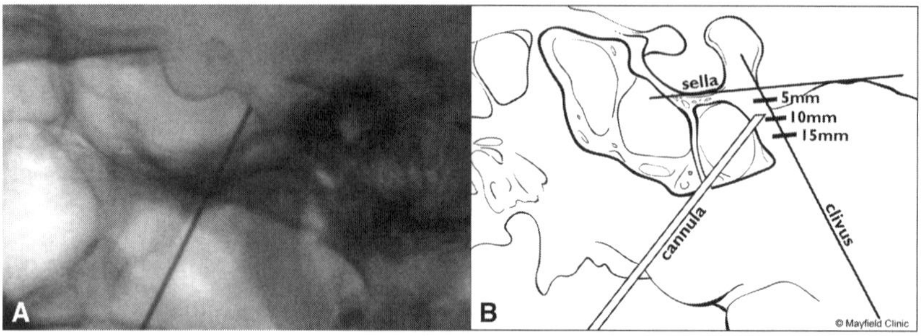

Figure 10.5 Lateral x-ray (A) and illustration (B) of the cannula inserted through the foramen ovale, with its tip intersecting the clivus at 5–15 mm below the floor of the sella.

Reprinted with permission Mayfield Clinic.

the smooth surface of the infratemporal fossa toward the superior-medial aspect of the foramen. Penetration of the medial aspect of the foramen ovale is ideal to best contact all of the trigeminal divisions. Lateral placement may elude the trigeminal cistern, thus missing contact with the maxillary or ophthalmic divisions. Reflex contraction of the jaw, caused by stimulation of the mandibular division of the motor root, signals successful entry into the foramen ovale.

Lateral fluoroscopy confirms accurate cannula positioning within the retrogasserian space. On fluoroscopy, the cannula should intersect the clivus about 5–15 mm below the sellar floor (Tew, Keller, & Williams 1978). Once positioning is confirmed, the stylet is removed from the cannula. If the cannula is within the trigeminal cistern, a flow of cerebrospinal fluid (CSF) occurs when the stylet is removed. However, previous surgical procedures or chemical injections may preclude the flow of CSF because adhesions have obliterated the subarachnoid space.

If satisfied with the position of the cannula and the flow of CSF, the surgeon removes the bite block and introduces the electrode into the cannula. The cable, connecting the electrode to the stimulator, should be connected to the electrode before its insertion. If connected after it is in the cannula, the electrode can vibrate within the trigeminal nerve root and elicit a trigeminal attack.

Electrode placement is confirmed with lateral fluoroscopy. The electrode depth determines which divisions of the trigeminal nerve are contacted. Characteristically, V_3 is contacted when the electrode is positioned 5 mm proximal to the clivus, V_2 when the electrode is positioned at the level of the clivus, and V_1 when the electrode is positioned 5 mm distal to the clivus (Fig. 10.6). In general, the needle should not extend beyond 10 mm of the clivus because of potential risk of cranial nerve (CN) IV or VI injury. The tip of a curved electrode can be reoriented to assist further in isolating a specific

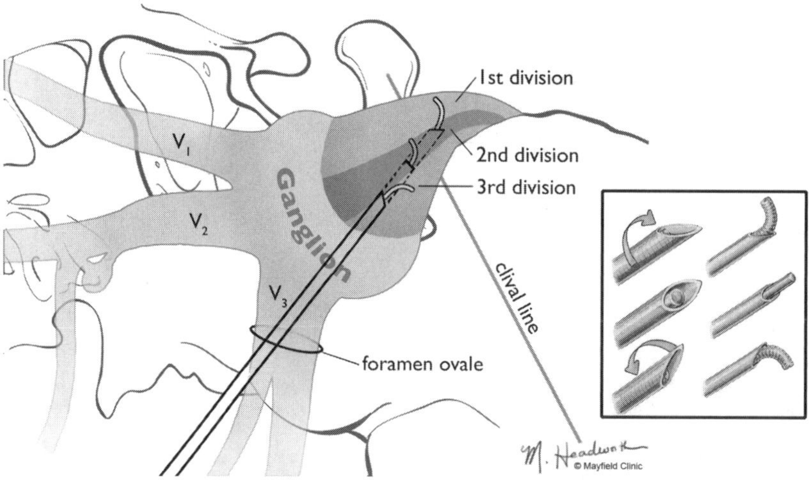

Figure 10.6 A curved electrode can be manipulated to target different regions of the trigeminal ganglion.

Depth is varied to target V_1 (5 mm beyond the clivus), V_2 (at the level of the clivus), or V_3 (5 mm before the clivus). Reprinted with permission Mayfield Clinic.

division of the trigeminal nerve. Before rotating a curved electrode, the surgeon should first retract it into the cannula to avoid damaging either the electrode tip or a portion of the trigeminal ganglion. Once correctly positioned, a small clamp at skin level holds the cannula in place, preventing its further advancement into the trigeminal ganglion (Fig. 10.7).

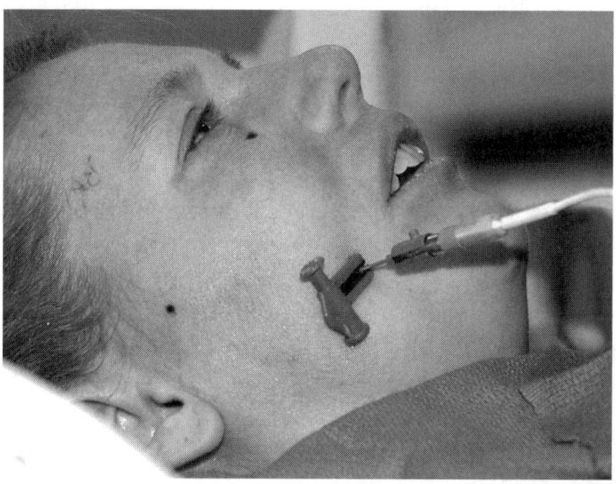

Figure 10.7 Small clamp around the cannula at skin level stabilizes its position.

Reprinted with permission Mayfield Clinic.

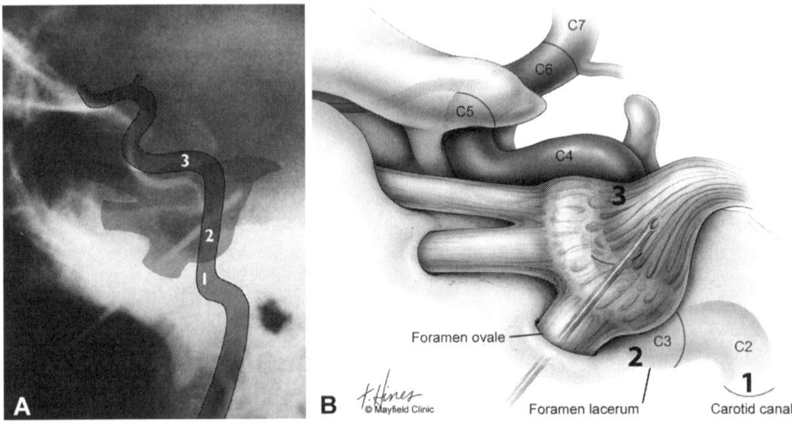

Figure 10.8 Lateral x-ray (A) and illustration (B) depict three danger points to the internal carotid artery (ICA) from cannula trajectory.

When targeting the foramen ovale, a trajectory angle either too posterior (1) can puncture the C2 portion of the carotid as it enters the petrous bone and too lateral and posterior (2) can puncture the C3 portion of the carotid where it lies within the foramen lacerum covered by a thin shell of bone. After penetration of foramen ovale, a trajectory too medial and anterior (3) can puncture the C4 segment in the cavernous sinus. Reprinted with permission Mayfield Clinic.

During cannulation of the foramen ovale, complications can and do occur. Therefore, the surgeon must completely understand the relationship between the retrogasserian ganglion, foramen ovale, and surrounding structures. Ischemic complications and carotid cavernous fistula have resulted from puncture of the internal carotid artery (ICA) (Rish 1976). During foramen ovale cannulation, the ICA is vulnerable in three locations, specifically, the C2–C4 segments (Fig. 10.8). Pulsatile blood from the cannula or rhythmic fluctuations in the temperature monitor indicates penetration of a significant vascular structure. If this happens, the cannula is removed, manual pressure is applied over the posterior pharyngeal space, and the procedure is discontinued until a later date,

Other structures can be encountered during cannula placement (Fig. 10.9). There are also aberrant foramina, which can be entered, such as the foramen of Vesalius medial to the foramen ovale, and the innominate canal of Arnold posterior to the foramen ovale. Entrance into either of these can penetrate the carotid artery and venous channels. Venous bleeding may occur and may require compression to avoid swelling.

Electrical Stimulation

Physiologic localization by electrical stimulation is the most reliable and precise method for accurate electrode-tip placement in the desired

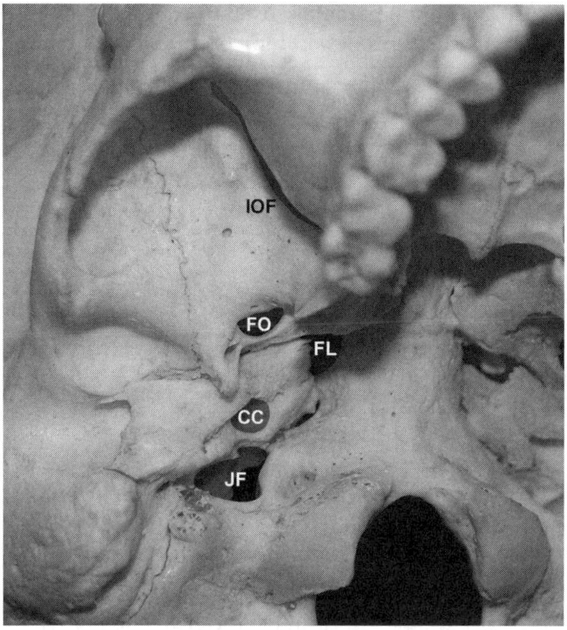

Figure 10.9 Skull base foramina can be punctured with a cannula when targeting the foramen ovale.

Inferior orbital fissure (IOF) can be hit by a cannula aimed too anterior and superior to the foramen ovale (FO). Jugular foramen (JF) can be hit by a cannula aimed too posterior and inferior. Internal carotid artery can be hit at the foramen lacerum (FL) or the carotid canal (CC). Reprinted with permission Mayfield Clinic.

division of the trigeminal root. First, stimulation precisely reproduces the patient's trigeminal pain pattern, thus confirming electrode contact with the targeted trigeminal fibers. Second, stimulation determines the intensity threshold required to simulate the facial pain; this provides insight into the duration and temperature required to generate an effective sensory lesion.

When the electrode is positioned in the trigeminal root, the patient is then awakened. Patient feedback is essential for this portion of the procedure. Starting stimulation settings are 0 volts (v) with 50 pulses/sec for 1 ms duration (Cosman Radiofrequency Generator); however, settings may vary based on stimulator. Stimulation voltage is gradually increased until the patient experiences paresthesias in the same general pattern of the TN. Typically, the 0.1–0.4 v required to reproduce the pain pattern is incrementally increased, repeating the stimulation voltage until the patient's pain pattern is reproduced. This threshold voltage is then translated into a temperature and duration for the initial lesion (Table 10.1). However, if 1.0 v is

Table 10.1 Cincinnati paradigm used to convert threshold stimulus into lesion temperature and duration

Stimulation intensity (volts)	Electrode temperature (°C)	Duration of lesion (seconds)
<0.1	60	60
0.2–0.3	65	60
0.3–0.4	70	60
0.5–0.6	75	60
0.7–0.8	80	60
>1.0	No lesion; reposition the electrode	

Reproduced with permission Mayfield Clinic.

reached without eliciting the typical pain pattern, stimulation is discontinued and the cannula repositioned.

During stimulation, the surgeon watches for any signs of unwanted CN stimulation, specifically CN III, IV, VI, or VII. Eye movement during stimulation indicates that the cannula is too near the nerves in the cavernous sinus. Facial contractions indicate that the cannula placement is either too deep or inclined too low on the clivus, or that the stimulation level is too high. Masseter contraction indicates that the cannula is too close to the motor division of CN V. If any of these signs occur, the cannula must be repositioned.

Because patient cooperation is so important at this step during the procedure, it is essential that the patient remains calm and not in pain. If a patient becomes very emotional or cannot comply, observation of the response to stimulation is often reliable.

Making the Radiofrequency Heat Lesion

Studies have shown a direct correlation between the degree of facial sensory deficit and the duration of trigeminal pain relief with PSR (Broggi et al. 1990; Kanpolat et al. 2001; Taha, Tew, & Buncher 1995), glycerol rhizolysis (Burchiel 1988; Ischia, Luzzani, & Polati 1990; Pickett, Bisnaire, & Ferguson 2005), and radiosurgery (Tawk et al. 2005). However, greater sensory deficits also lead to a higher incidence of complaints (e.g., problems eating) and dysesthesia. Our approach with PSR treatment, given that it can be repeated easily with minimal morbidity, is to create a lesion with moderate hypalgesia.

During lesion creation, the patient is put back to sleep with a minimal amount of intravenous methohexital (Brevital); importantly, the patient is awakened after the lesion is made to test its effectiveness. As most patients do not need additional sedation, sensory testing can be performed continuously during the lesioning process, allowing for precise titration of sensory loss.

The use of the parameters in Table 10.1 helps to determine the lesion temperature and duration, based on the patient's stimulus threshold. Exceptions to this paradigm include patients with a history of multiple sclerosis (MS), a low stimulus threshold, or previous RF ablation or MVD. In these exceptions, the lesions develop quickly, and a tendency exists to overshoot the intended sensory deficit. Consequently, for these patients, we recommend light or no anesthesia, if possible, to allow for continuous sensory testing and an initial 30-sec lesion duration.

Facial flush, secondary to antidromic release of vasodilatory neuropeptides (e.g., substance P, calcitonin gene-related peptide), is common during the lesioning process in the trigeminal division during RF ablation (Goadsby, Edvinsson, & Ekman 1988; Gonzalez, Onofrio, & Kerr 1975; Tran Dinh et al. 1992). This flush is not a concern, but rather signals that the correct trigeminal division is being targeted.

After the initial lesion, with the patient is fully awakened, sensory testing of the face is conducted to assess numbness. Testing follows a standard regimen, which includes both verbal feedback from the patient and observation by the surgeon. We begin by testing gross pinprick sensation in all three divisions on both sides of the face, marching a pin toward and then across midline. If a difference is noted between left and right sides, the patient rates on a 10-point scale the extent of numbness. We then test for the presence of analgesia by comparing pinprick to light touch. Because of overlap among the sensory distributions of the trigeminal nerve, a keen knowledge of the autonomous areas of sensory innervation is fundamental for proper sensory assessment (Fig. 10.10).

If the first lesion produced does not achieve the desired numbness, subsequent lesions can be made. In general, for each subsequent lesion, the surgeon increases the lesion temperature by 5° C. No additional intravenous anesthesia is administered. While the lesion is being made, the surgeon assesses the patient's response to pinprick in all trigeminal divisions.

When the desired numbness is reached, the surgeon observes the patient for an additional 15 minutes to ensure a fixed lesion, and then repeats the battery of sensory tests. As CN function may be affected, we specifically test the masseter, pterygoid, temporal, facial, and ocular muscles, as well as corneal reflex.

Postoperative Care

After the procedure, the patient is observed for at least 2 hours in an ambulatory surgery room. Postoperative care includes meticulous eye care and artificial tears if corneal sensation has been altered, and a temporary soft diet if oral sensation and/or motor function have been impaired. We recommend acetaminophen (Tylenol), if headache develops, which is common.

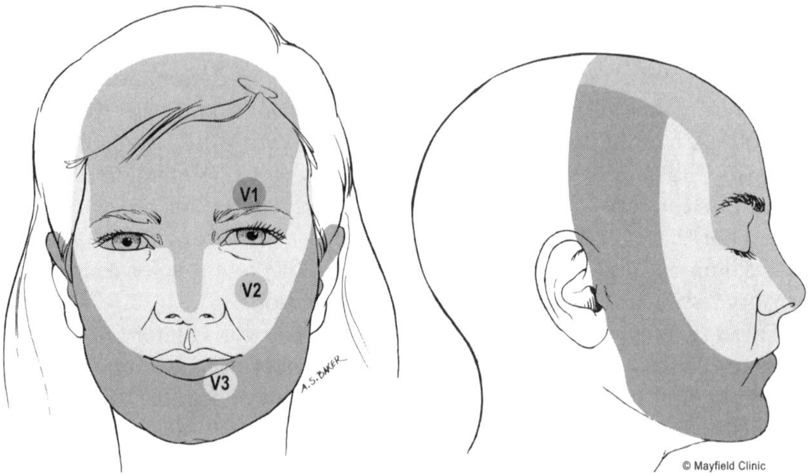

Figure 10.10 Dermatome distribution of the three divisions of the trigeminal nerve: ophthalmic division (V_1 = green), maxillary division (V_2 = blue), and mandibular division (V_3 = orange). Sensory testing by pinprick should begin in autonomous areas (slightly darker colored areas) where less innervation overlap occurs between divisions.

Reprinted with permission Mayfield Clinic.

After recovery from anesthesia, the patient is discharged with specific orders. Tapering of anticonvulsant medications begins on discharge and is completed by 1–2 weeks after surgery.

RESULTS AND COMPLICATIONS

Results

Of more than 3,000 patients with TN treated by PSR, we used a straight electrode in the initial 700 patients and a curved-tip electrode in the remaining. In our review of the first 1,200 patients, excellent or good results were reported in 93% at follow-up (mean 9 years, range 1–21 years) (Tobler et al. 1983). Of these 1,200 patients, 35% had undergone a previous operation (e.g., nerve avulsion, alcohol injection, PSR); in the 4% with MS, an 18% rate of bilateral involvement occurred. In our prospective study of 154 patients followed for 15 years, 95% achieved good or excellent pain relief (Taha et al. 1995).

Recurrence

In our prospective review, the recurrence rate at 15 years was 25% (Kaplan-Meier analysis) (Taha et al. 1995). Recurrence was 15% at 5 years, 7% at

Table 10.2 Inverse relationship between degree of sensory loss and pain recurrence

Outcome	Mild hypalgesia	Major hypalgesia	Complete analgesia
Median pain-free survival	<3 years	>15 years	>15 years
Recurrence	60%	25%	20%
Troublesome numbness	7% (lowest rate)	**15% (optimal rate)**	36% (worse rate)

Reproduced with permission Mayfield Clinic.

5–10 years, and 3% at 10–15 years. Recurrence was directly related to the degree of sensory loss. Specifically, recurrence affected 60% of patients with mild hypalgesia, 25% with dense hypalgesia, and 20% with analgesia. This inverse relationship between the degree of sensory loss and pain recurrence substantiates the need for a treatment endpoint of moderate hypalgesia (Table 10.2).

Side Effects

For our 3% of patients with corneal analgesia, 20% developed neurogenic keratitis, which highlights the importance of prophylactic eye care (Taha & Tew 1996). Transient (<4 months) diplopia that occurred in 1% of total patients was usually attributed to nerve injury, typically the abducens, and secondarily the trochlear or oculomotor, and this resolved spontaneously. Motor weakness (muscles innervated by the trigeminal nerve) occurred in 16% and resolved over time. The 3% rate of herpes simplex lesions that developed along the trigeminal cutaneous distribution (Blomstedt & Bergenheim 2002) may be low—most patients were not examined more than 48 hours after surgery and perhaps did not report this.

In our experience, use of a curved electrode and the surgeon's expertise are associated with marked reduction in all CN side effects associated with heating and positioning. However, some surgeons prefer a straight electrode. Therefore, in interpreting the success rates and complications associated with PSR, it is important to identify the type of electrode used, curved or straight.

Case Illustrations

In treating TN, our treatment protocol is guided principally by patient age and by presentation as new or recurrent. Yet many patients do not fit a typical model. The following atypical cases illustrate the nuances in selection of treatment, whether PSR or another, for this devastating disorder.

Case 1: Treatment of Trigeminal Neuralgia in Young, Healthy Patients

A 35-year-old otherwise healthy mother with a 4-year history of TN experienced pain triggered by eating, brushing teeth, and wind; she wore a scarf outside to block wind. Despite antiepileptic medications, her symptoms became more frequent and severe, making it difficult to care for her two young children.

Outcome: After MVD, her trigeminal pain resolved immediately, with normal facial sensation and intact hearing. Postoperatively, she developed a severe headache for some days and incisional pain, which improved after a short course of steroids and analgesics, respectively.

Surgeon's Notes

- *Treatment decision.* MVD is generally the treatment of choice in otherwise young, healthy patients because of its low recurrence rate (2% per year in the first 5 years, 1% per year after 10 years [Barker et al. 1996]) and a long life expectancy. As MVD is often associated with higher rates of complications for the elderly, patients older than 70 years are best treated with a percutaneous method or radiosurgery.
- *Prevention of incisional pain.* The incision type can affect postoperative incisional pain. In comparison with a traditional vertical, linear incision (Fig. 10.11A), an oblique, crescent-shaped incision (Fig. 10.11B) avoids most of the nerve innervations of the posterior neck and occiput, causes less muscle dissection.
- One or two doses of dexamethasone (Decadron) immediately after surgery nearly eliminates the persistent, severe headaches that patients may develop.

Case 2: Trigeminal Neuralgia in Patients with Multiple Comorbidities

A 60-year-old Vietnam veteran had a 3-year history of TN. He had other medical problems including colon cancer, congestive heart failure, previous myocardial infarction, hypertension, and diabetes. Pain was located mainly in the right V_2 with some involvement of V_1. After management with carbamazepine (Tegretol) and pregabalin (Lyrica), the patient had a severe, acute exacerbation that required hospitalization. With significant comorbidities, he was not a good candidate to undergo MVD, and would be better treated by a percutaneous treatment or radiotherapy.

Outcome: On admission, the patient received a morphine pump. After PSR on day 2, he had immediate pain relief, required no narcotics, and was discharged. Tegretol and Lyrica were tapered during the next 2 weeks.

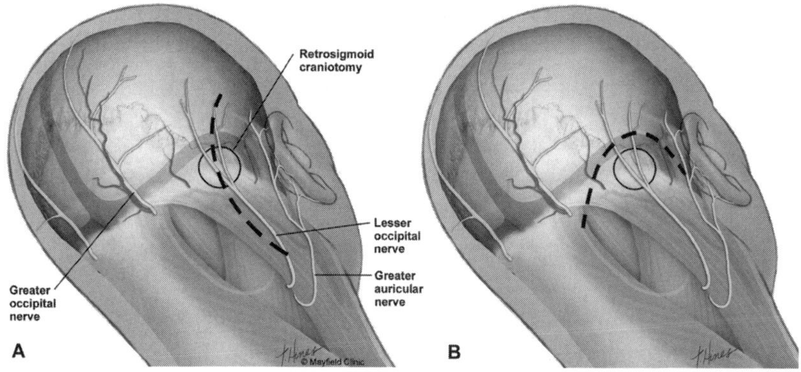

Figure 10.11 Postoperative headache following MVD can be caused by damage to the occipital nerves during skin incision and muscle retraction. Complete cutting of the nerve branches causes numbness of the posterior scalp. Conversely, partial injury or entrapment of the nerves from instruments and muscle retraction can cause neuroma formation, leading to headache pain. (A) The traditional straight skin incision for the retrosigmoid approach causes greater disruption to the lesser occipital nerve deep in the neck muscles. In addition, dissection of the muscles deep in the neck may lead to significant and protracted neck muscle pain. (B) The alternative high-arching curved skin incision crosses the nerve branches peripherally and avoids deep dissection of the neck muscles. This type of skin incision is less likely to cause postoperative headache.

Reprinted with permission Mayfield Clinic.

Surgeon's Notes

- *Treatment decision.* Radiotherapy is ineffective during acute exacerbation because its therapeutic effect requires from 3 weeks to 2 months (Brisman et al. 2002; Kondziolka et al. 1998; Kondziolka, Lunsford, & Flickinger 2002; Longhi et al. 2007; Pollock et al. 2000, 2001, 2002, 2005; Richards et al. 2005; Sheehan et al. 2005; Young, Vermulen, & Posewitz 1998). Balloon compression under general anesthesia was not considered because of the medical comorbidities. Thus, PSR offered a better long-term outcome than glycerol injection.

Case 3: Patients on Anticoagulants

A 64-year-old farmer with a history of left-sided V_3 TN underwent a balloon compression that resolved his pain. After a second balloon compression for recurrence 4 years later, he developed transient slurred speech, facial droop, and a severe worsening of his trigeminal pain. Management decisions were complicated; 30% of the pain was an atypical, dull, persistent pain. In addition to the severe exacerbation of pain, the patient had a recent transient ischemic attack. Anticoagulation therapy for a newly placed coronary stent had been discontinued 1 week earlier in anticipation of another balloon compression.

Outcome: After this patient underwent a PSR the same day, both the typical and atypical trigeminal pain completely resolved. He resumed his aspirin regimen the next day and clopidogrel (Plavix) 5 days later.

Surgeon's notes

- *Treatment decision.* With his medical history, neither MVD nor balloon compression was suitable for the acute pain, because both require anesthesia. Radiosurgery was not an option because of the acute nature of his pain. Thus, PSR was selected because of its superior long-term effects over glycerol injection and effectiveness for atypical pain.
- *Managing anticoagulation.* Anticoagulant or antiplatelet therapy must be discontinued 1 week before PSR. International normalized ratio (INR) and clotting studies are performed the day of the procedure to ensure that complete reversal has been achieved. After PSR, aspirin is resumed immediately and antiplatelet therapy 2 days later. For patients on Coumadin, a heparin drip is started 2 days after operation, with full anticoagulation resumed after 7 days.

Case 4: Trigeminal Neuralgia after a Failed MVD

A 62-year-old woman with right-sided V_2 and V_3 TN underwent an MVD when medications became ineffective; however, pain recurred 14 months later. Based on the operative report from that institution, venous compression was treated by mobilizing these vessels from the nerve, which was then cushioned by Teflon felt. The patient presented to us in severe pain from recurrent TN.

Outcome: She underwent a PSR as an outpatient procedure, experienced immediate relief of pain, and has remained symptom-free since.

Surgeon's Notes

- *Treatment decision.* When MVD has failed, our practice, irrespective of the patient's age, is to then treat with PSR. Consistent with the 40%–90% negative re-exploration rate reported in the literature (Bederson & Wislon 1989; Cho et al. 1994; Rath, Klein, & Richter 1996), we rarely perform re-exploration. After a repeat MVD, most patients had higher rates of complications and lower rates of initial success. Our findings are consistent with Barker et al. (1996), who reported higher rates of CN complications and

Rath et al. (1996), who reported twice the complication rate in repeat MVD procedures. In comparison with initial successes of 60%–85% after repeat MVD (Barker et al. 1996; Bederson and Wilson 1989; Cho et al. 1994), 98% of our patients had immediate pain relief after PSR, with 20% recurrence at 10 years.

- *Isolated venous compression.* With the risk of recurrence from isolated venous compression, our practice is to coagulate and cut these vessels, and then pad above and below the trigeminal nerve with a Teflon sponge (Barker et al. 1996; Hamlyn & King 1992; Klun 1992; Sun et al. 1994). If no compression is present and MVD has failed, we perform a partial sensory rhizotomy or a PSR the following day.

Case 5: Treatment after Failed Radiosurgery

A 56-year-old artist had TN involving V_1 and V_2 for many years. After initial treatment with medications, she sought different options because of side effects. Pain relief lasted for several months after radiosurgery. Two years later, she consulted with us because of a severe recurrence.

Outcome: The patient underwent a PSR. When the stimulus to reproduce her pain pattern was low (0.2 v), we used a low temperature (60° C) for a short duration (45 sec). She had immediate and continued pain relief.

Surgeon's Notes

- *Treatment decision.* Standard therapies after failed radiosurgery were MVD and PSR, and now repeat radiotherapy at some centers (Hasegawa et al. 2002; Herman et al. 2004; Pollock et al. 2001; Sheehan et al. 2005; Shetter et al. 2002). However, after a failed radiosurgery, we prefer, depending on the patient's age, either MVD or PSR. Repeat radiosurgery may be a poor option because the rates of facial sensory complaints are 32%–76% higher than after the initial radiosurgery (Hasegawa et al. 2002; Pollack et al. 2000). Recurrence after a repeat radiosurgery is up to 50% higher (Hasegawa et al. 2002; Herman et al. 2004; Pollack et al. 2000) occurring in one-quarter to one-third cases (Hasegawa et al. 2002; Pollack et al. 2000), and results in a higher incidence of ageusia (Nicol et al. 2000), reduced or absent corneal reflex (Matsuda et al. 2002), and injury to adjacent vasculature (Maher & Pollock 2000).

Case 6: Trigeminal neuralgia with Multiple Sclerosis

A 37-year-old woman had a 5-year history of TN and a history of MS. When symptoms worsened significantly, additional antiepileptics and higher doses made her feel drowsy and forgetful; caring for her children became more difficult.

Outcome: This patient underwent a PSR. Because lesions develop at lower temperatures and more quickly in MS, we were careful not to overshoot our sensory goal. A low temperature (60° C) for 50 seconds is used and sensory testing is performed during the lesioning process.

Surgeon's Notes

- *Treatment decision.* We treat patients with MS, regardless of age, with PSR. Kanpolat et al. (2000) reported initial pain control rates of 94.1% after PSR in MS patients. Although 29.4% of patients developed recurrences recurred over 25 months, PSR was easily repeated, with minimal complications; specifically, 82.4% achieved pain relief without medications, and 17.6% had pain relief with medication at 5 years.
- In comparison, initial failure rates after glycerol rhizotomy are as high as 25%, and only 59% of patients had long-term pain relief without medications (mean 36 months) (Kondziolka, Lunsford, & Bissonette 1994). In MS patients, MVD and radiosurgery are also associated with worse long-term pain relief: recurrence rates are as high as 15.3% (mean 13.5 months) (Broggi et al. 1999, 2000), with no pain relief in 40% (mean 24 months) after MVD, and as high as 41% (mean 17 months) after radiosurgery (Rogers et al. 2002).
- *Lesion production in patients with MS.* As the lesion develops more quickly in MS patients than in typical patients, a short-lesion period (about 30 sec) and sensory function testing during the lesioning process are imperative.
- *Considerations for bilateral disease.* About 20% of MS patients with TN have bilateral disease. In these cases, PSR is used to treat each side at separate times, especially when V_3 is involved bilaterally because bilateral V_3 sensory loss impairs eating.

Case 7: Treatment of Trigeminal Neuralgia in Patients with V_1 Involvement

A 45-year-old executive suffered an acute attack of TN isolated to the supraorbital branch of V_1; it was first treated by adding other antiepileptics to his normal long-term regimen of antiepileptic medications. When medications failed to provide relief, he sought a surgical treatment that would also enable him to attend an important business meeting later that week, without indications of having undergone an operation.

Outcome: In an outpatient setting, the patient underwent a supraorbital neurectomy via an eyebrow incision. The pain resolved immediately. He attended his meeting with no visible detriment to his appearance, and remains pain free 8 years later.

Surgeon's Notes

- *Treatment decision.* When treating V_1 pain, preservation of some sensory function is imperative to maintain the corneal reflex. In the absence of sensory function, neurogenic keratitis can affect up to 20% of patients with V_1 analgesia (Taha & Tew 1996). Although MVD is the treatment of choice in those more than 70 years old, 1% may lose facial sensation (Barker et al. 1996). We typically reserve a supraorbital neurectomy for patients older than 70 years and those with multiple comorbidities. However, it was ideal for our patient because it is an outpatient procedure with minimal morbidity.
- *Treatment paradigm for isolated V_1 pain.* Our treatment paradigm for isolated V_1 pain is based on patient age. Radiosurgery or balloon compression may be a poor alternative in patients younger than 70 years because of the incidence of facial dysesthesias or numbness, 8%–37% (Brisman 2004; Kondziolka et al. 2002; Pollack et al. 2005; Richards et al. 2005; Sheehan et al. 2005; Smith at al. 2003) and 17% (Brown & Pilitsis 2005), respectively, and the high rate of recurrence. Microvascular decompression is used in patients younger than 70 years, and radiosurgery or balloon compression is used in those older than 70 years or with multiple comorbidities. Our protocol generally recommends neurectomy in patients older than 70 years or PSR in those younger than 70 years with significant comorbidities.
- *Technique for supraorbital and infraorbital neurectomy.* We use local intravenous drugs for anesthesia. An eyebrow approach is used for supraorbital neurectomies, and a sublabial approach for infraorbital neurectomies.
- *Supra- and infraorbital approaches.* Standard dissection techniques are used to approach the respective foramina. Once the nerve is identified, we firmly grasp the nerve as close as possible to the foramen with a fine curved hemostat. The nerve is twisted by spinning the hemostat to avulse it for a maximal distance.
- *Closure.* The supraorbital approach is closed primarily with interrupted dermal sutures, followed by a running subcuticular stitch. The infraorbital approach is loosely closed with interrupted catgut sutures (usually one or two stitches).

Case 8: Modification of Infraorbital Neurectomy for Iatrogenic V_1 Neuralgia

A 65-year-old man had undergone operative resection of a basal cell carcinoma of the face 6 years earlier; a prosthesis was used to reconstruct the extensive erosion of the facial bone. Postoperatively, the patient developed sharp, lancinating pain in the distribution of the infraorbital nerve that was triggered by light facial touch.

Outcome: Because of the prosthesis, this patient underwent an infraorbital neurectomy by a direct percutaneous approach to the infraorbital foramen, rather than a sublabial approach. He tolerated the procedure well and had immediate postoperative pain relief.

Surgeon's Notes

- *Treatment decision.* Infraorbital nerve entrapment neuropathy is clinically similar to TN. Microvascular decompression and radiosurgery are ineffective treatments for this entrapment neuropathy because these treat proximal disease pathology. Infraorbital nerve entrapment must be treated locally with either a neurectomy or nerve injection (glycerol or alcohol). In our experience, recurrence develops more quickly after injection than after neurectomy.

Case 9: Bilateral Trigeminal Neuralgia

An 82-year-old woman with a long history of bilateral TN was first treated by PSR 14 years earlier and then again 6 months earlier for a recurrence in the left V_{1-2} distributions. When pain quickly recurred, the patient presented to us with severe left V_{1-2} pain and moderate right V_3 pain. Clinically, the patient was hypalgesic in the left V_1 with a diminished corneal reflex.

Outcome: The patient underwent a left MVD, which was well tolerated, followed by a PSR immediately for the right V_3 pain.

Surgeon's Notes

- *Treatment decision.* Patient age, involvement of the left V_1 distribution, and impaired corneal reflex on the left side were considerations in determining which treatment could best preserve the remaining sensation in this distribution. Neurectomy would be ideal for pain isolated to V_1, but not for V_2 involvement. Radiosurgery, although an option for left V_1 pain, was not effective for the acute exacerbation that necessitated immediate pain relief. Given the patient's diminished corneal reflex, PSR was not an option because it would cause further sensory loss in this distribution. Microvascular decompression was her best option, despite her age. After successful left-sided MVD was performed, a right-sided PSR was performed to relieve pain in the contralateral V_3 division.

Case 10: Trigeminal Neuralgia with V_3 Involvement

A 60-year-old opera singer had TN for 6 years that predominantly affected V_3 and somewhat V_2. She also had a history of hypertension, diabetes, and coronary artery disease. Trigeminal neuralgia symptoms that initially occurred several times monthly worsened—the patient had trouble brushing her teeth, kissing her husband, and singing. Being able to eat only soft foods, she had lost 40 pounds in 2 months.

Outcome: Following MVD, she had no loss of facial sensation and eventually resumed her singing career free of pain.

Surgeon's Notes

- *Treatment decision.* Although this patient had a number of comorbidities, as an opera singer she wanted a procedure with no risk of facial sensation loss. As any hypalgesia in V_3 would significantly affect her professionally, no percutaneous techniques or radiosurgery techniques were an option. She opted to undergo an MVD, despite her increased risk for postoperative complications.

Case 11: Treatment of Bilateral V_3 Trigeminal Pain

A 51-year-old woman with MS had a 6-year history of bilateral TN affecting V_3. After bilateral PSR procedures, she was pain free but hypalgesic in both V_3 distributions, had slight weakness in the masseter and pterygoid muscles on the left, but had no difficulty eating. Three years after these treatments, she consulted with us when pain recurred in the left V_3 distribution.

Outcome: The patient underwent a repeat PSR on the left side. With close monitoring of facial sensation while aiming to generate a focal lesion, we were very careful to not overshoot our intended lesion size because of her existing left masseter and pterygoid weakness. Left masseter and pterygoid motor weakness was unchanged postoperatively, and she was pain free.

Surgeon's Notes

- *Treatment decision.* As both V_3 sensation and muscle innervation are essential for eating, patients can tolerate some unilateral weakness and hypalgesia but not bilateral loss. Bilateral sensory loss interferes with sensing food and chewing. Treatment of bilateral V_3 disease is performed on separate days to carefully avoid causing analgesia and muscle weakness.

CONCLUSION

Trigeminal neuralgia is an extremely painful condition that debilitates those afflicted with the disease. Successfully treating patients who suffer from intractable TN is one of the most rewarding aspects of our experience as neurosurgeons. As can be ascertained from the illustrative cases, presentation and treatment results vary. Therefore, all surgeons should have the ability and experience of successful treatment with a variety of procedures. No single procedure or medication offers a satisfactory remedy for this disease, which has caused great pain for many.

REFERENCES

Barker FG, 2nd, Jannetta PJ, Bissonette DJ, et al. The long-term outcome of microvascular decompression for trigeminal neuralgia. *N Engl J Med* 1996;334: 1077–1083.

Bederson JB, Wilson CB. Evaluation of microvascular decompression and partial sensory rhizotomy in 252 cases of trigeminal neuralgia. *J Neurosurg* 1989;71: 359–367.

Blomstedt PC, Bergenheim AT. Technical difficulties and perioperative complications of retrogasserian glycerol rhizotomy for trigeminal neuralgia. *Stereotact Funct Neurosurg* 2002;79:168–181.

Brisman R. Gamma knife surgery with a dose of 75 to 76.8 Gray for trigeminal neuralgia. *J Neurosurg* 2004;100:848–854.

Brisman R, Khandji AG, Mooij RB. Trigeminal nerve-blood vessel relationship as revealed by high-resolution magnetic resonance imaging and its effect on pain relief after gamma knife radiosurgery for trigeminal neuralgia. *Neurosurgery* 2002;50:1261–1267.

Broggi G, Ferroli P, Franzini A, et al. Role of microvascular decompression in trigeminal neuralgia and multiple sclerosis. *Lancet* 1999;354:1878–1879.

Broggi G, Ferroli P, Franzini A, et al. Microvascular decompression for trigeminal neuralgia: comments on a series of 250 cases, including 10 patients with multiple sclerosis. *J Neurol Neurosurg Psychiatry* 2000;68:59–64.

Broggi G, Franzini A, Lasio G, et al. Long-term results of percutaneous retrogasserian thermorhizotomy for "essential" trigeminal neuralgia: considerations in 1000 consecutive patients. *Neurosurgery* 1990;26:783–787.

Brown JA, Pilitsis JG. Percutaneous balloon compression for the treatment of trigeminal neuralgia: results in 56 patients based on balloon compression pressure monitoring. *Neurosurg Focus* 2005;18:E10.

Burchiel KJ. Percutaneous retrogasserian glycerol rhizolysis in the management of trigeminal neuralgia. *J Neurosurg* 1988;69:361–366.

Cho DY, Chang CG, Wang YC, et al. Repeat operations in failed microvascular decompression for trigeminal neuralgia. *Neurosurgery* 1994;35:665–670.

Goadsby PJ, Edvinsson L, Ekman R. Release of vasoactive peptides in the extracerebral circulation of humans and the cat during activation of the trigeminovascular system. *Ann Neurol* 1988;23:193–196.

Gonzalez G, Onofrio BM, Kerr FW. Vasodilator system for the face. *J Neurosurg* 1975;42:696–703.

Hamlyn PJ, King TT. Neurovascular compression in trigeminal neuralgia: a clinical and anatomical study. *J Neurosurg* 1992;76:948–954.

Hartel F. Uber die intracranielle injektions behandlung der trimeninus-neuralgie. *Med Klin* 1914;10:582.

Hasegawa T, Kondziolka D, Spiro R, et al. Repeat radiosurgery for refractory trigeminal neuralgia. *Neurosurgery* 2002;50:494–500.

Herman JM, Petit JH, Amin P, et al. Repeat gamma knife radiosurgery for refractory or recurrent trigeminal neuralgia: treatment outcomes and quality-of-life assessment. *Int J Radiat Oncol Biol Phys* 2004;59:112–116.

Ischia S, Luzzani A, Polati E. Retrogasserian glycerol injection: a retrospective study of 112 patients. *Clin J Pain* 1990;6:291–296.

Kanpolat Y, Berk C, Savas A, et al. Percutaneous controlled radiofrequency rhizotomy in the management of patients with trigeminal neuralgia due to multiple sclerosis. *Acta Neurochir (Wien)* 2000;142:685–690.

Kanpolat Y, Savas A, Bekar A, et al. Percutaneous controlled radiofrequency trigeminal rhizotomy for the treatment of idiopathic trigeminal neuralgia: 25-year experience with 1,600 patients. *Neurosurgery* 2001;48:524–532.

Klun B. Microvascular decompression and partial sensory rhizotomy in the treatment of trigeminal neuralgia: personal experience with 220 patients. *Neurosurgery* 1992;30:49–52.

Kondziolka D, Lunsford LD, Bissonette DJ. Long-term results after glycerol rhizotomy for multiple sclerosis-related trigeminal neuralgia. *Can J Neurol Sci* 1994;21: 137–140.

Kondziolka D, Lunsford LD, Flickinger JC. Stereotactic radiosurgery for the treatment of trigeminal neuralgia. *Clin J Pain* 2002;18:42–47.

Kondziolka D, Perez B, Flickinger JC, et al. Gamma knife radiosurgery for trigeminal neuralgia: results and expectations. *Arch Neurol* 1998;55:1524–1529.

Longhi M, Rizzo P, Nicolato A, et al. Gamma knife radiosurgery for trigeminal neuralgia: results and potentially predictive parameters—part I: Idiopathic trigeminal neuralgia. *Neurosurgery* 2007;61:1254–1260.

Maher CO, Pollock BE. Radiation induced vascular injury after stereotactic radiosurgery for trigeminal neuralgia: case report. *Surg Neurol* 2000;54:189–193.

Matsuda S, Serizawa T, Sato M, et al. Gamma knife radiosurgery for trigeminal neuralgia: the dry-eye complication. *J Neurosurg* 2002;97:525–528.

Nicol B, Regine WF, Courtney C, et al. Gamma knife radiosurgery using 90 Gy for trigeminal neuralgia. *J Neurosurg* 2000; 93(Suppl 3):152–154.

Pickett GE, Bisnaire D, Ferguson GG. Percutaneous retrogasserian glycerol rhizotomy in the treatment of tic douloureux associated with multiple sclerosis. *Neurosurgery* 2005;56:537–545.

Pollock BE, Foote RL, Link MJ, et al. Repeat radiosurgery for idiopathic trigeminal neuralgia. *Int J Radiat Oncol Biol Phys* 2005;61:192–195.

Pollock BE, Foote RL, Stafford SL. Stereotactic radiosurgery: the preferred management for patients with nonvestibular schwannomas? *Int J Radiat Oncol Biol Phys* 2002;52:1002–1007.

Pollock BE, Foote RL, Stafford SL, et al. Results of repeated gamma knife radiosurgery for medically unresponsive trigeminal neuralgia. *J Neurosurg* 2000;93(Suppl 3):162–164.

Pollock BE, Phuong LK, Foote RL, et al. High-dose trigeminal neuralgia radiosurgery associated with increased risk of trigeminal nerve dysfunction. *Neurosurgery* 2001;49:58–62; discussion 62–54.

Pollock BE, Phuong LK, Gorman DA, et al. Stereotactic radiosurgery for idiopathic trigeminal neuralgia. *J Neurosurg* 2002;97:347–353.

Rath SA, Klein HJ, Richter HP. Findings and long-term results of subsequent operations after failed microvascular decompression for trigeminal neuralgia. *Neurosurgery* 1996;39:933–940.

Richards GM, Bradley KA, Tome WA, et al. Linear accelerator radiosurgery for trigeminal neuralgia. *Neurosurgery* 2005;57:1193–1200.

Rish BL. Cerebrovascular accident after percutaneous RF thermocoagulation of the trigeminal ganglion. Case report. *J Neurosurg* 1976;44:376–377.

Rogers CL, Shetter AG, Ponce FA, et al. Gamma knife radiosurgery for trigeminal neuralgia associated with multiple sclerosis. *J Neurosurg* 2002;97:529–532.

Sheehan J, Pan HC, Stroila M, et al. Gamma knife surgery for trigeminal neuralgia: outcomes and prognostic factors. *J Neurosurg* 2005;102:434–441.

Shetter AG, Rogers CL, Ponce F, et al. Gamma knife radiosurgery for recurrent trigeminal neuralgia. *J Neurosurg* 2002;97:536–538.

Smith ZA, De Salles AA, Frighetto L, et al. Dedicated linear accelerator radiosurgery for the treatment of trigeminal neuralgia. *J Neurosurg* 2003;99:511–516.
Sun T, Saito S, Nakai O, et al. Long-term results of microvascular decompression for trigeminal neuralgia with reference to probability of recurrence. *Acta Neurochir (Wien)* 1994;126:144–148.
Sweet WH, Poletti CE, Roberts JT. Dangerous rises in blood pressure upon heating of trigeminal rootlets; increased bleeding times in patients with trigeminal neuralgia. *Neurosurgery* 1985;17:843–844.
Taha JM, Tew JM Jr. Comparison of surgical treatments for trigeminal neuralgia: reevaluation of radiofrequency rhizotomy. *Neurosurgery* 1996;38:865–871.
Taha JM, Tew JM Jr., Buncher CR. A prospective 15-year follow up of 154 consecutive patients with trigeminal neuralgia treated by percutaneous stereotactic radiofrequency thermal rhizotomy. *J Neurosurg* 1995;83:989–993.
Tawk RG, Duffy-Fronckowiak M, Scott BE, et al. Stereotactic gamma knife surgery for trigeminal neuralgia: detailed analysis of treatment response. *J Neurosurg* 2005;102:442–449.
Tew JM, Jr., Keller JT, Williams DS. Application of stereotactic principles to the treatment of trigeminal neuralgia. *Appl Neurophysiol* 1978;41:146–156.
Tobler WD, Tew JM Jr., Cosman E, et al. Improved outcome in the treatment of trigeminal neuralgia by percutaneous stereotactic rhizotomy with a new, curved tip electrode. *Neurosurgery* 1983;12:313–317.
Tran Dinh YR, Thurel C, Cunin G, et al. Cerebral vasodilation after the thermocoagulation of the trigeminal ganglion in humans. *Neurosurgery* 1992;31:658–663.
Young RF, Vermulen S, Posewitz A. Gamma knife radiosurgery for the treatment of trigeminal neuralgia. *Stereotact Funct Neurosurg* 1998;70(Suppl 1):192–199.

11

Glycerol Rhizotomy

Douglas Kondziolka and L. Dade Lunsford

The problem of trigeminal neuralgia (TN) has many possible medical and surgical answers. Operation is usually considered for those patients who do not respond well to or tolerate medical treatment. Operative procedures include those aimed to address the cause of the pain, such as microvascular decompression (MVD), or those that address the nerve but ignore the cause of the pain (various rhizotomy procedures). Stereotactic radiosurgery, when performed at the anatomic location of vascular compression, may also work to treat the cause, but it is believed that the effect is more on selective axonal degeneration of the nerve. The various ablative procedures provide mechanical effects on the nerve (balloon microcompression, thermal-induced axonal degeneration by radiofrequency (RF) rhizotomy, radiation-induced degeneration produced by stereotactic radiosurgery, or chemical ablation via glycerol rhizotomy). Injection of chemical agents to peripheral nerve targets (i.e., alcohol injections) is also available.

Approaching the trigeminal nerve less invasively via a needle puncture through the face has a long history. Härtel is given credit for the accepted technique of spinal needle placement into the trigeminal cistern (Burchiel 1988). When absolute alcohol was injected into this location, multiple severe cranial neuropathies could be seen. Jefferson advocated the use of phenol mixed with glycerine rather than absolute alcohol (Jefferson 1963). Lars Leksell had long been interested in the use of focused radiation for the management of TN. His initial work in the early 1950s coupled an orthovoltage x-ray tube to a stereotactic frame in order to irradiate the trigeminal ganglion. The first-generation gamma knife was built in 1967. Leksell and Håkanson injected tantalum dust mixed with glycerol into the trigeminal cistern as a marker to localize the nerve for radiosurgery (Håkanson 1978, 1981). When the targeting solution was injected prior to performing radiosurgery, patients noted pain relief. Thus, percutaneous retrogasserian glycerol rhizotomy (PRGR) was created.

In our care of patients with TN, we seek the goals of rapid-onset and long-lasting pain relief, together with preservation of trigeminal nerve function. Percutaneous retrogasserian glycerol rhizotomy offers distinct advantages over other percutaneous procedures. These include the lack of need for intraoperative confirmatory sensory testing (patient cooperation is not necessary) or a RF generator. The patient simply need not participate during the procedure and can be more deeply anesthetized. Precise anatomic localization of the target is performed using intraoperative cisternography, rather than having the patient describe RF-induced sensory changes. Glycerol is associated with a lower risk of facial sensory loss compared to either RF rhizotomy or balloon microcompression. This feature significantly reduces the risk of deafferentation pain. The choice of the procedure is related to the factors of patient age, medical condition, symptom severity, and personal preference. Glycerol rhizotomy remains our preferred primary surgery for patients with multiple sclerosis-related TN (Kondziolka, Lunsford, & Bissonette 1994; Pickett, Bisnaire, & Ferguson 2005).

PATIENT SELECTION

As with all surgery for TN, only patients with typical TN pain should be selected for glycerol rhizotomy. The correct diagnosis is validated by a careful history that elucidates the quality, character, and distribution of pain. In patients with atypical TN (who usually have a lingering pain without triggers), rhizotomy can be used to manage any severe lancinating component, but has little effect on more constant pain. We rarely perform rhizotomy in this setting, except in patients who have previously undergone a successful procedure for prior typical TN symptoms.

After the appropriate diagnosis is made, we recommend initial medical treatment with appropriate doses of carbamazepine, Trileptal, gabapentin, phenytoin, baclofen, or perhaps Lamictal. Selected additional medications also may be used. High-resolution brain imaging should be performed to exclude a skull base lesion, a vascular anomaly, or basal tumor that might alter the regional anatomy or be the cause of TN. At our center, glycerol rhizotomy is offered as one first-line therapy in patients with idiopathic TN. However, we typically recommend gamma knife radiosurgery first, unless the patient cannot eat or drink and requires more rapid pain relief. For such patients, the possible latent interval associated with gamma knife radiosurgery is not acceptable (Lunsford 1982). As a minimally invasive strategy, PRGR is used as a second-line approach in patients who have not responded adequately to radiosurgery. Finally, PRGR is an excellent first choice for patients with TN in the setting of multiple sclerosis (Kondziolka et al. 1994; Pickett et al. 2005), which seems to occur at an earlier age than in patients without idiopathic neuralgia. It is an appropriate second-line therapy in those who have failed other surgical options, such as MVD. It is important to note that the technique of glycerol rhizotomy can vary from institution to institution. Some surgeons do not perform a contrast cisternogram, and others do not directly visualize the injection of glycerol into the trigeminal cistern with metallic markers such as tantalum. Thus, if PRGR was said to have failed due to technical difficulties, we may repeat the procedure in an attempt to confirm that glycerol was in fact injected into the appropriate location. We think that injection of contrast to identify the trigeminal cistern is the only way to truly know that the best target has been reached.

Finally, preoperative testing to rule out a bleeding diathesis, electrocardiogram, and chest x-ray are obtained as indicated. All antiplatelet agents (such as aspirin or ticlopidine) must be discontinued 1 week before PRGR. If patients must remain on warfarin or other anticoagulants, then gamma knife radiosurgery is a better surgical choice.

Anesthetic Technique

At our institution, PRGR is performed with the patient under continuously monitored intravenous sedation in the operating room setting. The anesthesiologist monitors blood pressure, heart rate, oxygen saturation, and respiratory function. They are requested to provide adequate sedation for the patient and to quickly respond to any cardiovascular changes that might occur during the procedure. Because PRGR does not require intraoperative verbal patient responses to guide the surgeon, deeper sedation is allowed. Patients often receive intravenous propofol or other rapidly acting agents, together with a narcotic. Some patients, especially younger men, may benefit from preadministration of 0.4 mg atropine sulfate, an anticholinergic agent that serves to blunt the occasional vasovagal response that may be seen during the procedure. Most of the discomfort during the procedure occurs when the 20-gauge spinal needle is passed through the foramen ovale, and it is thus important that patients are adequately sedated during this time. A deep injection of local anesthetic is as important as making sure that the skin surface is anesthetized.

Both the surgeon and anesthesiologist should be aware that up to 20% of patients can have a vasovagal response to foramen ovale needle penetration or to the glycerol injection. Administration of an intravenous anticholinergic agent is important at the first sign of bradycardia. Other patients may have a hypertensive response to needle placement, usually due to pain or anxiety. Such a response can be lessened by the administration of hydralazine or β-blockers. The systolic blood pressure should be kept below 160 mm Hg, since higher blood pressures can be associated with facial hematomas from needle placement. Because the procedure is begun with the patient supine but completed in the semi-sitting position during glycerol injection, a balance of pain control, blood pressure management, and respiratory care must be maintained by the surgeon and anesthesiologist.

OPERATIVE TECHNIQUE

The patient is placed supine on an operating room table that allows control of head, leg, and body position. The patient's head is suspended in a Mayfield cerebellar head rest, so that the arm of the rest does not interfere with fluoroscopic imaging in the lateral or anterior-posterior (AP) direction.

Initially, a C-arm fluoroscopic image intensifier is positioned in the AP projection. The value of a competent radiology technologist cannot be overestimated. The operator works to align the head, such that the petrous ridge is at the same level as the inferior orbital rim. The foramen ovale can often be visualized just inferior and lateral to the junction of the inferior and medial orbital rims. We clean the patient's face with 70% ethanol solution, and towels are placed around the neck and upper chest as the area is draped.

We mark an entry point using an ink marker. This point is located 2.5 cm lateral to the corner of the mouth on the side of pain. We also mark trajectories toward a point that is in line with the medial ipsilateral pupil and at a point 2.5 cm anterior to the external auditory canal. We use 1% lidocaine with a 25-gauge needle to create a small intradermal injection, and then use a 21- or 23-gauge needle to inject lidocaine into the deep structures of the cheek. A gloved finger is placed inside the patient's oral cavity to prevent penetration of the mucosa either by the anesthetic needle or by the 20-gauge spinal needle used for the rhizotomy (Lunsford & Bennett 1984). The 20-gauge needle is then inserted along the marked trajectory under fluoroscopic guidance toward the skull base. This is placed using an AP projection. Using a lateral projection, the needle tip is directed at a point about 1 cm behind the posterior clinoid along the angle of the clivus.

Penetration of the foramen ovale can sometimes be uncomfortable, and thus administration of a short-acting barbiturate or propofol is administered immediately prior to puncture. Penetration of the needle through the foramen ovale can be felt by the surgeon. The stylet of the needle should be removed to check for flow of cerebrospinal fluid (CSF) (Fig. 11.1). If no CSF is encountered, then the needle with the stylet replaced is advanced at

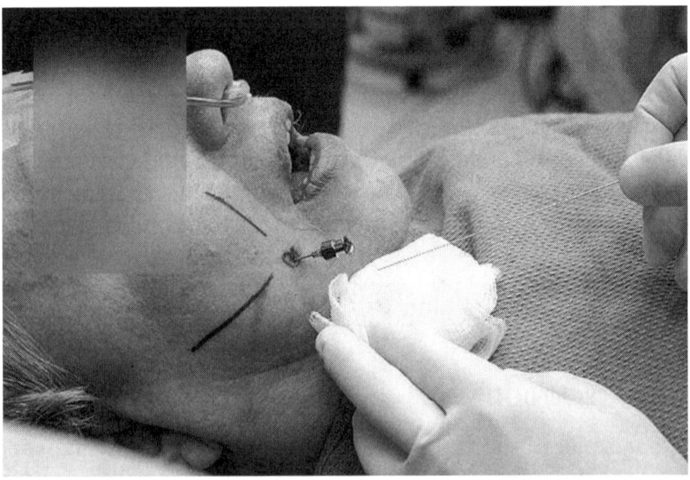

Figure 11.1 After placement of the transovale spinal needle, cerebrospinal fluid is seen to drip out from the trigeminal cistern.

1 mm increments under fluoroscopic guidance until the trigeminal cistern is entered; CSF flow should then be confirmed. If the needle is placed past the clival line without flow of spinal fluid, it may require adjustment. The most common problem is that the needle may either be too medial or too lateral in the cistern. If too lateral within the foramen ovale, the tip of the needle may be in the subdural or subtemporal space. Although the finding of CSF flow is desirable, its absence does not always preclude identification of the trigeminal cistern. This is particularly true in repeated cases. In our experiences, chances for CSF flow are maximized when the needle hub is directed medially (Fig. 11.2). If spinal fluid flow is identified, or the needle is believed to be within the trigeminal cistern, the patient is placed into the sitting position for a contrast cisternogram. Cisternography is required to assess the volume of the trigeminal cistern and to select the proper amount of glycerol. With the needle in the cistern, the head of the bed is elevated to put the patient in the semi-sitting position, with the neck slightly flexed. We use a tuberculin syringe to inject sterile iohexol in 0.05 ml increments, under fluoroscopic guidance, until the contrast is seen to overflow out of the cistern. The average volume of the trigeminal cistern is 0.25 mL and rarely exceeds 0.4 mL. The contrast is then allowed to evacuate from the cistern by spontaneous drainage, which may require that the patient be placed again into the recumbent position. If full evacuation of the contrast is desired (particularly important for patients with lower division pain), the patient can be returned to the supine position (Lunsford 1984). It should

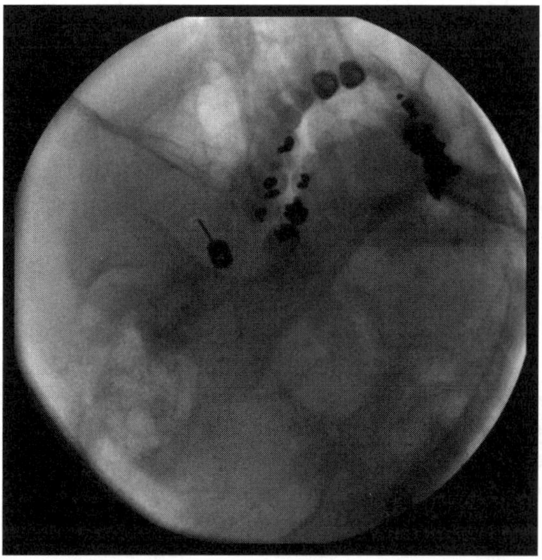

Figure 11.2 The transovale fluoroscopic view, showing the spinal needle tip within the medial aspect of the foramen ovale.

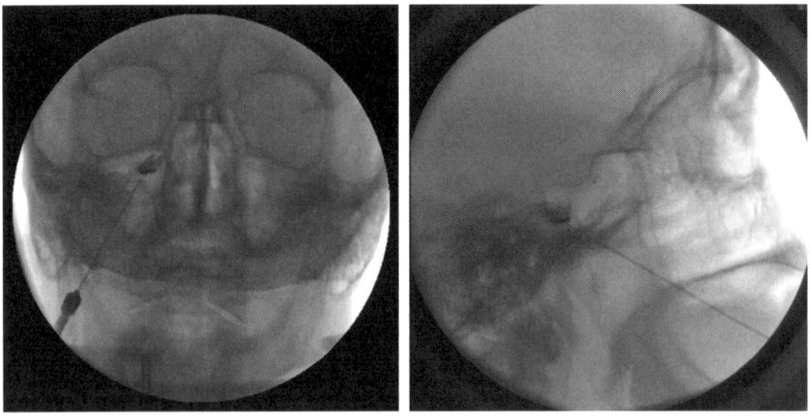

(a) (b)

Figure 11.3 Intraoperative anterior-posterior (a) and lateral (b) fluoroscopic images showing glycerol mixed with tantalum dust within the trigeminal cistern.

be noted that some surgeons do not inject contrast (Pickett et al. 2005), relying on fluoroscopic findings and CSF return. We continue to advocate contrast injection because it is the only way to directly confirm that the trigeminal cistern has been entered (Fig. 11.3).

The glycerol injection is performed in the same manner as injection of contrast medium, under fluoroscopic guidance. Again, the patient is placed into a semi-sitting position. We mix 99.9% anhydrous glycerol with radiopaque tantalum powder. The final volume of glycerol injected is dependent upon the cisternal volume measured and the nerve distributions affected. There are different techniques for a glycerol injection, which vary from filling the entire cistern for patients with multidivisional pain to leaving approximately one-third of the contrast material still in the cistern and "floating" the glycerol on top of the contrast in those patients with isolated V_1 pain. Because of its lighter density, the glycerol mixture floats above the residual contrast medium, exerting its effect mainly on upper-division fibers. During the injection, some patients experience ipsilateral periorbital discomfort and sometimes facial flushing. After the glycerol is injected, the needle is removed, and a small bandage is placed on the skin entry point. We keep the patient at a semi-sitting position for 2 hours to prevent escape of glycerol into the posterior fossa. Most patients are kept in the hospital overnight and discharged home the next day.

OPERATIVE RESULTS

Numerous studies have confirmed the value of PRGR in the management of TN (Håkanson 1981; Jho & Lunsford 1997; Lunsford & Bennett 1984;

North et al. 1990; Pickett et al. 2005; Pollock 2005; Saini 1987; Slettebo Hirschberg, & Lindegaard 1993; Young 1988). However, comparative assessments can be difficult because of the variations in surgical techniques. As mentioned earlier, some centers do not perform cisternography, and others instill larger glycerol volumes. Most centers report that initial pain relief is seen in the majority of patients, with pain improvements in the range of 90%. We usually tell patients that half of those who respond will do so within the first day of the procedure, and in half it may take up to 2 or 3 weeks for the full effect. Confusion does exist as to the definition of recurrence rates, depending on the time frame of evaluation, the need for concomitant medication, and the degree of pain control.

At the University of Pittsburgh, glycerol rhizotomy was performed in 1,174 patients up to 2004. Immediate or early complete pain relief occurred in 90% of patients. An initial report that evaluated 112 patients demonstrated 90% pain relief at 2 years, with 60% having complete relief after glycerol rhizotomy alone, and 23% requiring some additional yet reduced drug therapy. A subsequent analysis of 376 patients with follow-up to 7 years found the long-term pain control rate of 85% (Jho & Lunsford 1994). Sixty percent had complete relief after glycerol rhizotomy alone, although in some patients repeat procedures were necessary. A longer-term assessment up to 11 years found long-lasting relief of pain in 77% of patients, with 55% off all medications and 22% requiring some drug usage (Jho & Lunsford 1994). It should be emphasized that TN is not a static disease but is characterized by remissions and recurrences, some mild and some severe. This challenge is known by all experienced groups. Pollock (2005) recently reported 98 patients and found that 73% were without pain at some point after surgery; the numbers of these patients who were found to have remained pain-free off medications at 1 and 3 years were 61% and 50%, respectively. Mild paresthesias or numbness was noted in 53%, and 12% developed herpes simplex perioralis with full recovery.

Other than the perioperative blood pressure or cardiac changes noted earlier, other complications are relatively rare. Some days after their first procedure approximately 10%–20% of patients will have detectable but usually mild reduction in light touch or pain (pinprick) perception. With repeated glycerol procedures, the incremental sensory dysfunction assessment goes up, so that by two or three procedures, 50%–70% of patients will have detectable sensory changes of a mild to moderate degree. Deafferentation pain, in our experience, has been extremely unusual and most likely occurs in the context of a complication, as noted below.

Many patients have chronic herpes simplex perioralis virus dormant in the gasserian ganglion. With percutaneous therapies, the subsequent development of cold sores is common. For patients who have a history of repeated cold sore attacks, we place them prophylactically on acyclovir and give them acyclovir ointment in the perioperative interval. Early aseptic meningitis (1–2 days) is an extremely rare event, occurring in approximately two out of 1,000 cases. Although spinal fluid analysis must be repeated on an urgent basis to confirm the absence of bacterial meningitis, patients can be placed on corticosteroids if the CSF Gram stain is negative. The pleocytosis may be profound when it occurs, and can be very hard to differentiate from true bacterial meningitis. The risk of bacterial meningitis is minimized by making sure the spinal needle does not penetrate the oral mucosa.

In our experience of more than 1,000 patients with glycerol rhizotomy, we have had one perioperative death. This patient sustained a myocardial infarction about 1 hour after the procedure. We regard any operative intervention as potentially stressful, but consider this 0.1% surgical mortality risk to be low in a higher-risk population. The risk of developing delayed corneal dysfunction is extremely low, especially with an initial procedure.

REFERENCES

Burchiel KJ. Percutaneous retrogasserian glycerol rhizolysis in the management of trigeminal neuralgia. *J Neurosurg* 1988;69:361–366.

Håkanson S. Transoval trigeminal cisternography. *Surg Neurol* 1978;10:137–144.

Håkanson S. Trigeminal neuralgia treated by the injection of glycerol into the trigeminal cistern. *Neurosurgery* 1981;9:638–646.

Jefferson A. Trigeminal root and ganglion injections using phenol in glycerin for the relief of trigeminal neuralgia. *J Neurol Neurosurg Psychiatry* 1963;26:345–352.

Jho HD, Lunsford LD. Percutaneous retrogasserian glycerol rhizotomy. *Neurosurg Clin N Amer* 1997;8:63–74.

Kondziolka D, Lunsford LD, Bissonette DJ. Long-term results after percutaneous retrogasserian glycerol rhizotomy for trigeminal neuralgia in patients with multiple sclerosis. *Can J Neurol Sci* 1994;21:137–140.

Kondziolka D, Lunsford LD, Flickinger JC, et al. Stereotactic radiosurgery for trigeminal neuralgia: A multi-institution study using the gamma unit. *J Neurosurg* 1996;84:940–945.

Lunsford LD. Treatment of tic douloureux by percutaneous retrogasserian glycerol injection. *JAMA* 1982;248:449–453.

Lunsford LD, Bennett MH. Percutaneous retrogasserian glycerol rhizotomy for tic douloureux. Part 1: Technique and results in 112 patients. *Neurosurgery* 1984; 14:424–430.

North RB, Kidd DH, Piantadosi S, et al. Percutaneous retrogasserian glycerol rhizotomy. *J Neurosurg* 1990;72:851–856.

Pickett, GE, Bisnaire D, Ferguson GG. Percutaneous retrogasserian glycerol rhizotomy in the treatment of tic douloureux associate with multiple sclerosis. *Neurosurgery* 2005;56:537–545.

Pollock BE. Percutaneous retrogasserian glycerol rhizotomy for patients with idiopathic trigeminal neuralgia: a prospective analysis of factors related to pain relief. *J Neurosurg* 2005;102:223–228.

Saini SS. Retrogasserian anhydrous glycerol injection therapy in trigeminal neuralgia: observations in 552 patients. *J Neurol Neurosurg Psych* 1987;50:1536–1538.

Slettebo H, Hirschberg H, Lindegaard KF. Long-term results after percutaneous retrogasserian glycerol rhizotomy in patients with trigeminal neuralgia. *Acta Neurochir* 1993;122:231–235.

Young R. Glycerol rhizolysis for treatment of trigeminal neuralgia. *J Neurosurg* 1988;69:39–45.

12

Percutaneous Balloon Compression

Jeffrey A. Brown

Neurosurgeons treating trigeminal neuralgia (TN) do so based on the sound philosophy of minimizing surgical risk while maximizing the quality of their surgical outcome. I have often quoted the maxim "less is more," used to describe the architectural approach of the Bauhaus-turned-Chicagoan architect Ludwig Mies van der Rohe. Trigeminal neuralgia being a nonfatal disease should be treated so as to minimize the risk to life from any effort to cure it, with debate existing regarding the benefit accrued from performing a microvascular decompression (MVD). Each day, a patient faces his treating neurosurgeon with the decision of how best to deal with his electric shock–like, intermittent, jabbing facial pain that no longer responds adequately to medication or pain management injections.

Sean Mullan conceived of percutaneous trigeminal nerve balloon compression as a minimalist approach toward trigeminal ablation (Mullan & Lichtor 1983). (Years earlier, Dr. Mullan had introduced a percutaneous ablative technique to replace the frequently performed open cervical cordotomy for the neuropathic pain associated with invasive lung cancer [Mullan 1966].)

During the 1950s, the concept arose that TN occurred because the trigeminal nerve is compressed by the middle fossa. Taarnhoj believed the dural canal over the margin of the petrous ridge could be a source of trigeminal compression (1952). Shelden and colleagues (1955) reviewed the results of a series of patients on whom they had operated by decompressing either the maxillary or mandibular divisions at their exiting foramina or at the root level. Love and Svien noted that the results of such procedures were better when facial numbness was present after surgery (Love & Svien 1954; Svien & Love 1959). Thereafter, patients were often treated by a middle fossa craniotomy, after which the surgeon would rub or compress the ganglion (Brown & Preul, 1989).

Percutaneous treatments for TN had already emerged in the early 20th century. Harris first injected the gasserian ganglion with alcohol percutaneously in 1910 (Stookey & Ransohoff 1959). Haertel detailed the percutaneous technique for injection through the foramen ovale in 1914 (Stookey & Ransohoff 1959). Kirschner then built an apparatus for locating the foramen in order to coagulate the ganglion electrically (Crawford 1951). Sweet built on Kirschner's coagulation technique by describing the percutaneous technique of injection with radiographic control in 1950, then created selective controlled percutaneous radiofrequency (RF) thermocoagulation lesions with an RF generator (Sweet & Wepsic 1974). Sean Mullan had first developed a percutaneous means of creating a cervical cordotomy lesion by using a strontium needle (Mullan 1966). In 1983, he first described the percutaneous modification of Taarnhoj's operation using a balloon to injure the trigeminal fibers (Mullan & Lichtor, 1983). The results of more than 1,000 cases have been evaluated in the literature since this first report (Brown & Pilitsis 2005).

Trigeminal neuralgia, *tic douloureux*, or in the past, *spasme cinique*, is a neuropathic pain syndrome (André 1756; Brown, Coursaget, Preul, & Sangvai 1999). It is unique among neuropathic pain syndromes because it is treatable by an ablative surgical technique, and it is not associated with easily detectable numbness. Doctor Jannetta has found, however, that in one-third of the patients, usually some loss of light touch is present if the examination is performed carefully. More reasonable is the concept that the trigger point represents a region of hyperesthesia located at the site of vascular compression. A peripheral ablation is effective because it acts as a distal anesthetic block. When the trigeminal pain becomes truly neuropathic—that is, when the compression is sufficient to cause demonstrable numbness or significant constant burning, peripheral ablation is no longer indicated. Additional nerve injury, even if peripheral, at this point may add to the dysesthetic quality of pain. This is especially true if the pain no longer has an intermittent, severe electric shock element, triggered by a peripheral stimulus.

If TN is conceptualized as a progressive disease, then percutaneous ablation is best done during the early disease phase, before permanent nerve injury is clinically expressed by the presence of constant burning dysesthesia. The burning sensation may be quite bothersome, but is not like the sudden lightning bolts felt during the hyperaesthetic early phase.

Biopsy specimens of trigeminal roots at the site of compression obtained during MVD surgery for clinical TN show axonal loss, demyelination and dysmyelination, myelin debris, excess collagen, and closely opposed axons without intervening glial processes. Such findings support a hypothesis that TN occurs as a result of changes in the electrical excitability of abnormal afferent trigeminal root axons. Thus, the data are consistent with the idea that TN is neuropathic in nature (Devor, Govrin-Lippmann, & Rappaport 2002).

Balloon compression has unique elements that derive from the anatomic basis of the injury created by mechanical compression, which is different from thermal or chemical injuries. These unique anatomic elements, in turn, can guide the surgeon in his decision-making process to select the most appropriate surgical option available to the patient. This chapter reviews the history of the development of balloon compression, the scientific basis for performing it, details regarding the current technique, results, pitfalls, and morbidity associated with the surgery.

ANATOMY OF INJURY CAUSED BY MECHANICAL BALLOON COMPRESSION OF THE TRIGEMINAL NERVE ROOT

Trigeminal balloon compression in New Zealand rabbits causes a trigeminal depressor response similar to that observed in humans during compression. This suggests that the New Zealand rabbit is a suitable model for studying the histopathological changes that occur after balloon compression in humans. There is no difference in the perikaryonal distribution of neurofilaments between compressed and control trigeminal ganglia. Focal demyelination and Schwann cell proliferation preceding remyelination are present in the trigeminal sensory root at 84 days. Cell size measurements and immunocytochemical studies show that there is no specific loss of small ganglion cells or fine-caliber primary afferents. Fink-Heimer staining of the trigeminal subnucleus caudalis reveals that transganglionic degeneration is most dense in the deeper layers, which are the sites of termination of large myelinated fibers. Injured areas of the nerve have higher ratios of small (<3 μm diameter) to large-diameter axons, compared to control. Differential injury of axons, compared to sparing of trigeminal ganglion cell bodies, suggests that axonal regeneration is possible and may contribute to the recovery of motor and sensory function in patients after percutaneous balloon compression (Brown et al. 1996; Preul et al.1990). Sparing of unmyelinated, pain-responsive fibers, although appearing to be an unlikely result for an operative treatment designed to treat pain, is easily explained if the neuropathic nature of TN is understood. These data lead to the hypothesis that balloon compression relieves trigeminal pain by injuring the myelinated axons involved in the sensory trigger. Unmyelinated pain fibers mediate nociceptive pain transmission. Preservation of unmyelinated fibers by balloon compression, while alleviating TN pain, is also consistent with the neuropathic pain hypothesis for the mechanism operant in TN.

PATIENT SELECTION

Those patients with Burchiel type 1 TN (TN1) are candidates for percutaneous balloon compression (Burchiel 2003). Usually, patients will undergo a period of treatment with anticonvulsant therapy using carbamazepine, gabapentin, diphenylhydantoin, or oxcarbazepine. Pain relief using an anticonvulsant at appropriate dosage helps to confirm the diagnosis of TN. How long medical therapy should continue before one considers an ablative procedure depends on the patient's tolerance for the medication or for the concept of a lifetime of medical treatment. Trigeminal neuralgia does not resolve with medical treatment. If medication is discontinued, pain recurs. Usually, because of disease progression, dose escalation is necessary, with the concomitant onset of disturbing additional effects from the anticonvulsant medication. Such effects include signs of cognitive dysfunction such as drowsiness, inattention, and diminished reaction time and speed of information processing (Hessen, Losius, Reinvang, & Gjerstad 2006).

Balloon compression requires that patients must be able to tolerate a light general anesthesia. Because the median age at diagnosis of TN is 65 years, many of these patients are taking aspirin, warfarin, or clopidogrel (Plavix). All such blood thinners should be discontinued or their effects reversed preoperatively and for several days afterward. Those patients at highest risk for cardiac arrhythmia, cardiac valvular dysfunction, and stroke because their blood thinners are being stopped may not be able to undergo balloon compression. Contralateral jaw weakness is not a contraindication, despite the expectation of temporary masseter and pterygoid muscle weakness.

Brief bradycardia occurs during compression. Also, there may be hypertension after compression. Preoperative evaluation should include an electrocardiogram to identify those patients with cardiac arrhythmias. Untreated hypertension should be medically stabilized. Patients with a history of cold sores or fever blisters may take oral acyclovir to alleviate a postoperative outbreak. There is no clinical evidence to support the effectiveness of such therapy, however.

OPERATIVE TECHNIQUE

For a neurosurgeon, the operation is easiest to perform in the operating suite using a portable fluoroscope for imaging. It may also be done in the angiography suite, taking advantage of multiplanar imaging capabilities. Oral anticonvulsant agents used to treat pain should be continued, and intravenous antibiotic prophylaxis may be used, although the likelihood of oral contamination is low. In my experience, it has happened on only one occasion in 25 years.

Induce a light general anesthesia, and then place an external pacemaker. Set the pacemaker to trigger automatically should the heart rate drop to less than 45 bpm during compression. The anesthesiologist should confirm capture by the pacemaker before proceeding. The external pacer blocks the bradycardia quicker than intravenous atropine. If the bradycardia persists during compression, administer 0.4 mg atropine intravenously. The atropine should be drawn into a syringe awaiting infusion for this situation. This depressor response consists of both bradycardia and brief hypotension, often with reflexive hypertension after triggering the pacemaker. Preoperative atropine inhibits the depressor response, but does not allow its use as an indicator of successful nerve compression.

Position the patient supine and, after induction, place a cloth roll under the shoulders, allowing approximately 15 degrees of neck extension. Some surgical tables have a steel bar at the head of the table that is used to adjust the angle of the table head. Remove this table piece. The bar may interfere with the modified submental image, obstructing visualization of the foramen ovale. Rotate the head 15–30 degrees to the opposite side.

Because older patients often have degenerative cervical spondylosis, further extension and rotation may be limited. Prepare the perioral region with a sterile solution, lubricate and tape the eyes shunt, then surround the entrance site with plastic drapes. Mark the entry point on the cheek 2.5 cm lateral to the angle of the lip in a skin crease. For V_1 pain treatment, this mark is set slightly more lateral. Position a digital pressure monitor (Merit Medical, South Jordan, Utah) on an adjacent intravenous pole located at waist level opposite the surgeon. Drape the fluoroscope imaging units on the side away from the surgeon. Place a half-sized drape over the unit on the side of surgery. It will not remain sterile because of the need for submental and anterior-posterior images. Fill the insufflation syringe with several cubic centimeters of radiographic dye.

A U.S. Food and Drug Administration (FDA)-approved kit for this procedure is available that includes sharp and blunt trocars, an introducing cannula, curved and straight guiding stylets, and a No. 4 balloon. (Cook Vascular, Inc., Leechburg, Pennsylvania). The insufflation syringe connects to the balloon catheter and measures intraluminal pressures in atmospheres. The target intraluminal pressure is 1.3–1.5 atm. Intraluminal

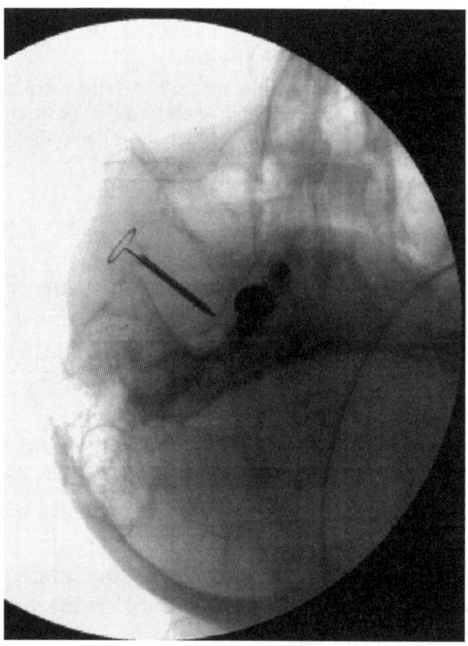

Figure 12.1 Modified submental image demonstrating the 14-gauge cannula with a straight inner stylet penetrating the right foramen ovale.

The foramen is visible superior to the petrous ridge, medial to the mandible and below the maxillary sinus.

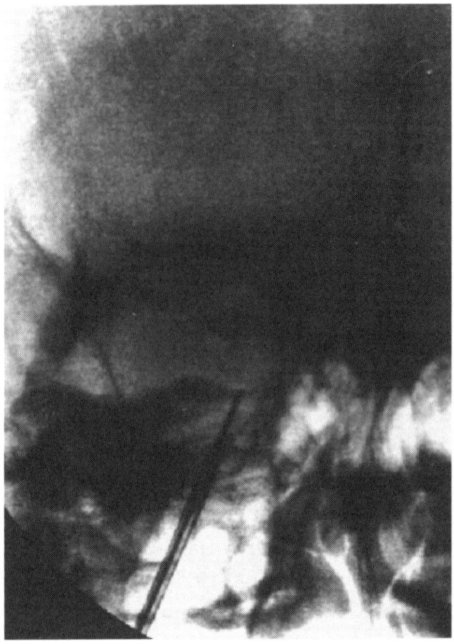

Figure 12.2 Anterior-posterior radiographic intraoperative image showing position of the straight inner guiding stylet within the 14-gauge cannula when properly positioned for treatment of V_2 pain.

The tip of the stylet is placed at the center of the dip in the petrous bone representing the entrance to Meckel's cave. The balloon catheter will be positioned along the same path, with its tip approximately 2 mm beyond the petrous bone edge, as seen through the orbit on the image intensifier.

pressure need not be measured. The No. 4 balloon catheter may be inflated with 0.75–1.0 mL of contrast until a pear shape is observed. The appearance of the pear shape may be variable, however. Pressure measurement provides an additional guide to measure the appropriate degree of compression delivered to the trigeminal nerve root.

The first fluoroscopic image to be used is the lateral view. The entry point of the cannula should be designed so that the cannula approaches the floor of the middle fossa and the foramen ovale, nearly parallel to the slope of the petrous bone for V_3 pain. For maxillary division pain, a more oblique angle is selected. For V_1 pain, the oblique angle is even greater. Hold the No. 14-gauge cannula with the sharp obturator inserted against the cheek and obtain a lateral fluoroscopic image. Adjust the superior–inferior site of insertion to obtain an insertion path consistent with the targeted division. Once this is accomplished, nick the cheek with a No. 11 blade. This incision should accommodate the cannula easily without requiring a suture at the end of the procedure. Slide the 45-degree sharp obturator

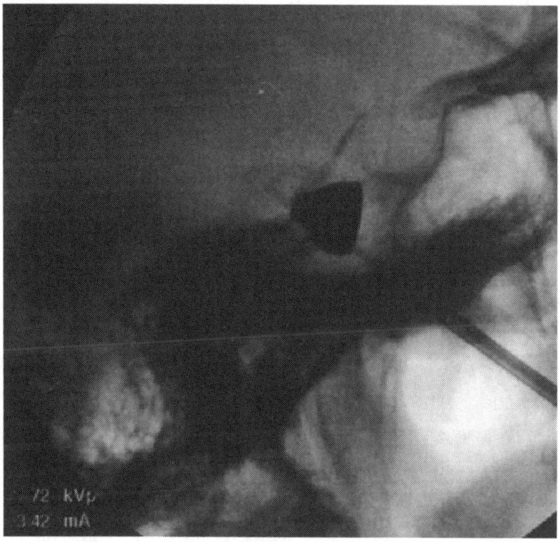

Figure 12.3 Lateral intraoperative radiograph showing the correctly inflated balloon forming a pear shape at a pressure of 1.5 atm.

This image corresponds to the shape of the balloon when the catheter tip is located at the center of the porus trigeminus, as seen in anterior posterior image of the previous figure.

that is included in the kit into the cannula and use it to puncture the skin of the cheek. Replace the sharp with the blunt obturator. Ensure that the No. 14-gauge cannula *does not pass beyond the foramen ovale.* Only the guiding stylets and balloon catheter pass into the cranial cavity.

Obtain a submental view once the cannula has reached the skull base. First, identify the foramen ovale on the image intensifier, then advance the cannula using repeated fluoroscopic images of the submental view. The approach angle should be essentially parallel to the fluoroscopy. In this modified submental view, the anteroposterior (AP) imaging unit is directed at an angle of about 29 degrees under the chin. The neck is slightly extended, and the head laterally rotated 15 degrees to the opposite side. In this view, the foramen ovale is seen medial to the mandible, lateral to the maxilla, and directly above the petrous bone. The view provides direct visualization of the foramen ovale. When the foramen is engaged, the depressor response may briefly occur. The surgeon should feel some resistance on the cannula, as though its sides were gripped, while it engages. The cannula should not penetrate any further. No cerebrospinal fluid will be obtained, since the cannula has not entered the subarachnoid space surrounding the trigeminal ganglion. This is different from the expectations regarding appropriate positioning that occurs with glycerol and thermal rhizotomy. Once the cannula has engaged the foramen ovale, the blunt obturator is removed and a straight guiding stylet is inserted. Venous bleeding may occur from the epidural venous complex. If so, it will stop when the cannula is advanced slightly more so as to engage the foramen ovale. Insert a straight guiding stylet until it just passes beyond the edge of the cannula and the inner aspect of the foramen ovale. The surgeon may feel a characteristic "pop," similar to the tactile feeling noted when performing a lumbar puncture. If excessive resistance to advancement of the stylet occurs, the cannula may not be correctly positioned at the foramen ovale.

Next, obtain an AP fluoroscopic view. On the AP view, the petrous bone is centered in the ipsilateral orbit. The medial dip in the petrous bone is the proximal entrance to Meckel's cave, the porus trigeminus. Direct the stylet to the center of the porus for V_2 pain or multidivisional pain; direct toward the lateral porus for V_3 pain, and toward the medial porous for V_1 pain. In patients with predominantly V_1- pain, aim toward a more lateral to medial position to enable the stylet to pass into the medial segment of porous. The entrance to the porus is located approximately 17 mm beyond the foramen ovale. The cannula system is designed so that when the cannula is placed at the foramen ovale, it is not possible to pass the guiding stylet beyond the porus trigeminus into the posterior fossa.

The curved stylet may be used to allow mobility within the porus to reach the medial or central aspect. Its curve should be directed caudally during passage through the cannula. The tip is rotated superomedially after it is beyond the cannula. This maneuver decreases risk of dural perforation. If the dura is perforated, the stylet should be redirected to remain interdural, so that balloon compression may occur. The only indication that dural perforation has occurred may be that a pear shape fails to appear during inflation despite the AP and lateral images indicating appropriate positioning of the balloon.

Obtain a lateral view. In order to position the balloon catheter at the best angle for V_3, multidivisional, or V_1 pain, it is most helpful to position the fluoroscopy imaging beam parallel to the skull base. The planum sphenoidale and posterior clinoids, when superimposed in the fluoroscopic images, also provide the best image of the sella turcica. This view will then show the cannula tip at the base of the middle fossa. The lateral view is then used for the balloon compression. For V_2 or V_3 pain, the stylet should remain parallel and adjacent to the petrous bone. For V_1 pain, the stylet should be visualized more superiorly, above the petrous bone. Once the proper trajectory has been established, the stylet is removed. The balloon catheter is then placed in the same place as the guiding stylet. The catheter has a thin inner wire that identifies its position.

For V_3 pain, use the AP image intensifier view to place the tip of the balloon catheter approximately 2 mm beyond the edge of the petrous bone. For V_1 pain, insert the catheter slightly farther. This is because the catheter is positioned superomedial in the nerve in order to reach the V_1 fibers. These fibers are in the superior portion of the trigeminal root. V_3 fibers are in the inferior trigeminal root. The balloon is traversing the root obliquely from the fixed entry site at the foramen ovale.

Once properly positioned radiographically, remove the stylet within the catheter and slide the blocking device, firmly securing it on the balloon at the edge of the cannula. This maneuver prevents the balloon from sliding into the posterior fossa when it is inflated. Evacuate air from the balloon with a tuberculin syringe connected to a three-way stopcock. The balloon is then connected to the insufflation syringe and then to the monitor, which is allowed to stabilize at a zeroed pressure.

Slowly inflate the balloon while repeatedly monitoring blood pressure and observing intermittent lateral fluoroscopic images. When the balloon inflates within the porus, the characteristic pear shape is seen on the lateral view. If the catheter tip is not within the porus, then the characteristic pear is not visualized, numbness is less, and mild pain relief is limited to the V_3. At the porus, the distal balloon lifts the dura off the ganglion. Proximally, within the porous, it compresses the retrogasserian fibers against the firm edge of the dura and the petrous ridge as the dura splits, allowing the nerve to pass into Meckel's cave. If the balloon ruptures, there have been no sequelae. If the patient is known to be allergic to the dye used, premedication with steroid is suggested.

When properly inflated, using a No. 4 French balloon catheter, the intraluminal balloon pressure should be raised to 1.3–1.6 atm. Once you reach the target pressure and you see a pear shape, leave the balloon inflated for 1 minute longer if you seek more numbness. The depressor response is usually present, and the pacemaker may be briefly triggered. There may be a secondary elevation of blood pressure, especially after triggering the pacemaker. This hypertensive response should be controlled by using additional anesthetic. After deflation, the balloon and catheter are removed together. If the catheter is inadvertently removed separately, cerebrospinal fluid may drip through the cannula, because the subarachnoid space surrounding the ganglion in Meckel's cave has now been opened. Compress the cheek against the maxilla for 5 minutes. Close the entry point with a sterile tape and small bandage.

POSTOPERATIVE MANAGEMENT

Transfer the patient to the recovery room, where mild analgesics may be given for surgical pain. Place an ice pack against the cheek to reduce postoperative swelling. The patient may be discharged home a few hours after the procedure or remain hospitalized until the next day. Postoperatively, the patient should be evaluated for the adequacy of his pain relief. Typically, the patient awakens without pain, except for local discomfort at the needle entry site. Trigeminal pain may persist for a day or two postoperatively, and then subside if the compression has been mild. The degree of sensory loss should also be assessed. A decrease in touch and pinprick perception occurs in two-thirds of patients. Patients may find the associated subjective numbness slightly uncomfortable at first, but usually adjust in the first 3–4 weeks. The numbness generally decreases substantially by 3–6 months. Pain relief tends to persist even after the numbness resolves. Decreased sensation is most common in the V_3, and sometimes occurs in patients being treated for V_1 or V_2 pain. Despite this absence of sensory change, the patient may have complete pain relief. Rarely, patients report dysesthesia, unpleasant hypalgesia (decreased sensitivity to pain), and hypoesthesia (decreased sensitivity to touch).

The corneal reflex is usually not decreased, perhaps because compression selectively preserves A-δ and C fibers, and the corneal reflex is mediated by these unmyelinated fibers (Cruccu, Berardelli, & Manfredi 1987). This selectivity makes balloon compression especially useful as a percutaneous treatment of patients with V_1 TN pain. By contrast, thermal rhizotomy injures all fiber types nonselectively at temperatures required to create a clinical lesion; gamma knife radiosurgery has similar effects; and glycerol rhizotomy is not easily performed selectively.

Patients who have a history of herpes simplex may develop a labial eruption within days of operation. Mild ipsilateral temporal and masseter muscle weakness occurs in two-thirds of patients, but usually is of minimal

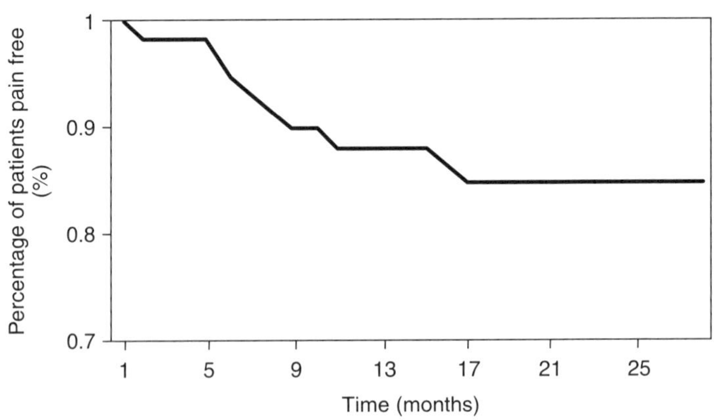

Figure 12.4 Kaplan-Meier analysis of pain recurrence following balloon compression for trigeminal neuralgia in patients who experienced initial pain relief.

The mean time until recurrence was 13 months. Results are expressed as the mean values +/− standard error of the mean. Reprinted from Brown JA, Pilitsis JG. Percutaneous balloon compression for the treatment of trigeminal neuralgia: results in 56 patients based on balloon compression pressure monitoring. *Neurosurg Focus* 2005;18:E10.

clinical relevance, as patients generally have avoided using that side of their mouths for years. If temporomandibular joint pain develops because of muscular imbalance created by the masseter muscle weakness, it is treated with oral anti-inflammatory medication until resolution.

RESULTS

One study of this procedure using Kaplan-Meier curves found a recurrence rate of 26% following balloon compression, with a mean time until recurrence of 18 months (Brown & Preul 1989; Brown, McDaniel, & Weaver 1993). The recurrence rate is 30% at 10 years (Mullan & Lichtor 1983). Recurrence rates are higher in patients with multiple sclerosis and may reach 50%. Recurrences are generally managed with carbamazepine or other anticonvulsants. If medical therapy fails, the patient may have a repeat procedure. Repeat procedures are generally well tolerated and do not present increased technical difficulty. Lopez et al. (2004) summarized morbidity seen in three of the largest series of patients reviewed after balloon compression treatment for TN. There was a 1.5% incidence of cranial nerve deficits, 2.6% incidence of meningitis, 2% incidence of vascular complications, and 10% incidence of troublesome dysesthesias.[21] The vascular complications were noted early in the history of the procedure, before development of an FDA-approved kit that included a blunt obturator. Patients responding to a questionnaire designed to determine how they valued the results of their surgery for TN noted that balloon compression led to the most optimal opportunity for improved quality of life when compared to other ablative procedures (Spatz, Zakrzewska, & Kay 2007).

Numerous series have been published over the last two decades and have recognized other infrequent complications (Abdennebi, Bouatta, Chitti, & Bougatene 1997; Belber & Rak 1987; Brown & Gouda 1997; Connelley 1982; Correa & Teixeira 1998; Fiume et al. 1985; Lee & Chen 2003; Lobato, Rivas, Sarabia, & Lamas 1990; Meglio, Cioni, Moles, & Visocchi 1990; Mizuno, Saito, Takayasu, & Yoshida 2000; Natarajan 2000; Skirving & Dan 2001; Urculo et al. 2004; Zanusso & Columbo 1990). One case report described balloon compression causing subarachnoid hemorrhage leading to death. In that case, the surgeon used a sharp obturator that passed through the foramen ovale (Spaziante, Cappabianc, Peca, & de Divitis 1988). A carotid cavernous fistula and an external carotid fistula have also been reported (Revuelta et al. 1993). Because of these cases, only a cannula with a blunt obturator should be used to reach the foramen ovale after penetrating the soft tissue of the cheek.

CONCLUSION

Percutaneous balloon compression is a simple and effective treatment for TN that has been used successfully for more than two decades. It is especially useful in patients with V_1 pain because it does not injure the myelinated fibers that mediate the blink reflex. It is most helpful in patients with pain that has spread across multiple division because it does not require multiple lesions. It also useful in patients with whom it would be difficult to communicate with during selective thermal rhizotomy. It is relatively easy to perform once the principles of the technique are understood.

REFERENCES

Abdennebi B, Bouatta F, Chitti M, Bougatene B. Percutaneous balloon compression of the Gasserian ganglion in trigeminal neuralgia. Long-term results in 150 cases. *Acta Neurochir (Wien)* 1995;136:72–74.

Andre N. Observations pratiques sur les maladies de l'urethre et sur plusieurs faits convulsifs, et la guerison de plusieurs maladies chirurgicales, avec la decomposition d'un remede propre a reprimer la dissolution gangreneuse et cancereuse et a la reparer, ... par M. Andre. Texte imprime. Paris: Delaguette; 1756.

Belber CJ, Rak RA. Balloon compression rhizolysis in the surgical management of trigeminal neuralgia. *Neurosurgery* 1987;20:908–913.

Brown JA, Coursaget C, Preul MC, Sangvai D. Mercury water and cauterizing stones: Nicolas Andre and tic douloureux. *J Neurosurg* 1999;90:977–981.

Brown JA, Gouda JJ. Percutaneous balloon compression of the trigeminal nerve. *Neurosurg Clin N Am* 1997;8:53–62.

Brown JA, Hoeflinger B, Long PB, et al. Axon and ganglion cell injury in rabbits after percutaneous trigeminal balloon compression. *Neurosurgery* 1996;38: 993–1003; discussion 1004.

Brown JA, McDaniel MD, Weaver MT. Percutaneous trigeminal nerve compression for treatment of trigeminal neuralgia: results in 50 patients. *Neurosurgery* 1993;32:570–573.

Brown JA, Pilitsis JG. Percutaneous balloon compression for the treatment of trigeminal neuralgia: results in 56 patients based on balloon compression pressure monitoring. *Neurosurg Focus* 2005;18:E10.

Brown JA, Preul MC. Percutaneous trigeminal ganglion compression for trigeminal neuralgia. Experience in 22 patients and review of the literature. *J Neurosurg* 1989;70:900–904.

Burchiel KJ. A new classification for facial pain. *Neurosurgery* 2003;53:1164–1166; discussion 6–7.

Connelley TJ. Balloon compression and trigeminal neuralgia. *Med J Aust* 1982;2:119.

Correa CF, Teixeira MJ. Balloon compression of the Gasserian ganglion for the treatment of trigeminal neuralgia. *Stereotact Funct Neurosurg* 1998;71:83–89.

Crawford JVW. Surgery for Pain. In: Walker AE, ed. *A history of neurological surgery*. Baltimore: Williams and Wilkins, 1951.

Cruccu G, Berardelli A, Manfredi M. Afferents for the human corneal reflex. *J Neurol* 1987;234:64.

Devor M, Govrin-Lippmann R, Rappaport ZH. Mechanism of trigeminal neuralgia: an ultrastructural analysis of trigeminal root specimens obtained during microvascular decompression surgery. *J Neurosurg* 2002;96:532–543.

Fiume D, Scarda G, Natali G, Della Valle G. [Percutaneous microcompression of the gasserian ganglion. New treatment for trigeminal neuralgia]. *Riv Neurol* 1985;55:387–391.

Hessen E, Lossius MI, Reinvang I, Gjerstad L. Influence of major antiepileptic drugs on attention, reaction time, and speed of information processing: results from a randomized, double-blind, placebo-controlled withdrawal study of seizure-free epilepsy patients receiving monotherapy. *Epilepsia* 2006;47: 2038–2045.

Lee ST, Chen JF. Percutaneous trigeminal ganglion balloon compression for treatment of trigeminal neuralgia, part II: results related to compression duration. *Surg Neurol* 2003;60:149–153; discussion 153–154.

Lobato RD, Rivas JJ, Sarabia R, Lamas E. Percutaneous microcompression of the gasserian ganglion for trigeminal neuralgia. *J Neurosurg* 1990;72:546–553.

Lopez BC, Hamlyn PJ, Zakrzewska JM. Systematic review of ablative neurosurgical techniques for the treatment of trigeminal neuralgia. *Neurosurgery* 2004;54: 973–982; discussion 82–83.

Love JG, Svien HJ. Results of decompression operation for trigeminal neuralgia. *J Neurosurg* 1954;11:499–504.

Meglio M, Cioni B, Moles A, Visocchi M. Microvascular decompression versus percutaneous procedures for typical trigeminal neuralgia: personal experience. *Stereotact Funct Neurosurg* 1990;54–55:76–79.

Mizuno M, Saito K, Takayasu M, Yoshida J. Percutaneous microcompression of the trigeminal ganglion for elderly patients with trigeminal neuralgia and patients with atypical trigeminal neuralgia. *Neurol Med Chir (Tokyo)* 2000;40: 347–350; discussion 350–351.

Mullan S, Lichtor T. Percutaneous microcompression of the trigeminal ganglion for trigeminal neuralgia. *J Neurosurg* 1983;59:1007–1012.

Mullan S. Percutaneous cordotomy for pain. *Surg Clin North Am* 1966;46:3–12.

Natarajan M. Percutaneous trigeminal ganglion balloon compression: experience in 40 patients. *Neurol* India 2000;48:330–332.

Preul MC, Long PB, Brown JA, et al. Autonomic and histopathological effects of percutaneous trigeminal ganglion compression in the rabbit. *J Neurosurg* 1990;72:933–940.

Revuelta R, Nathal E, Balderrama J, et al. External carotid artery fistula due to microcompression of the gasserian ganglion for relief of trigeminal neuralgia. Case report. *J Neurosurg* 1993;78:499–500.

Shelden CH, Pudenz RH, Freshwater DB, Crue BL. Compression rather than decompression for trigeminal neuralgia. *J Neurosurg* 1955;12:123–126.

Skirving DJ, Dan NG. A 20-year review of percutaneous balloon compression of the trigeminal ganglion. *J Neurosurg* 2001;94:913–917.

Spatz AL, Zakrzewska JM, Kay EJ. Decision analysis of medical and surgical treatments for trigeminal neuralgia: how patient evaluations of benefits and risks affect the utility of treatment decisions. *Pain* 2007;131:302–310.

Spaziante R, Cappabianca P, Peca C, de Divitiis E. Subarachnoid hemorrhage and "normal pressure hydrocephalus": fatal complication of percutaneous microcompression of the gasserian ganglion. Case report. *Neurosurgery* 1988; 22:148–151.

Stookey BRJ, Ransohff J. *Trigeminal neuralgia: It's history and treatment.* Springfield IL: Charles C. Thomas, 1959.

Svien HJ, Love JG. Results of decompression operation for trigeminal neuralgia four years plus after operation. *J Neurosurg* 1959;16:653–655.

Sweet WH, Wepsic JG. Controlled thermocoagulation of trigeminal ganglion and rootlets for differential destruction of pain fibers. 1. Trigeminal neuralgia. *J Neurosurg* 1974;40:143–156.

Taarnhoj P. Decompression of the trigeminal root and the posterior part of the ganglion as treatment in trigeminal neuralgia; preliminary communication. *J Neurosurg* 1952;9:288–290.

Urculo E, Alfaro R, Arrazola M, et al. Trochlear nerve palsy after repeated percutaneous balloon compression for recurrent trigeminal neuralgia: case report and pathogenic considerations. *Neurosurgery* 2004;54:505–508; discussion 508–509.

Zanusso M, Colombo F. Percutaneous microcompression for trigeminal neuralgia. *J Neurosurg* 1990;73:804–805.

13

Stereotactic Radiosurgery

Mark E. Linskey

Stereotactic radiosurgery (SR) along with radiofrequency lesioning (RFL), glycerol rhizotomy (GR), and percutaneous balloon compression (BC), is one of the four most commonly utilized palliative destructive procedures for classic trigeminal neuralgia (Mathews MS et al. (in press); Zakrzewska JM et al., 2008; Zakrzewska JM et al., 2009). Palliative destructive procedures do not attempt to cure the syndrome by addressing its likely cause (vascular compression). Rather, the goal is to attempt to ameliorate the symptom through controlled damage to the trigeminal ganglion or nerve root. In essence, one trades relief of the symptom for risk of trigeminal deficits from the nerve subtotal damage purposefully inflicted. With all of these four procedures, the surgeon purposely damages the trigeminal nerve root or ganglia in a controlled and partial manner. With RFL, the damage is thermocoagulation using an electrode. With GR, the damage is chemical using alcohol (glycerol). With BC, the damage is mechanical, stemming from crushing the nerve against rigid dural reflections or bone. With SR, the damage is a single very high dose of focused radiation (Zakrzewska and Linskey 2008).

DEFINITION AND TECHNIQUES

According to the definition agreed upon by the American Association of Neurological Surgeons (AANS), Congress of Neurological Surgeons (CNS), and the American Society for Therapeutic Radiology and Oncology (ASTRO) (Barnett, et al. 2007):

> Stereotactic radiosurgery is a distinct discipline that uses externally generated ionizing radiation in certain cases to inactivate or eradicate (a) defined target(s) in the head or spine without the need to make an incision. The target is defined by high-resolution stereotactic imaging. To assure quality of patient care, the procedure involves a multidisciplinary team consisting of a neurosurgeon, radiation oncologist, and medical physicist.
>
> Stereotactic radiosurgery typically is performed in a single session, using a rigidly attached stereotactic guiding device, other immobilization technology, and/or a stereotactic image-guidance system, but can be performed in a limited number of sessions up to a maximum of five.

Technologies that are used to perform stereotactic radiosurgery include linear accelerators, particle beam accelerators, and multisource Cobalt 60 units. In order to enhance precision, various devices may incorporate robotics and real-time imaging.

When it comes to functional lesioning neurosurgery such as TN SR, the procedure is performed in a single session at very high single dose in order to maximize lesioning effect on normal tissue. By far and away, the most commonly used technology for TN SR has been the Gamma Knife® (Håkanson S, Leksell L. 1977) (GK; Elekta AB, Stockholm) delivery system. With the GK 201- (older U, B, and C units), or 192- (newer Perfexion unit) Cobalt 60 sources are collimated onto a 4 mm diameter focal point (isocenter) that is targeted stereotactically. In a small number of cases so far, rotational linear accelerator (LINAC) technology has been utilized to collimate down to a 5 mm focal point using various LINAC devices (Chen 2004, 2008; De Salles et al. 2008; Gorgulho & De Salles 2006; Gorghulo et al. 2006; Pusztaszeri et al. 2007; Rahimian et al. 2004). Also in a small number of cases, a robotic step-and-shoot technique using the CyberKnife® (Accuray, Sunnyvale, California) has been used in either isocentric technique, and even more recently in a non-isocentric volume target manner to treat patients with TN (Adler et al. 2009; Fariselli et al. 2009; Lim et al. 2005; Patil et al. 2007; Romanelli et al. 2003; Tarricone et al. 2008; Villavicencio et al. 2008). So far, particle beam SR technology has not been applied to TN.

HISTORY

Radiofrequency lesioning is the oldest of the four currently popular palliative destructive procedures, having been developed by Sweet in the late 1960s (Sweet & Wepsic 1970). Glycerol rhizotomy was developed by Håkanson in the late 1970s and reported in 1981 (Håkanson 1981). Balloon compression was developed by Mullan in the early 1980s and published in 1983 (Mullan & Lichtor 1983).

Stereotactic radiosurgery was conceived by Lars Leksell prior to all these procedures in 1951 (Leksell 1951). However, it took him until 1967 to develop and perfect the GK delivery system, which he first applied to patients in 1967 (Linskey & Kuo in press). Trigeminal neuralgia was an early concern for application, and the first report of GKSR came out in 1971 (Leksell 1971). It is a curious piece of TN history that GR was actually accidently discovered in the 1970s while trying to develop a way to target the trigeminal ganglia for GKSR (Håkanson S et al., 1977). Glycerol was initially chosen as a carrier to deliver tantalum dust in suspension to the trigeminal cistern, so that the ganglion could be seen on plain x-ray. Patients became pain-free prior to SR, and GR went on to supplant SR at the Karolinska institute. Stereotactic radiosurgery did not reemerge as a treatment for TN until accurate targeting could be solved in the post-magnetic resonance imaging (MRI) era, with the preganglionic trigeminal nerve root chosen as the target.

The key milestone in reassessing SR as a potential treatment for TN was the development of high-resolution volumetric MRI, which allowed the trigeminal nerve to be directly visualized and accurately targeted in three dimensions. This targeting technique also allowed the target site to be moved behind the ganglion, onto the trigeminal nerve root. With this advance, a multi-institution pilot study investigating GKSR for TN was initiated in the early 1990s and published in 1996 (Kondziolka et al. 1996). This landmark study showed very promising results, and the use of GKSR for TN literally exploded over the next 10 years (Fig. 13.1). By the end of 2006, with only 80% of the worldwide gamma units reporting their data,

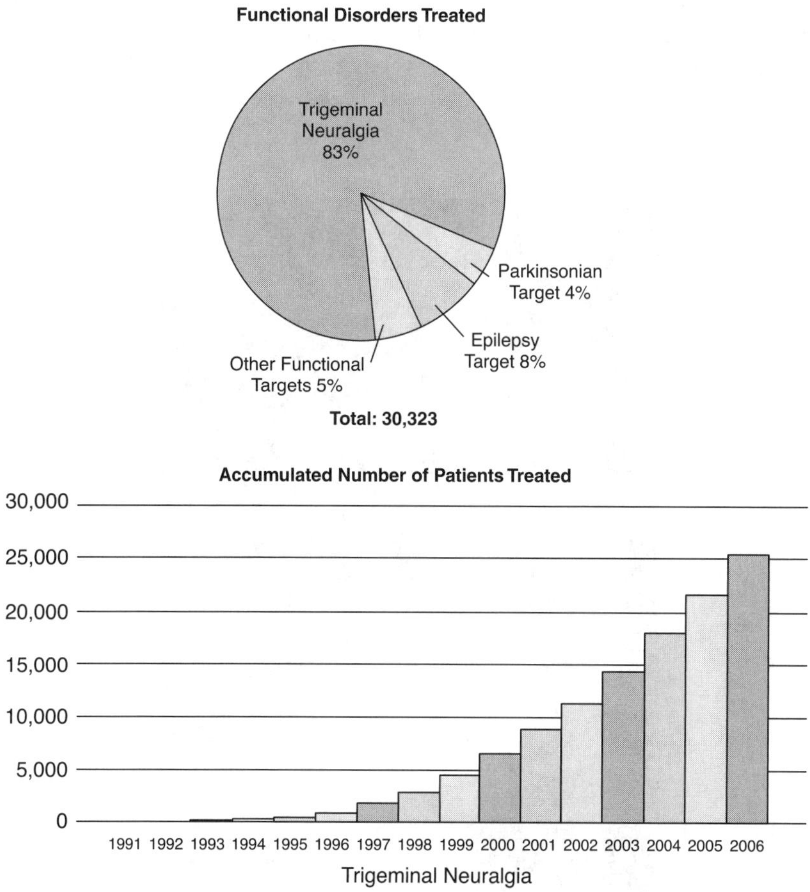

Figure 13.1 Graph depicting rise in frequency of gamma knife stereotactic radiosurgery (GKSR) for trigeminal neuralgia 1996–2006.

With only 80% of active gamma units reporting, by 2006 more than 4,000 cases were being treated per year worldwide. http://www.elekta.com/assets/gamma_knife_surgery/pdfs/ww06_us.pdf

more than 25,000 TN patients had been treated worldwide, and the annual treatment rate exceeded 4,000 TN patients per year (http://www.elekta.com/assets/gamma_knife_surgery/pdfs/ww06_us.pdf). By the end of 2006, GKSR has surpassed all surgical interventions in number of TN patients treated per year.

TECHNIQUE

With GKSR, a Leksell model G stereotactic frame (Elekta AB, Stockholm) is affixed to the patients head under local anesthesia with four-point percutaneous fixation (Fig. 13.2). A contrast-enhanced volumetric, fine-cut, targeting MRI data set is then obtained with the MR stereotactic localizer attached to the coordinate frame. For patients with pacemakers, computed tomography (CT) cisternography is utilized for targeting purposes (Fig. 13.3). Any point inside the patient's head can now be precisely defined in three dimensions by an X-, Y-, and Z- coordinate on the stereotactic frame.

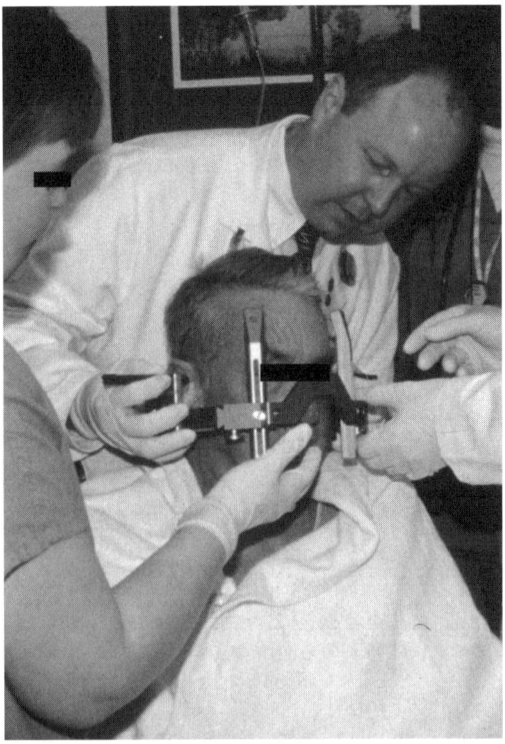

Figure 13.2 A patient undergoing percutaneous Leksell model G stereotactic frame placement under local anesthesia in preparation for gamma knife stereotactic radiosurgery for trigeminal neuralgia.

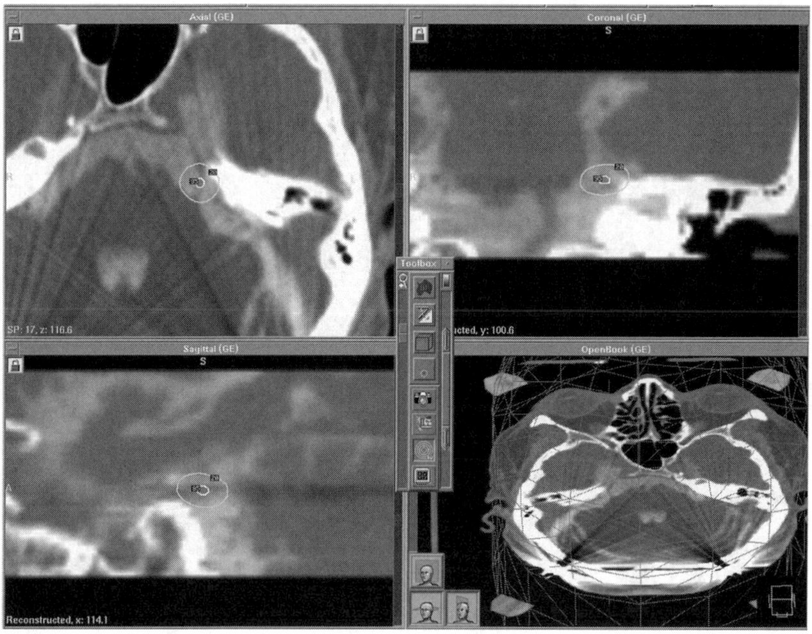

Figure 13.3 An example of a computed tomography cisternogram utilized for trigeminal nerve root targeting for patients with pacemakers with the SR treatment plan indicated.

Once the targeting imaging dataset is reconstructed on the computer targeting workstation, Leksell GammPlan® software is used to place the maximum dose point of the 4 mm isocenter directly within the trigeminal nerve root, confirming placement in all three planes. In my practice, I intentionally move the isocenter as close to the brainstem surface as allowable, while keeping the maximum brainstem surface dose no higher than 16 Gy. Depending on the length of the cisternal course of the trigeminal nerve root and the angle of take-off of the nerve, this leads to the need for custom source-blocking patterns in approximately 50% of cases, to custom sculpt the steepness and angle of the radiation fall-off at the brainstem surface interface (Figs. 13.4 and 13.5). For patients with classic TN, we use a maximum dose of 80 Gy. For patients with at least some atypical features or who have multiple sclerosis, we prescribe 90 Gy as the maximal dose.

Once planning is complete, the patient is placed on the gamma unit couch with the frame docked in position (Fig. 13.6). For U-, B-, and some C-units, the docking is performed at the isocenter coordinates. For the 4C- and the Perfexion unit, the couch robotically moves to the correct coordinate position automatically. For the U-, B-, C-units, the 4 mm collimator is preselected and put into place before docking the patient, and any source

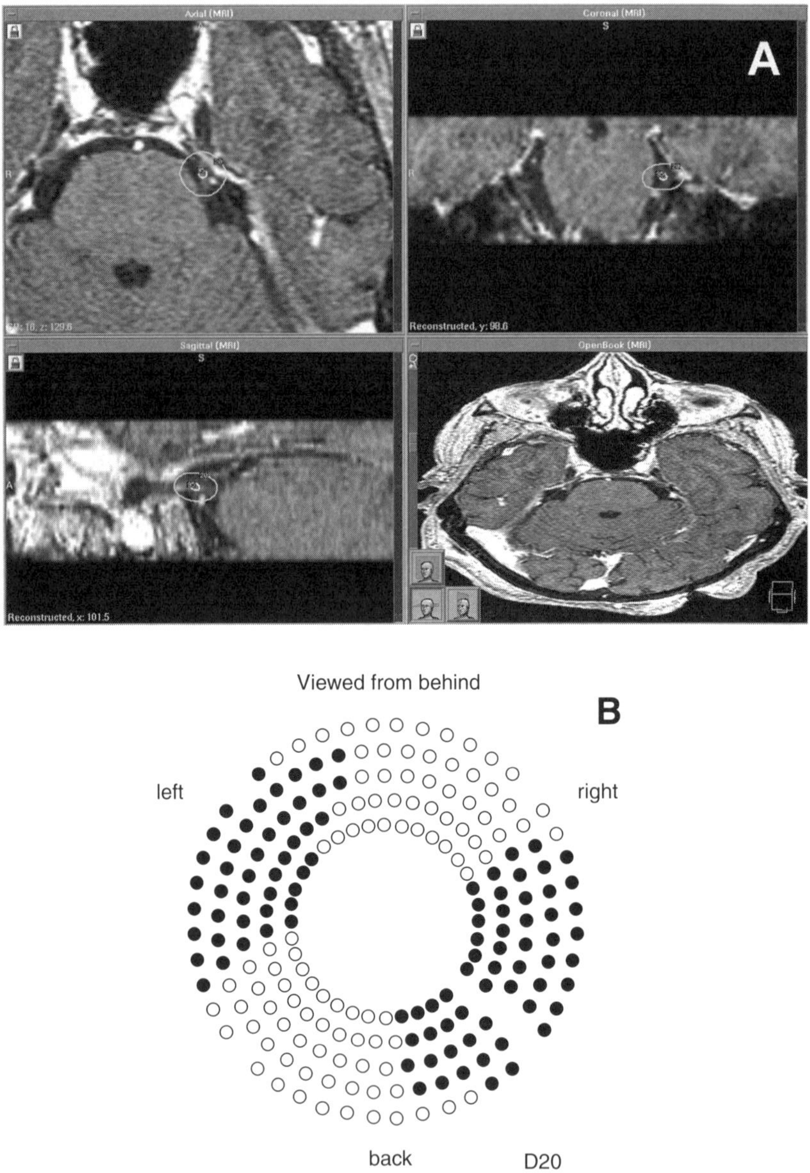

Figure 13.4a,b Examples of magnetic resonance stereotactic targeting of the trigeminal nerve root with an unblocked plan, a custom isocenter beam blocking pattern, and the resultant SR treatment plan using the beam blocking plan for a patient treated with a gamma knife B-unit.

Maximum dose is 80 Gy and the 20% isodose line indicated corresponds to 16 Gy, which is set flush with the surface of the brainstem.

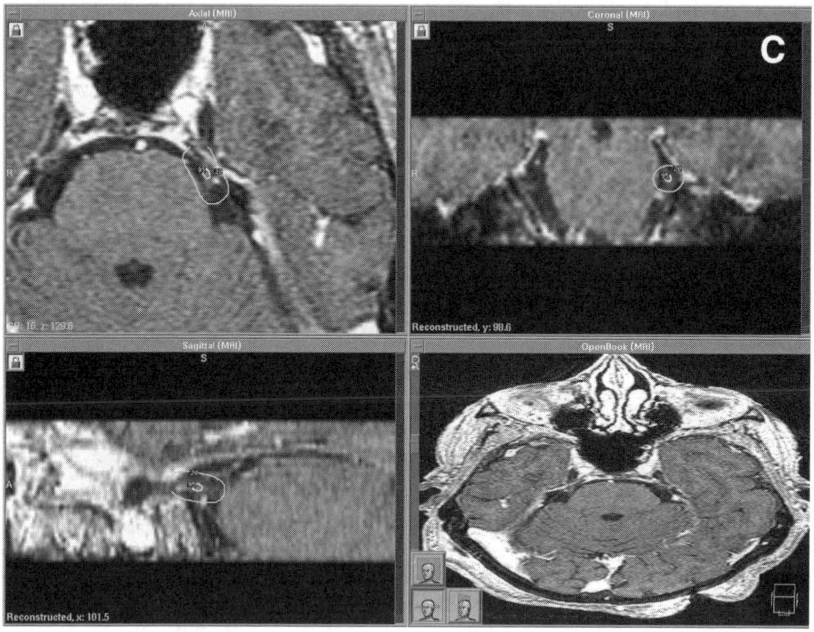

Figure 13.4c (Continued)

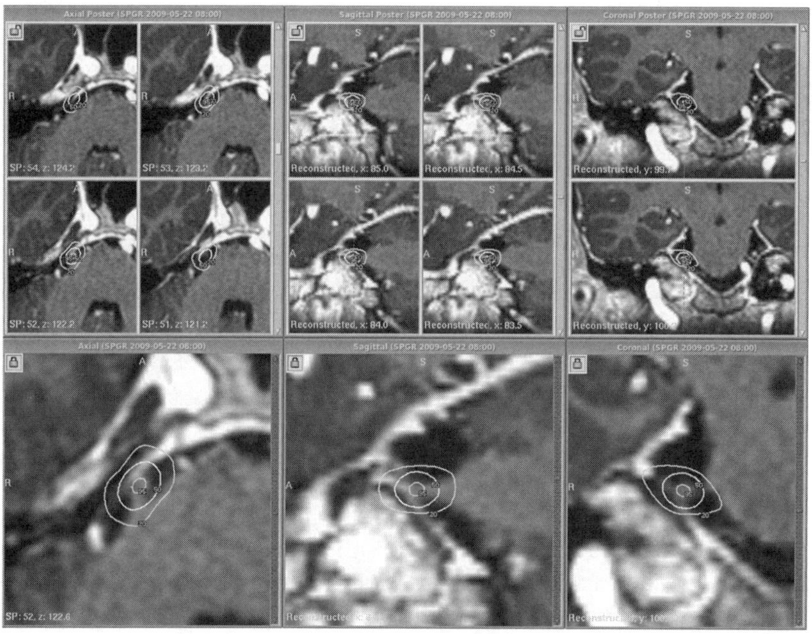

Figure 13.5 Examples of magnetic resonance stereotactic targeting of the trigeminal nerve root with an unblocked plan, and the resultant customized SR treatment plan using the two sector blocks for a patient treated with a Gamma Knife Perfexion unit.

Maximum dose is 80 Gy and the 20% isodose line indicated corresponds to 16 Gy, which is set flush with the surface of the brainstem.

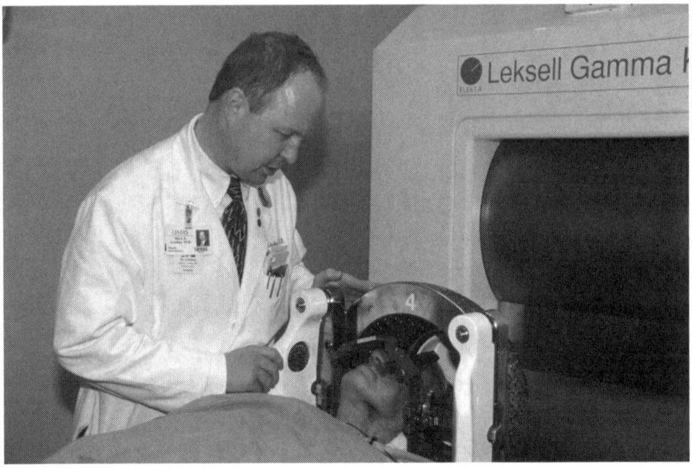

Figure 13.6 A patient placed on the Gamma Knife B-unit gantry with his frame set at the proper coordinates and the 4 mm collimator in place in preparation for gamma knife stereotactic radiosurgery for trigeminal neuralgia.

blocking is performed and checked manually. With the Perfexion unit, the collimator size and any sector blocking is performed automatically by the computer control unit through an automatic electronic switch mechanism. Depending on the need for blocking pattern and the age of the Cobalt 60, treatment time ranges from 20 minutes to approximately 90 minutes. The patient enters the unit for treatment delivery, which is painless. At the conclusion of the treatment, the patient is removed from the unit, the frame removed, the pin sites dressed, and the patient sent home after a brief period of observation. The procedure is performed on an outpatient basis.

RESULTS

The results of GKSR have now been published and confirmed from multiple gamma units worldwide, representing several thousand published cases. Table 13.1 shows the compilation results of 14 selected published series representing 1,295 treated cases, with sufficient case numbers, length of follow-up and treatment and results documentation to extract and compare results (Brisman 2000, 2007; Brisman & Mooij 2000; Dellaretti et al. 2008; Huang et al. 2008; Knafo, Kenny, & Mathieu 2009; Kondziolka et al. 1996; Linskey, Ratanatharathorn, & Penagaricano 2008; Longhi et al. 2007; Maesawa et al. 2001; Nicol et al. 2000; Pollock 2002; Pollock 2005; Régis et al. 2006; Rogers et al. 2000; Young, Vermulen, & Posewitz 1998).

Table 13.1 Compilation table of selected published results utilizing GKSR to treat trigeminal neuralgia

Institution	Year	No. Patients	Dose (Gy)	Median Follow-up (range)	Pain free, no medications	Significantly improved ± medications (threshold criteria)
Universite de Sherbrooke, Canada (Knafo 2009)	2009	67	80	6 months	34.3%	32.6% (pain-free) 77.6% (≥50% pain free)
University of Arkansas, USA (Linskey 2008)	2008	44	80*	2.9 years (.17–6.9 years)	45.5%	68.2% (≥75% pain free) 86.4% (≥50% pain free)
Chun-Shan Medical University, Taiwan (Huang 2008)	2008	89	79 (60–90)	5 years (2.7–7.25 years)	56%	62% (pain free +/– medications) 69.8% (≥50% pain free
Santa Casa Hospital, Brazil (Dellaretti 2008)	2008	76	85.1 (75–90)	1.7 years (0.5–3.5 years)	Not Reported	62% (Pain free +/– medications at 3 years, actuarial)
Verona University Hospital, Italy (Londhi 2007)	2007	160	(75–95 Gy)	3.1 years (0.5–12 years)	61%	89% (Pain free +/– medications)
Timone University Hospital, France (Regis 2006)	2006	100	85 (70–90)	1 year (1 Year)	58%	83% (pain free +/– medications)
Columbia University, USA (Brisman 2006)	2006	61	75	1.5 years (.25–2.5 years)	24%	48% (≥90% pain free +/– medications)
Mayo Clinic, USA (Pollock 2002)	2002	117	80–90	2.2 years (.08–4 years)	59%	75% (≥50% pain free)
University of Pittsburgh, USA (Maeswawa 2001)	2001	220	60–90	2.0 years (0.5–6.5 years)	40%	69.1% (≥50% pain free)
Columbia University, USA (Brisman 2000)	2000	105	75	6 months (0.5–1 year)	Not Reported	80–81.1% (≥50% pain free)
Barrows Neurological Institute, USA (Rogers 2000)	2000	54	70–80	1 year (.25–2 years)	35%	89% (some relief)
University of Kentucky, USA (Nicol 2000)	2000	42	90	1.2 years (.17–2.5 years)	66.7%	95.2% (≥50% pain free)
Northwest Neuroscience Institute, USA (Young 1998)	1998	110	70–80	1.7 years (.33–4.1 years)	54%†	88.2% (≥50% pain free)
Multi-Institution GK Study, USA (Kondziolka 1996)	1996	50	60–90	1.5 years (.72–3 years)	58%‡	94% (≥50% pain free)

*42/44 cases utilized 80 Gy, only 2/44 utilized 90 Gy

†76% initially pain free off all medication. However, 34% of the 88.2% with ≥50% pain relief had a recurrence of pain by follow-up. Assuming an equal distribution among those pain-free off all medication versus those partially improved, the calculated percentage of patients pain-free off all meds at latest follow-up would be 54%

‡No distinction made between those pain free-off medication and those pain-free requiring medication

Time to Pain Relief

Patients need to be counseled that GKSR does not work right away. It takes time for a radiation-induced lesion to develop and mature. In my series, the median time to pain relief is 4 weeks (mean, 7.5 weeks; range, 1 week–6 months) (Linskey et al. 2008). We generally keep patients on their preoperative TN medications until they become pain-free, assessing them at 3 and 6 months after SR. If they become pain-free, the TN medications are then weaned off over several weeks. We do not consider GKSR to have failed until 6 months after SR.

Definition of Success and Rates of Pain Relief

Reported success rates after GKSR are critically dependent upon the definition of success applied. In pharmaceutical trials of new drugs for TN, the standard success endpoint used is 50% or greater pain improvement. On the other hand, in surgical trials, such as those for microvascular decompression (MVD), the gold standard endpoint is a patient who is pain-free, off all medications. As depicted in Table 13.1, SR results have been reported using endpoints that vary across a wide spectrum (some pain relief, ≥50% pain improvement, >75% pain improvement, ≥90% pain improvement, pain-free with medications, pain-free without medications).

If one utilizes the strictest endpoint of pain-free, no medications, it is clear from Table 13.1 that GKSR achieves this goal in an average of 49% of patients (range of result, 24%–66.7%), over an average mean follow-up period of 2 years (range, 0.08–7.25 years). On the other hand, if one uses 50% or greater pain improvement as the criteria, GKSR achieves this goal in an average of 81.8% of patients (range of result, 69.1%–95.2%), over the same average follow-up interval.

Unfortunately, these results are not stable over time, but steadily deteriorate with increasing time from the date of treatment. In a report critiquing published reports of TN treatments, Zakrzewska and Lopez emphasized the need for independent assessment of pain relief results, as well as the critical importance of actuarial life table analysis (Zakrzewska & Lopez 2003). The latter is especially important for palliative destructive procedures for classic TN, which appear to have a steady rate of recurrence, given that the vascular compression is not addressed by the intervention. Zakrzewska and Lopez went on to survey the literature to perform a meta-analysis of those TN SR reports that did include life table analysis through the end of 2003 (Lopez, Hamlyn, & Zakrzewska 2004a, 2004b). Although they only identified three studies that met this criteria, the results were important. Given an endpoint of pain-free +/− medications (a looser definition than pain-free off all medications), the success rate of GKSR in these three studies was 66% at 1 year, falling off to 59% by 2 years and 56% by 3 years (Lopez et al. 2004a).

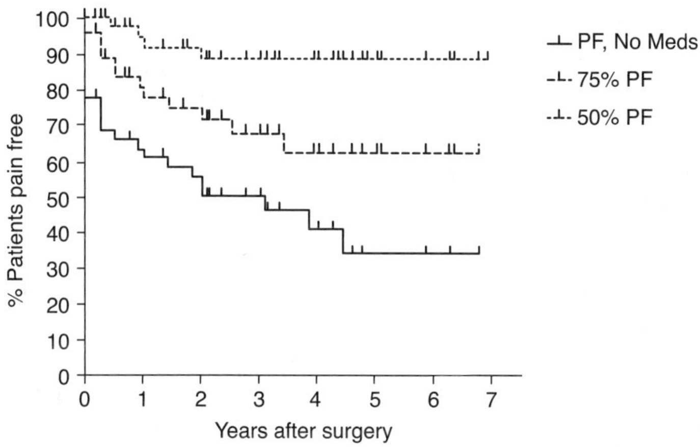

Figure 13.7 Kaplan-Meier life table analysis plots of pain control rates after gamma knife stereotactic radiosurgery for trigeminal neuralgia using three different outcome endpoints.

All three lines represent results from the same prospective cohort of patients, but each utilizes a different pain control outcome measure. The upper line depicts ≥50% pain free rates, which are 100%, 98%, 92%, and 88%, initially, at 1 year, at 2 years, and at 3 years after stereotactic radiosurgery. The middle line depicts >75% pain-free rates, which are 96%, 83%, 72%, and 62%, initially, at 1 year, at 2 years, and at 3 years after stereotactic radiosurgery. The lowest line depicts pain-free, off all medication rates, which are 78%, 66%, 50%, and 33%, initially, at 1 year, at 2 years, and at 3 years after stereotactic radiosurgery. From Linskey ME, Ratanatharathorn V, Penagaricano J. A prospective cohort study of microvascular decompression and Gamma Knife surgery in patients with trigeminal neuralgia. *J Neurosurg* 2008;109:160–172.

In our own series, using the strictest pain-free, off all medication endpoint, we experienced a GKSR success rate of 78% initially, 66% at 1 year, 50% at 2 years, and 33% at 3 years after treatment (Fig. 13.7). If we loosened the criteria to greater than 75% pain relief, we found a GKSR success rate of 96% initially, 83% at 1 year, 72% at 2 years, and 62% at 3 years after treatment. If we loosened the criteria all the way to 50% or greater pain relief, we found a GKSR success rate of 100% initially, 98% at 1 year, 92% at 2 years, and 88% at 3 years after treatment (Linskey et al. 2008).

Clearly, defining the endpoint definition, as well as the time of assessment after SR, is critical when assessing SR results. Many Internet websites for SR units only refer to unqualified percentage success rates in their content, usually defaulting to 50% or greater pain relief results. Unqualified, quoted success rates of 80%–95% are extremely attractive, and seductive to patients. Unfortunately, we also find that patients have often been presented unqualified percentages for SR success rates when treatment options are discussed prior to referral to our clinic for second opinion. These are areas in which we must improve patient counseling and preoperative education.

Complications

In our GKSR series (Linskey et al. 2008), there has been no mortality or major morbidity. One patient experienced transient headache and a second transient nausea the evening after GKSR, which subsequently resolved. Cranial nerve complications have been restricted to the trigeminal nerve. Four patients (9.1%) experienced transient facial paresthesias that subsequently completely resolved 2–6 months after onset. Three patients (6.8%) experienced permanent new mild paresthesias or numbness. One patient (2.3%) experienced more severe permanent sensory numbness. Thus, the overall incidence of any trigeminal symptom was 18.8%, the overall incidence of permanent trigeminal symptom was 9.1%, and for significant permanent trigeminal symptom 2.3%. There was no case of trigeminal motor weakness or anesthesia dolorosa. Mean onset of trigeminal symptoms was 3.8 months after GKSR (range, 1 day–9 months; SD, 2.8 months).

Our results are similar to those reported at most GKSR centers, where, with maximal doses of 90 Gy or less (new 4 mm collimator output factor) and a single isocenter treatment, permanent mild trigeminal numbness rates are 10% or less, and permanent significant numbness rates are less than 5% (Brisman 2000, 2007; Brisman & Mooij 2000; Dellarettti et al. 2008; Huang et al. 2008; Knafo et al. 2009; Kondziolka et al. 1996; Linskey et al. 2008; Longhi et al. 2007; Maesawa et al. 2001; Nicol et al. 2000; Pollock et al. 2002, 2005; Régis et al. 2006; Rogers et al. 2000; Young et al. 1998). Contrary to popular belief, corneal ulceration and painful dysesthesias have occurred after GKSR; however, these findings are associated with doses of 100 Gy or more (≥90 Gy old 4 mm collimator output factor), as well as with repeat GKSR (Pollock et al. 2001, 2005). There is also at least one case report of subsequent posterior fossa exploration after GKSR, suggesting the potential for atherosclerotic changes in adjacent blood vessels (Maher & Pollock 2000). This observation has yet to be confirmed by others in the field.

Unlike other percutaneous palliative destructive procedures such as RFL, GR, and BC, motor trigeminal weakness and the reflex autonomic effects (bradycardia, tachycardia, hypotension, hypertension, and/or arrhythmias) often experienced during lesioning (which can be dangerous in elderly patients with cardiac conditions), as well as the rare instances of meningitis, subarachnoid hemorrhage, or carotid-cavernous fistula occasionally seen with percutaneous procedures, have not been reported.

Although induction of neoplasia is a theoretical possibility after any radiation exposure, including SR (Loeffler, Niemierko, & Chapman 2003; McIver & Pollock 2004), it has yet to be reported after GKSR for TN.

Failure, Recurrence and Retreatment

Almost all patients initially respond to GKSR if one uses a 50% or greater pain relief criteria. However, if the strictest criteria of pain-free off all medication is the criteria applied, in our experience 12% of patients fail to respond at any time to GKSR (Linskey et al. 2008). In addition, the observation that pain control continues to deteriorate over time with GKSR, just as with any other palliative destructive procedure, implies that recurrence rates will critically depend on the measurement point after SR, and will likely continue to increase over time. If you eliminate those patients who never responded from consideration, our 1-, 2-, and 3-year recurrence rates after successful GKSR (pain-free off all medication) are 12%, 28%, and 45%, respectively. If we use the loosest 50% or greater pain-free endpoint, our 1-, 2-, and 3-year recurrence rates after successful GKSR are 2%, 8%, and 12%, respectively. Depending on the patient's perception and interpretation of the desirability of retreatment for these endpoints, anywhere from 12% to 45% of initially successful GKSR patients may opt for retreatment of some sort, versus living with their partial result, by 3 years after treatment. Our subjective impression is that this figure is approximately 25% at 3–5 years.

Retreatment after GKSR carries greater risks of trigeminal numbness, corneal ulceration, and painful dysesthesias (Gellner et al. 2008; Pollock et al. 2005). In our practice, we wait a minimum of 12 months after initial GKSR before considering exposure to a second lesion, to allow for maximal biological recovery before submitting the nerve to a potentially cumulative dose. Repeat GKSR warrants a lower dose, given the cumulative effect of radiation dose over time. If the retreatment is performed within 5 years of the initial SR, we generally deliver a maximum dose of 60 Gy. If the time period is longer, higher doses can be considered.

Patient Satisfaction

The main drawback to GKSR for TN from most patient's perspective is the latency of therapeutic effect, requiring the patient to remain on TN medications while both patient and physician await response. On the other hand, the outpatient and minimally invasive nature of the procedure, with avoidance of the percutaneous foramen ovale needle, are very attractive to patients.

In our study (Linskey et al. 2008), we performed patient satisfaction surveys at 5 and 8 years into the prospective cohort study. We asked two basic questions at each interval. First: Were patients satisfied with the procedure and, if they found themselves in similar circumstances, would they still make the same choice? Second: If a friend or relative found themselves in similar circumstances, would they recommend GKSR? The answers to the two questions were yes for 100% of GKSR patients 5 years into the study, but fell off to 75% for both questions 8 years into the study. Thus, patients are initially extremely satisfied with GKSR as an operative procedure for TN, but this level of satisfaction falls off in parallel to loss of pain control. A similar drop was not seen for MVD patients, who remained 100% yes for both questions at the 8 year mark. Ultimately, pain control influences patient satisfaction more than degree of surgical invasiveness and temporary need for hospitalization (Linskey et al. 2008).

COMPARISON WITH OTHER PALLIATIVE DESTRUCTIVE PROCEDURES

Percutaneous procedures can provide immediate pain relief. The main implication for a balanced multimodality TN treatment approach is that there remains a place for percutaneous palliative destructive procedures for patients who cannot, or prefer not, to undergo MVD and are clinically in extremis from their pain. In our algorithm, this role is filled by GR, with reversion to RFL if a technically satisfactory contrast cisternogram cannot be obtained. Fortunately, the majority of patients achieve enough partial control from antiepileptic drugs to allow the time for the GKSR lesion to mature and have full effect.

The rapid and enthusiastic preference for GKSR as the currently most popular palliative destructive procedure appears to be predominantly related to: (1) a lower risk of numbness, unpleasant dysesthesia, or exposure keratitis; (2) a lower risk of motor trigeminal weakness; (3) elimination of the invasive percutaneous needle; (4) elimination of the need for pulse anesthesia during foramen ovale needle transit and actual lesioning; (5) elimination of the reflex autonomic effects (bradycardia, tachycardia, hypotension, hypertension, and/or arrhythmias) often experienced during lesioning, which can be dangerous in elderly patients with cardiac conditions; (5) elimination of the rare risks of meningitis, subarachnoid hemorrhage or carotid-cavernous fistula occasionally seen with percutaneous procedures; and (6) the relative newness, novelty, and high-technology aspects of GKSR compared with other palliative destructive procedures. In my practice, GKSR took over the first, or primary, palliative destructive procedure position from GR in our multimodality treatment algorithm for TN in 1999.

COMPARISON WITH MICROVASCULAR DECOMPRESSION

Currently, in addition to our own report, two publications in the literature compare the results of MVD versus GKSR performed by the same surgeon (Pollock et al. 2005; Brisman 2007; Linskey et al. 2008). One is a retrospective studies (Pollock et al. 2005), and the other two are prospective cohort clinical trials (Brisman 2007; Linskey et al. 2008). As such, the latter studies represent Class II evidence-based medicine (EBM) data, whereas the former study qualifies as Class III evidence (Linskey 2006).

Pollock retrospectively reviewed his experience over a 5-year period with 77 patients less than 70 years old, 49 of whom underwent MVD, and 28 of whom were treated with GKSR (Pollock et al. 2005). With a mean follow up of 2.15 years, actuarial rates of pain-free status at 1 and 3 years were 75% and 72% for MVD and 59% and 59% for GKSR ($p = 0.01$). Brisman performed a prospective cohort study of MVD versus GKSR in a series of

85 patients (24 MVD and 61 GKSR). With very short clinical follow-up, he reported 12- and 18-month pain-free rates of 68% and 68% for MVD and 58% and 24% for GKSR. These results did not achieve statistical significance ($p = .089$) and suffered from an unusually low success rate with MVD (68% pain-free vs. an average of 75%–80% in most large MVD experiences), as well as an unusually low GKSR treatment dose (75 Gy) and resultant pain-free success rate (24% vs. an average of 49% in Table 13.1).

Our study represents the largest prospective cohort comparative study with the longest clinical follow-up published to date. The results for achieving pain-free status are highly significant at $p = 0.0002$ (Fig. 13.8), and the relative risk for losing pain-free status by 5 years after surgery is 3.35 for GKSR compared with MVD. Using EBM criteria (Linskey 2006), this study represents Class II evidence for the superiority of MVD over GKSR for patients with typical TN. A disingenuous approach to comparing GKSR and MVD would be to use percentages from a different endpoint for GKSR as opposed to MVD. However, even comparing greater than75% pain-free rates after GKSR with pain-free, off all medication, rates for MVD (Fig. 13.9), the trend strongly favors MVD ($p = 0.0892$). It is not until one compares 50% or greater pain-free rates after GKSR with pain-free, off all medication, rates for MVD that the two operative interventions appear equivalent (Fig. 13.9).

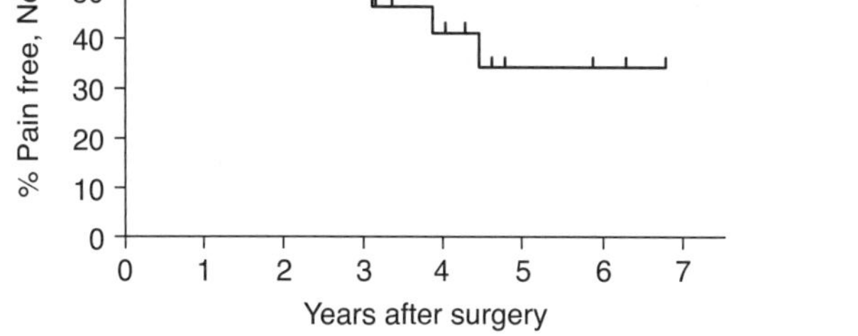

Figure 13.8 Kaplan-Meier life table analysis plots of pain free off all medication rates for microvascular decompression (MVD) versus gamma knife stereotactic radiosurgery (GKSR).

MVD significantly provided superior pain control over all times measured ($p = 0.0002$). From Linskey ME, Ratanatharathorn V, Penagaricano J. A prospective cohort study of microvascular decompression and Gamma Knife surgery in patients with trigeminal neuralgia. *J Neurosurg* 2008;109:160–172.

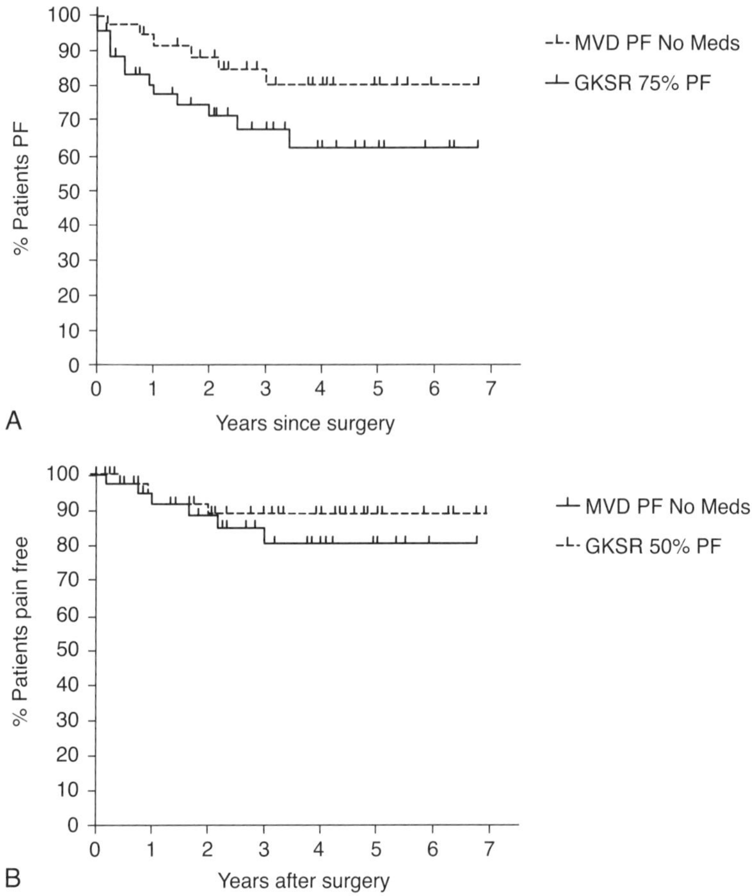

Figure 13.9 Kaplan-Meier life table analysis plots comparing different microvascular decompression (MVD) versus gamma knife stereotactic surgery (GKSR) pain control end points.

In (A) pain-free, off all medication rates for MVD are compared against >75% pain free rates for GKSR. A strong trend favors MVD even with this asymmetric comparison, but does not reach statistical significance ($p = 0.0892$). It is only when pain-free, off all medication rates for MVD are compared against ≥50% pain free rates for GKSR (B) that the two surgical treatments appear equivalent in outcome for patients with TN.

In interpreting and comparing treatment results of surgical procedures for TN, keeping careful track of the endpoint definitions remains imperative. The most objectively verifiable and desirable endpoint from a purist view point is becoming completely pain-free off of all medication. However, many patients may be completely satisfied if they are able to be completely pain-free on small doses of medication that do not cause any side effects. Lesser degrees of pain relief are much more difficult to assess objectively and may not be as significant for the patient as they appear to be for the surgeon. Thresholds for a "good" result of 50% or greater pain relief +/− need for medications would appear to be extremely generous from the patient's viewpoint. Indeed, several of our GKSR patients initially achieved pain-free off all medication status but had a minor recurrence in which they became 80%–90% pain-free on medications. While this would have been considered a "good" response in most GKSR reports, these patients actually opted for a second GKSR procedure and were able to reachieve a pain-free, off all medication state.

COST-EFFECTIVENESS CONCERNS

Although extremely popular and attractive to TN patients, there are concerns regarding applying expensive SR technology toward treating TN when compared against the other effective, but relatively lower-technology intensive palliative destructive procedures. Given the differential TN outcomes of GKSR and MVD over time and the greater need for repeated procedures with GKSR, there is even concern for the relative cost of GKSR versus MVD when assessed by overall lifetime cost per quality-adjusted pain-free life year.

The best study investigating this so far was by Pollock and Ecker from the Mayo Clinic (Pollock et al. 2005). In their 2004 cost-effectiveness comparison of GR, MVD, and GKSR, the cost per quality-adjusted pain-free year for 126 patients (51 GR, 33 MVD, and 69 GKSR) was $6,342, $8,174, and $8,269, respectively. The results more strongly reflected the greater cost-effectiveness of GR versus GKSR at a mean follow-up of only 20.6 months. GKSR and MVD were similar in cost-effectiveness for an average of less than 2-year follow-up, but given the predictable ongoing loss of pain control with palliative destructive procedures, one wonders what the results would look like at 5–10 years after initial treatment.

LINAC DATA

The data outlined earlier are valid for GKSR for TN. One must be cautious in assuming that LINAC SR technologies will achieve equivalent results when one is creating such a small normal tissue functional lesion on such a small target. Although photons of roughly equivalent energy (whether a gamma ray or an x-ray) are equal in lesioning potential, the practical application requires equivalent targeting and focusing. Ultimately, equivalence claims must be judged on empiric data demonstrating and confirming equivalent therapeutic results and complication rates.

Unfortunately, although through December 1, 2008, there have been 236 papers published and listed in Medline on GKSR for TN, there have only been 22 LINAC papers over the same period (Fig. 13.10). If one breaks the LINAC papers down in an attempt to assess individual LINAC technologies

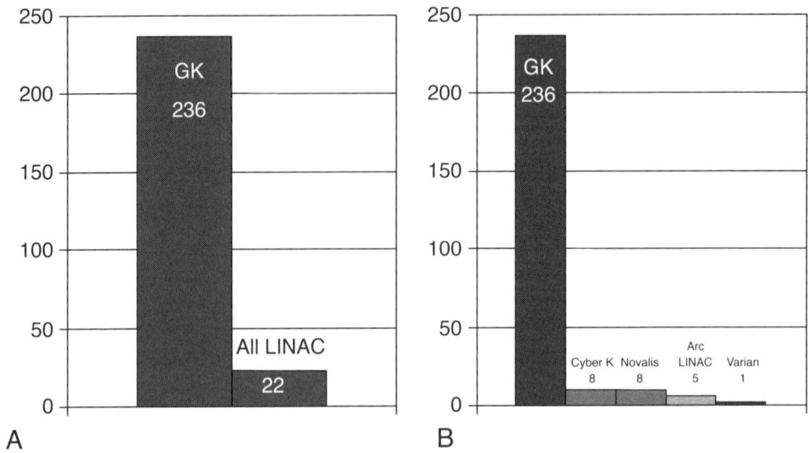

Figure 13.10 Listing of publications listed in Medline for stereotactic radiosurgery for trigeminal neuralgia through 12/31/08.

(A) GKSR publications versus all LINAC SR publications. (B) GKSR publications versus LINAC SR publications broken down by technology.

such as CyberKnife®, Novalis® (BrainLAB AG, Feldkirchen, Germany), X-Knife® (Integra Radionics, Burlington, Massachusetts), Varian Trilogy® (BrainLAB AG, Feldkirchen, Germany), or other units, the numbers all drop into the single digits.

What limited LINAC SR TN data we have would suggest that similar pain control results can be achieved (Adler 2009; Broggi, Ferroli, & Franzini 2008; Chen et al. 2004, 2008; De Salles et al. 2008; Deinsberger & Tidstrand 2005; Fariselli et al. 2009; Gerbi, Higgins, Cho, & Hall 2004; Gorgulho & De Salles 2006; Gorgulho et al. 2006; Goss et al. 2003; Kubicek et al. 2005; Lim et al. 2005; Pagni, Fariselli, & Zeme 2008; Patil et al. 2007; Pusztaszeri et al. 2007; Rahimian et al. 2004; Richards et al. 2005; Romanelli et al. 2003; Stern et al. 2008; Tarricone et al. 2008; Villavicencio et al. 2008). Unfortunately, these results appear to be associated with permanent trigeminal numbness results that exceed those reported after GKSR, and in some cases approach 47% (Villavicencio 2008). Reasons for the apparent higher numbness risk rates have yet to be fully worked out. However, two observations may shed some light.

The first is that neuroimaging after GKSR for TN reveals that the focal damage induced is limited by neuroimaging criteria to the nerve root itself (Alberico, Fensternmaker, & Lobel 2001), whereas imaging after at least Novalis® SR for TN has reveled MR contrast enhancement and T2 signal changes that extend well into the pons at the level of the trigeminal nerve (Gorgulho et al. 2006). In our own region of southern California, we have seen individual cases of similar neuroimaging changes after

CyberKnife® SR for TN. We await further reports and analysis of imaging changes after LINAC SR for TN and their potential relation to trigeminal numbness rates.

The second has been a shift, with CyberKnife® SR for TN, from isocentric treatment to a non-isocentric nerve root volume dosing approach, which appears to still be in evolution (Adler et al. 2009; Romanelli et al. 2003; Villavicencio et al. 2008). As a step-and-shoot technology rather than an arc rotational technology, CyberKnife® is uniquely positioned to treat a larger trigeminal nerve root volume at a lower maximum dose. Therapeutic effect versus toxicity will likely be a dose–volume function that will have to be empirically calculated. It would appear that early efforts in this technique included either too large a nerve root volume or too high a dose for that volume, as reported numbness rates were quite high (Villavicencio et al. 2008). It is our understanding that the technique continues to evolve, so that, currently, 4–6 mm of the nerve root is targeted with a mean marginal dose of 58 Gy (Adler et al. 2009; Fariselli et al. 2009). The final form and subsequent long-term results of this technique have yet to be defined.

CAUTIONS

Recommending GKSR as the initial treatment for young healthy patients with classic TN must be considered with caution and careful informed consent. Common misconceptions that are often heard in our clinic after initial consultations elsewhere, include: "There is no downside to beginning with the least invasive procedure first and then moving on to those with increased risk if this fails," and "If GKSR doesn't work, you can always do more, you haven't lost anything." Both of these are seductive arguments, with significant implications for the patient.

First, it must be kept in mind that time is a very important factor in success for MVD for TN. Jannetta's observation that MVD results significantly diminish after 8 years of suffering with TN (Barker et al. 1996) have now been confirmed and augmented by Burchiel's results, suggesting that the statistically significant cut point for worsened outcome may be as soon as 3 years (Burchiel et al., presented at the Western Neurosurgical Society, September 2007, and the Congress of Neurological Surgeons, September 2007).

Second, major MVD series have clearly shown that prior history of a palliative destructive procedure significantly worsens outcome of subsequent MVD (Barker et al. 1996). It would seem that a structural lesion in the trigeminal system, whether derived from nascent pathology, such as multiple sclerosis plaque or lacunar infarction, or iatrogenic trigeminal lesion from palliative destructive therapeutic intervention, predisposes the patient to worse outcome regardless of the subsequent procedure attempted. It must be kept in mind that a patient will never be younger, will never be a better risk for general anesthesia, and will never have a greater chance for a positive therapeutic result than at the present.

CONCLUSION

GKSR is a safe, important, and effective treatment tool to help patients with TN. It is the least invasive of the four palliative destructive procedures (GKSR, GR, RFL, and BC). Among the four, it carries the least risk of facial numbness, while achieving equivalent early results. Although it is not appropriate for a patient in acute extremis, it has become the most popular palliative destructive procedure because it avoids the percutaneous trans-foramen ovale needle, the pain of the lesioning process, reflex autonomic changes on the heart and cardiovascular system, risk of trigeminal motor weakness, and rare needle complications of hemorrhage, stroke, and meningitis. There is currently no other SR technology with the proven accuracy, experience, safety, and efficacy of GKSR. LINAC SR technologies are early in validation of results. So far, they appear to be able to achieve similar levels of pain relief, but also appear to carry a greater risk of facial numbness.

Microvascular decompression achieves significantly better pain control results for TN than GKSR. However, not all patients are candidates for MVD, or choose to undergo the procedure. In our practice, GKSR is the TN surgical procedure of choice for patients who are elderly, medically infirm, or at high risk for general anesthesia; have surgical contraindications; or who have extremely low up-front risk tolerance. Microvascular decompression remains our preferred procedure recommendation for young, healthy patients, willing to accept the anesthetic and microsurgical risk.

The truth is that both MVD and palliative destructive procedures are needed for the optimal care of our full spectrum of TN patients. Improving pain control and lowering the dose of cognitively and functionally debilitating medicines in our elderly and infirm patient pool is a very laudable endpoint, even when complete or permanent relief of pain is not a realistic goal.

REFERENCES

Adler JR Jr., Bower R, Gupta G, et al. Nonisocentric radiosurgical rhizotomy for trigeminal neuralgia. *Neurosurgery* 2009;64(2 Suppl):A84–90.

Alberico RA, Fenstermaker RA, Lobel J. Focal enhancement of cranial nerve V after radiosurgery with the Leksell gamma knife: experience in 15 patients with medically refractory trigeminal neuralgia. *AJNR Am J Neuroradiol* 2001;22(10): 1944–1948.

Barker FG II, Jannetta PJ, Bissonette DJ, et al. The long-term outcome of microvascular decompression for trigeminal neuralgia. *N Engl J Med* 1996;334: 1077–1083.

Barnett Gene H, Linskey Mark E, et al., and The American Association of Neurological Surgeons/Congress of Neurological Surgeons Washington Committee Stereotactic Radiosurgery Task Force. Stereotactic radiosurgery—an organized neurosurgery-sanctioned definition. *J Neurosurg* 2007;106:1–5.

Brisman R. Gamma knife radiosurgery for primary management for trigeminal neuralgia. *J Neurosurg* 2000;93(Suppl 3):159–161.

Brisman R. Microvascular decompression vs. gamma knife radiosurgery for typical trigeminal neuralgia: preliminary findings. *Stereotact Funct Neurosurg* 2007; 85:94–98.

Brisman R, Mooij R. Gamma knife radiosurgery for trigeminal neuralgia: dose-volume histograms of the brainstem and trigeminal nerve. *J Neurosurg* 2000;93(Suppl 3): 155–158.

Broggi G, Ferroli P, Franzini A. Treatment strategy for trigeminal neuralgia: a thirty years experience. *Neurol Sci* 2008;29(Suppl 1):S79–82.

Chen JC, Girvigian M, Greathouse H, et al. Treatment of trigeminal neuralgia w ith linear accelerator radiosurgery: initial results. *J Neurosurg* 2004;101 (Suppl 3):346–350.

Chen JC, Greathouse HE, Girvigian MR, et al. Prognostic factors for radiosurgery treatment of trigeminal neuralgia. *Neurosurgery* 2008;62(5 Suppl):A53–60.

De Salles AA, Gorgulho AA, Selch M, et al. Radiosurgery from the brain to the spine: 20 years experience. *Acta Neurochir Suppl* 2008;101:163–168.

Deinsberger R, Tidstrand J. LINAC radiosurgery as a tool in neurosurgery. *Neurosurgery* 2005;28(2):79–88.

Dellaretti M, Reyns N, Touzet G, et al. Clinical outcomes after Gamma Knife surgery for idiopathic trigeminal neuralgia: review of 76 consecutive cases. *J Neurosurg* 2008;109(Suppl):173–178.

Fariselli L, Marras C, De Santis M, et al. CyberKnife radiosurgery as a first treatment for idiopathic trigeminal neuralgia. *Neurosurgery* 2009;64(2 Suppl):A96–101.

Gellner V, Kurschel S, Kreil W, et al. Recurrent trigeminal neuralgia: long term outcome of repeat gamma knife radiosurgery. *J Neurol Neurosurg Psychiatry* 2008;79(12):1405–1407.

Gerbi BJ, Higgins PD, Cho KH, Hall WA. Linac-based stereotactic radiosurgery for treatment of trigeminal neuralgia. *J Appl Clin Med Phys* 2004;5(3):80–92, 2004; Epub 2004 Jul 1.

Gorgulho AA, De Salles AA. Impact of radiosurgery on the surgical treatment of trigeminal neuralgia. *Surg Neurol* 2006;66(4):350–356. Review.

Gorgulho A, De Salles AA, McArthur D, et al. Brainstem and trigeminal nerve changes after radiosurgery for trigeminal pain. *Surg Neurol* 2006;66(2):127–135.

Goss BW, Frighetto L, DeSalles AA, et al. Linear accelerator radiosurgery using 90 gray for essential trigeminal neuralgia: results and dose volume histogram analysis. *Neurosurgery* 2003;53(4):823–828.

Håkanson S. Trigeminal neuralgia treated by the injection of glycerol into the trigeminal cistern. *Neurosurgery* 1981;9:638–646, 1981

Håkanson S, Leksell L. Stereotactic radiosurgery in trigeminal neuralgia. [Abstract]. *Excerpta Med Int Cong Series* 1977;418:57, 1977

Huang CF, Tu HT, Liu WS, et al. Gamma Knife surgery used as primary and repeated treatment for idiopathic trigeminal neuralgia. *J Neurosurg* 2008;109(Suppl):179–184.

Knafo H, Kenny B, Mathieu D. Trigeminal neuralgia: outcomes after gamma knife radiosurgery. *Can J Neurol Sci* 2009;36(1):78–82.

Kondziolka D, Lunsford LD, Flickinger JC, et al. Stereotactic radiosurgery for trigeminal neuralgia: a multi-institutional study using the gamma unit. *J Neurosurg* 1996;84:940–945.

Kubicek GJ, Hall WA, Orner JB, et al. Long-term follow-up of trigeminal neuralgia treatment using a linear accelerator. *Stereotact Funct Neurosurg* 2004;82(5–6): 244–249; Epub 2005 Jan 5.

Leksell Gamma Knife Society. Indications Treated December 2006: 202 units out of 249 reporting. Elekta website. Accessed 26 June 2009, at http://www.elekta.com/assets/gamma_knife_surgery/pdfs/ww06_us.pdf.

Leksell L. The stereotaxic method and radiosurgery of the brain. *Acta Chir Scand* 1951;102:316–319.

Leksell L. Stereotaxic radiosurgery in trigeminal neuralgia. *Acta Chir Scand* 1971;137:311–314.

Lim M, Villavicencio AT, Burneikiene S, et al. CyberKnife radiosurgery for idiopathic trigeminal neuralgia. *Neurosurg Focus* 2005;18(5):E9.

Linskey ME. Evidence-based medicine for neurosurgeons: introduction and methodology. *Prog Neurol Surg* 2006;19:1–53, 2006

Linskey ME, Kuo J. General and Historical Considerations of Radiotherapy and Radiosurgery. In Winn HR, ed. *Youmans textbook of neurological surgery*, 6th ed. Philadelphia: Saunders (in press).

Linskey ME, Ratanatharathorn V, Penagaricano J. A prospective cohort study of microvascular decompression and Gamma Knife surgery in patients with trigeminal neuralgia. *J Neurosurg* 2008;109:160–172.

Loeffler JS, Niemierko A, Chapman PH. Second tumors after radiosurgery: tip of the iceberg or a bump in the road? *Neurosurgery* 2003;52(6):1436–1440.

Longhi M, Rizzo P, Nicolato A, et al. Gamma knife radiosurgery for trigeminal neuralgia: results and potentially predictive parameters–part I: Idiopathic trigeminal neuralgia. *Neurosurgery* 2007;61(6):1254–1260.

Lopez BC, Hamlyn PJ, Zakrzewska JM. Stereotactic radiosurgery for primary trigeminal neuralgia: state of the evidence and recommendations for future reports. *J Neurol Neurosurg Psychiatry* 2004a;75(7):1019–1024.

Lopez BC, Hamlyn PJ, Zakrzewska JM. Systematic review of ablative neurosurgical techniques for the treatment of trigeminal neuralgia. *Neurosurgery* 2004b; 54(4):973–982.

McIver JI, Pollock BE. Radiation-induced tumor after stereotactic radiosurgery and whole brain radiotherapy: case report and literature review. *J Neurooncol* 2004;66(3):301–305.

Maesawa S, Salame C, Flickinger JC, et al. Clinical outcomes after stereotactic radiosurgery for idiopathic trigeminal neuralgia. *J Neurosurg* 2001;94:14–20, 2001

Maher CO, Pollock BE. Radiation induced vascular injury after stereotactic radiosurgery for trigeminal neuralgia: case report. *Surg Neurol* 2000;54(2):189–193.

Mathews MS, Binder DK, Linskey ME. Trigeminal Neuralgia: Diagnosis and Non-Operative Management. In Winn HR, ed., *Youmans Textbook of Neurological Surgery*, 6th ed. Philadelphia: Saunders (in press).

Mullan S, Lichtor T. Percutaneous microcompression of the trigeminal ganglion for trigeminal neuralgia. *J Neurosurg* 1983;59:1007–1012.

Nicol B, Regine WF, Courtney C, et al. Gamma knife radiosurgery using 90 Gy for trigeminal neuralgia. *J Neurosurg* 2000;93(Suppl 3):152–154.

Pagni CA, Fariselli L, Zeme S. Trigeminal neuralgia. Non-invasive techniques versus microvascular decompression. It is really available any further improvement? *Acta Neurochir Suppl* 2008;101:27–33.

Patil CG, Veeravagu A, Bower RS, et al. CyberKnife radiosurgical rhizotomy for the treatment of atypical trigeminal nerve pain. *Neurosurg Focus* 2007;23(6):E9.

Pollock BE. Comparison of posterior fossa exploration and stereotactic radiosurgery in patients with previously nonsurgically treated idiopathic trigeminal neuralgia. *Neurosurg Focus* 2005;18:E6.Links, 2005

Pollock BE, Ecker RD. A prospective cost-effectiveness study of trigeminal neuralgia surgery. *Clin J Pain* 2005;21(4):317–322.

Pollock BE, Foote RL, Link MJ, et al. Repeat radiosurgery for idiopathic trigeminal neuralgia. *Int J Radiat Oncol Biol Phys* 2005;61(1):192–195.

Pollock BE, Phuong LK, Foote RL, et al. High-dose trigeminal neuralgia radiosurgery associated with increased risk of trigeminal nerve dysfunction. *Neurosurgery* 2001;49(1):58–62.

Pollock BE, Phuong LK, Gorman DA, et al. Stereotactic radiosurgery for idiopathic trigeminal neuralgia. *J Neurosurg* 2002;97:347–353.

Pusztaszeri M, Villemure JG, Regli L, et al. Radiosurgery for trigeminal neuralgia using a linear accelerator with BrainLab system: report on initial experience in Lausanne, Switzerland. *Swiss Med Wkly* 2007;137(47–48):682–686.

Rahimian J, Chen JC, Rao AA, et al. Geometrical accuracy of the Novalis stereotactic radiosurgery system for trigeminal neuralgia. *J Neurosurg* 2004;101(Suppl 3): 351–355.

Régis J, Metellus P, Hayashi M, et al. Prospective controlled trial of gamma knife surgery for essential trigeminal neuralgia. *J Neurosurg* 2006;104:913–924.

Richards GM, Bradley KA, Tomé WA, et al. Linear accelerator radiosurgery for trigeminal neuralgia. *Neurosurgery* 2005;57(6):1193–1200.

Rogers CL, Shetter AG, Fielder JA, et al. Gamma knife radiosurgery for trigeminal neuralgia: the initial experience of the Barrow Neurological Institute. *Int J Radiat Oncol Biol Phys* 2000;47:1013–1019.

Romanelli P, Heit G, Chang SD, et al. Cyberknife radiosurgery for trigeminal neuralgia. *Stereotact Funct Neurosurg* 2003;81(1–4):105–109.

Stern RL, Perks JR, Pappas CT, et al. The option of LINAC-based radiosurgery in a Gamma Knife radiosurgery center. *Clin Neurol Neurosurg* 2008;110(10): 968–972, 2008; Epub 2008 Jul 9.

Sweet WH, Wepsic JG. Relation of fiber size in the trigeminal posterior root to conduction of impulses for pain and touch: Production of analgesia without anesthesia in the effective treatment of trigeminal neuralgia. *Trans Neurol Assoc* 1970;95:134–139.

Tarricone R, Aguzzi G, Musi F, et al. Cost-effectiveness analysis for trigeminal neuralgia: Cyberknife vs microvascular decompression. *Neuropsychiatr Dis Treat* 2008;4(3):647–652.

Villavicencio AT, Lim M, Burneikiene S, et al. Cyberknife radiosurgery for trigeminal neuralgia treatment: a preliminary multicenter experience. *Neurosurgery* 2008;62(3):647–655; discussion 647–655.

Young RF, Vermulen S, Posewitz A. Gamma knife radiosurgery for the treatment of trigeminal neuralgia. *Stereotact Funct Neurosurg* 1998;70(Suppl 1):192–199.

Zakrzewska JM, Linskey M. Trigeminal neuralgia. *BMJ Clin Evid* 2008; 2(1207):1–9.

Zakrzewska JM, Linskey M. Trigeminal neuralgia. In Zakrzewska JM, ed., *Orofacial Pain*. New York: Oxford University Press, 2009, 119–134.

Zakrzewska JM, Lopez BC. Quality of reporting in evaluations of surgical treatment of trigeminal neuralgia: recommendations for future reports.*Neurosurgery* 2003;53(1):110–120.

14

Microvascular Decompression

Peter J. Jannetta, Mark R. McLaughlin, and Raymond F. Sekula, Jr.

Many of the enigmas due to limited information which were inherent in the thinking about trigeminal neuralgia (TN) have passed into oblivion. Despite astute reasoning by superb neurosurgeons and multiple theories regarding TN's etiology, clarification of the mechanism and development of advanced treatment were beyond the ken of the best investigators of several generations.

Much of this was due to inadequate technology. It has been observed by some that the more technically astute neurosurgeons of the pre-microscopic era were high myopes, who had some natural magnification and could see better than their colleagues. But this was not enough. A further part of the problem was that the status of neurosurgery was shaky. Operative results were not wonderful. Operative complication rates were such that, if an operative procedure for a particular problem was developed that had moderate morbidity and acceptable mortality, virtually everyone in the then-small group of active clinicians adopted it. There was little or no room for deviation of thought or practice and hardly any capacity for creative thinking.

The rather restrictive thinking surrounding the operative treatment of TN was such that only replacement of one symptom (lancinating facial pain) by another (numbness) was acceptable. All treatments injured the nerve, whether through section in the middle fossa (Spiller-Frazier 1901, 1919, 1925), peripheral section of the trigeminal branches, or alcohol injection of the peripheral branches. Starting in the 1920s, however, one productive deviant*, Walter Dandy, began to operate safely in the cerebellopontine angle. He sectioned the portio major of the trigeminal nerve at the pons, and his patients usually had prolonged pain relief, along with loss of pain perception with relative retention of light touch perception. Dandy observed a progressively higher incidence of arteries, benign extra-axial tumors, and bony enostoses around or on the trigeminal nerve in his patients (Dandy 1932, 1934). He never completed the syllogism by moving the impinging blood vessel, although he did excise tumors when he found them. In reviewing his operative drawings, it appears that he did not

* An IBM company term for people who are just that: productive and deviant.

always have a clear look at the entire trigeminal nerve with his approach. It remained for another neurosurgeon, W. James Gardner (Gardner & Milkos 1959), to attempt to mobilize arteries away from the trigeminal nerve (and also of the facial nerve in patients with hemifacial spasm [HFS]). In a careful review of his contributions, it is clear that Gardner was close to the brass ring. And yet, just like Dandy, he could not see well enough. He saw what he thought of as pathological arteries in about half of a small series of patients, but he did not clearly look at the junctional area of the nerve and the pons. He traumatized the nerve as the treatment in all cases. Some of the arteries were anterior inferior cerebellar arteries pushing on the auditory nerve. Last, Gardner did not use the operating microscope for this work. This limited him.

It was my [PJJ] privilege to know and spend considerable time with Dr. Gardner, who personally reiterated the above statements to me. He was a good and great man, ahead of his time, open minded, lucid in thought, and kind to members of my generation.

So, the stage was set for the development of microvascular decompression (MVD) for cranial nerve vascular compression syndromes. I spent considerable time as a National Institutes of Health (NIH) fellow working with neurophysiologist Solomon D. Erulkar in the Department of Pharmacology at the University of Pennsylvania. We worked on the spinal cord projections of the vestibular system in cats (Erulkar et al., 1966). We used the binocular microscope almost daily in experiments that might run for 30 hours or more. I was planning a career in academic neurosurgery, and it seemed to me that the microscope was particularly applicable to neurosurgery. I was unaware of the work of Theodore Kurze and his Boswell scholar, Robert W. Rand. I wrote to my future chief of neurosurgery asking for a microscope for the department (cost $1,800), but was denied. When I arrived in Los Angeles in 1963, I found that Kurze had first used the binocular microscope in surgery in 1957. It took 34 years from Nylen's use of the dissecting microscope to drain infected ears (Nylen 1923) to Kurze's leap from the laboratory across the hall to the operating room. Rand had a microscope, and he allowed me access to it.

Young, naive people do new things. Some of this is because they do not know that a certain fact cannot be true or that a task cannot be done. Kurze had developed several ways of approaching cerebellopontine angle tumors, specifically acoustic neuromas (vestibular schwannomas), while working with members of the House clinic. He left that group. He published little. House published a lot. When I arrived in Los Angeles Kurze and Rand were working together on these tumors, treating large lesions using laborious techniques. The beginning of anything new in surgery is often laborious. I, captivated by the application of the microscope, spent lots of time with these two bright and interesting men. I usually closed a big unilateral horseshoe incision late in the evening after the tumor had been removed.

Subsequently, I was asked to do a little job that changed my life, added spice to my professional life, and pushed me outside the political mainstream of neurosurgery for some time. Rand asked me to dissect the cranial nerves so that we could demonstrate the anatomy using the microscope and a black-and-white closed-circuit television system to the first-year dental students at our institution. We never know the importance (or unimportance) of what we do.

On a Wednesday night in the early spring of 1965, I do not recall the date, but I know that it was 11:30 p.m., I had dissected the first four cranial nerves and was working on the trigeminal. I saw some nerve fascicles that were not supposed to be there. I found that Dandy (Dandy 1934) had partly described the extra fascicles, calling them "accessory sensory fascicles." He preserved them when doing his selective portio major section for TN relief. Using the microscope, I was able to clarify these fascicles more clearly (Jannetta and Rand 1966, Jannetta 1967). I had help from Lawrence Kruger and Carmine Clemente, from the Brain Research Institute, as well as from W. Eugene Stern who, although he did not look favorably upon the microscope, gave me access to his laboratory, animals, and his laboratory director, Roy Jones.

I dissected a large series of trigeminal nerves and developed a technique for microsurgical selective section of the portio major for TN relief. I performed 17 selective sections of the portio major on the left side in cadavers. A case of right-sided TN became available through the auspices of John Alksne, the chief of service at one of our allied hospitals (and subsequent chief of neurosurgery at University of California San Diego). Mr. W.P. had a 10-year history of right-sided TN. He had rubbed all the hair off the right side of his head because it eased his pain. He was having about 200 attacks of severe lancinating pain per day, and his wife had left him. An operation was indicated. I was forbidden to operate at our major hospital. I was forbidden to operate through a retromastoid exposure by my faculty, because it was felt to be dangerous to operate in the cerebellopontine angle. This was a heritage from the pre-microsurgical era. Not enough thought was given to the dangers of posterior temporal lobe retraction and venous injury. So we operated. Dr. Alksne assisted me, and Dr. Rand was present. We used Rand's microscope, which I brought to the hospital in my old 1957 Ford station wagon.

A magic moment! We exposed the trigeminal nerve through an opening in the tentorium cerebella. An artery, the superior cerebellar artery, was cross-compressing the trigeminal nerve. "That's the cause of the tic," I said. It was very convincing to me. Alksne understood immediately. I performed a selective portio major section of the nerve. Mr. W.P. was relieved of his pain (although his wife would not return). It had taken over 20 years to arrive at a generalized understanding of the vascular etiology in TN and, worse yet, to conceive an operation based on this vascular etiology, and—the obvious next move—to surgically move the offending blood vessel away from the nerve and hold it away. I performed the first MVD on a patient with hemifacial spasm in February 1966. The first MVD for TN followed 4 months later. During this period, I saw and operated upon several patients with TN, sectioning the nerve in all but one. The latter had a small unexpected meningioma pushing into the nerve. I excised the tumor, and the pain was relieved without deficit. (This was, of course, in the pre-imaging era.)

Into the residents' clinic came Mr. H.H., a 41-year-old precision mechanic with progressive left-sided HFS. He had severe tonus phenomenon, so severe that the contractions were transmitted to his hands and he could not perform his work. I remember standing near him as he sat on the examining table. I said, "Mr. H., you have an artery pressing on your facial nerve causing the spasm." It was an effortless extrapolation. I operated upon him through a retromastoid craniotomy (I had not yet given it this name). The faculty members who had forbidden me to do this were away and the supervising neurosurgeon, Paul Crandall, agreed to my doing this procedure. I had easy access to the facial and auditory nerves, so I spent considerable time fussing with the anterior inferior cerebellar artery as it coursed distally around the seventh and eighth nerve bundle. For some reason, I was not convinced that this artery was causal of the spasm. At last I saw a small vein running across the facial nerve, anteriorly on the pons. I divided the vein and coagulated the cut ends with forceps using the Bovie—we had no bipolar coagulation in 1966, no Greenfield, no Malis. Mr. H.H. had a good night, but developed spasm early in the morning; this lasted a matter of hours and ceased, never to return. If I had remained interested in the artery and had not seen the vein, I do not know if I ever would have had the temerity to persist with the MVD. Definition of the vascular etiology of glossopharyngeal neuralgia, vertigo, tinnitus, Ménière disease, and disabling positional vertigo all followed.

Let us now return to TN. I had moved to New Orleans and was finally free of restrictions. I began in early 1967 to operate on TN via a retromastoid craniectomy. It was progressively more reasonable to assume, as our experience evolved, that TN is due to vascular compression of the trigeminal nerve in the cerebellopontine angle. Compressing vessels were frequently multiple and often distal. Anatomical studies, echoing the early work of Haven and Davis in 1923, showed that the central myelin extended far distally in the portio major, with the core of the central myelin sometimes going out to Meckel's cave. The 100 or so fascicles penetrate the so-called fibrous cone of the portio major, each fascicle a junctional area, "a root entry zone" (Fig. 14.1).

The significant question was, "Am I good enough to find and treat all the blood vessels?" Not, "Is there a blood vessel here which could be causing the TN?" Many of the vessels are small, too small for even the best of contemporary imaging techniques. Also, a blood vessel may seem to be causal on a magnetic resonance imaging (MRI) scan, but another smaller

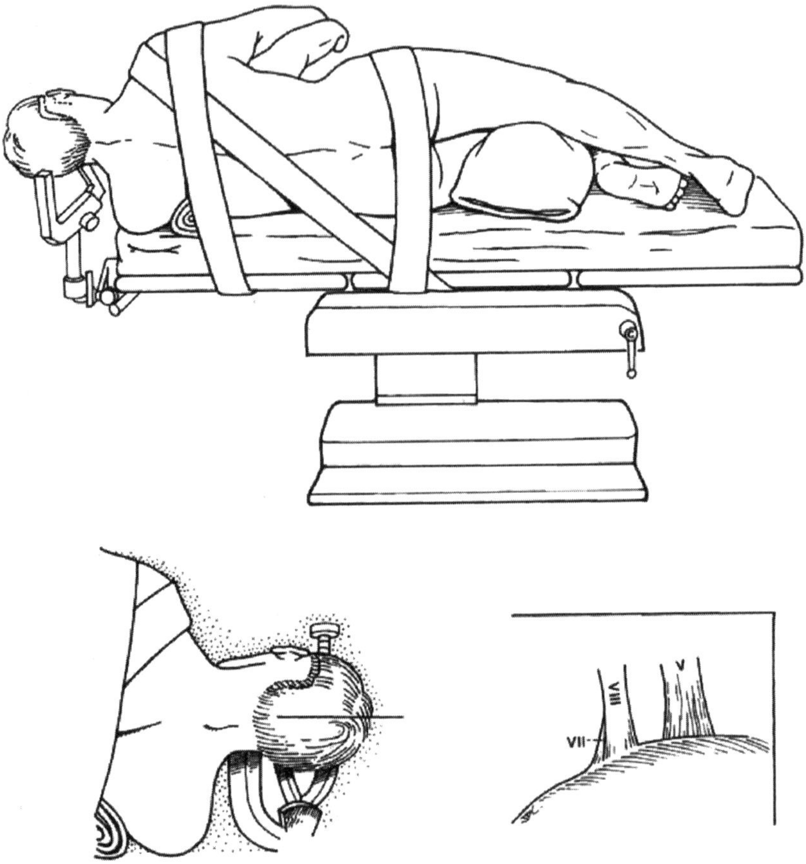

Figure 14.1 Patient placement.

Upper: Drawing showing the patient's head placed at the foot of the operating table to allow more leg room for the surgeon during the microsurgical portion of the procedure. The head is secured with three-point fixation, and the patient is turned in the lateral decubitus position. The head is rotated slightly away from the affected side and flexed to approximately two finger breadths from the sternum. *Lower*: For trigeminal nerve approach, the vertex of the head is kept parallel to the floor to keep the seventh–eighth cranial nerve complex at a more inferior position with respect to the trigeminal nerve.

artery, arteriole, vein, or venule is found to be causative. Peculiar thinking has led some to state that if no offending blood vessel is seen on an imaging study, there is no vascular compression and a destructive procedure is indicated. This is not very bright. Pity the poor person, especially the young person, who has such an operation. Some vascular compression is extremely subtle. I have seen four patients with a large vein totally inside the trigeminal nerve, many with a vein under the ala of the cerebellum (not clearly on the nerve when the cerebrospinal fluid (CSF) is drained and the cerebellum supported by a self-retaining retractor). Distal crossing veins coming up the pons and entering the dura mater above Meckel's cave, and the aberrant trigeminal vein (Dandy 1932, 1934) are frequently missed, especially in dolichocephalic patients.

In cases of TN, a clinical pathologic relationship exists which is generally operant: The superior cerebellar artery, looping down from above, causes V_3 pain. As it elongates, it compresses the side of the nerve, causing V_2 pain. If the artery stretches the nerve, as it does over time, it may cause numbness. Numbness is not only present after many years of TN but may occur early on, during severe exacerbations of pain. Despite solid evidence to the contrary, I was taught as a resident that facial numbness was not found in TN. Lewy and Grant, using von Frei hairs, had clearly shown that 20% of TN patients had facial numbness predominantly in the area of the pain (Lewy & Grant 1938). My colleagues and I found sensory abnormalities in over 30% of patients. Bennett et al. in our laboratories found that trigeminal evoked potentials (TEP) in V_2 and V_3 were abnormal in 86% of TN patients (Bennett & Jannetta, 1980, 1983). After MVD, the evoked potentials returned to normal in 83% of patients. This evoked potential, the TEP, is a more sensitive measure of trigeminal sensory function than is clinical sensory examination. Isolated V_2 pain is usually venous, and frequently is found in young women due to lateral or medial trigeminal nerve compression. V_1 pain is due to caudal compression, frequently due to dolichoectatic arteries in elderly men who have been heavy smokers.

The differentiation of atypical TN (ATN) from nervus intermedius neuralgia (NIN) is usually challenging. If ATN has responded well to medical therapy with total relief of pain, even for a short time, it is more likely to be trigeminal in origin, caused by vascular compression of the motor-proprioceptive fascicles distally. With little or no response to medications, especially carbamazepine (Tegretol) or gabapentin (Neurontin), the pain is more likely due to nervus intermedius dysfunction.

STEP 1: PREOPERATIVE PREPARATION OF THE PATIENT.

An intravenous catheter is placed in the arm, the patient is given anesthesia, and long alternating pressure stockings are placed on the lower extremities.

Step 2: Positioning the Patient

The position of the vertex dictates cranial nerve exposure.

The patient is placed on the operating room table with his head at the foot of the bed to maximize the surgeon's comfort during the microsurgical portion of the procedure. A second intravenous catheter and a radial artery line are placed. Following induction of anesthesia and intubation, a three-point head-fixation device is applied, and the patient is placed in the lateral decubitus position with appropriate padding of pressure points and an axillary roll. The neck is flexed slightly, with the chin approximately two finger breadths from the sternum (Fig. 14.1). The head is rotated approximately 10 degrees away from the affected side. The vertex is kept parallel to the floor, to keep the seventh and eighth cranial nerve complex at a more inferior position in relation to the trigeminal nerve. The head holder is secured in the proper position. The patient is taped securely to the table at the hips and chest to allow rotation of the table during the operation. The patient's shoulder is taped down out of the way.

STEP 3: OPERATIVE INCISION

The placement of the incision is variable, depending on the size and thickness of the patient's neck.

A 3 × 5 cm area behind the ear is clipped and bone landmarks are identified by palpation before the patient is prepared for surgery. The mastoid eminence, digastric groove, and inion are identified, and an iniomeatal line drawn to define the transverse sinus. A second line is drawn laterally over the digastric groove. The intersection of these lines reveals the junction of the transverse and sigmoid sinuses. This allows the surgeon to place a burr hole properly. These external landmarks guide the surgeon, minimize the length of the incision, and allow adequate exposure for burr hole placement (Fig. 14.2). A vertical incision is drawn 3 to 5 cm long, approximately 0.5 cm posterior (medial) and parallel to the hair line. Identical incisions are used for both upper and lower cranial nerve exposures. A slightly shorter incision is required for thin- and long-necked patients. For short- and thick-necked patients, the incision should be slightly longer, placed a bit more posteriorly, with the inferior aspect angled more posteriorly (medially). This incision requires slightly more extensive muscle dissection over the mastoid and digastric groove, but positions the thicker neck musculature posteriorly (medially), allowing freer movement of the surgeon's hands and instruments while performing the microsurgery (Fig. 14.2). Three-quarters of the incision should be drawn inferior to the junction of the transverse and sigmoid sinuses, and one-quarter should be above. The area is prepared and draped in the usual fashion, and the incision is made down to the occipital bone using monopolar cautery. The soft tissues are dissected using a periosteal elevator and electrocautery where necessary. The initial periosteal dissection should proceed anteriorly (laterally) before completing the posterior (medial) dissection. This provides better fixation with an angled or straight Weitlaner retractor. The posterior aspect of the mastoid eminence must be cleared of soft tissue. The nuchal muscles are dissected with electrocautery. The transverse occipital artery is identified, ligated, and divided. The mastoid emissary vein is usually identified and must be waxed in its fossa. The Weitlaner retractor is put in place. In thin-necked patients, a straight retractor often gives adequate exposure and takes up less room within the incisional opening.

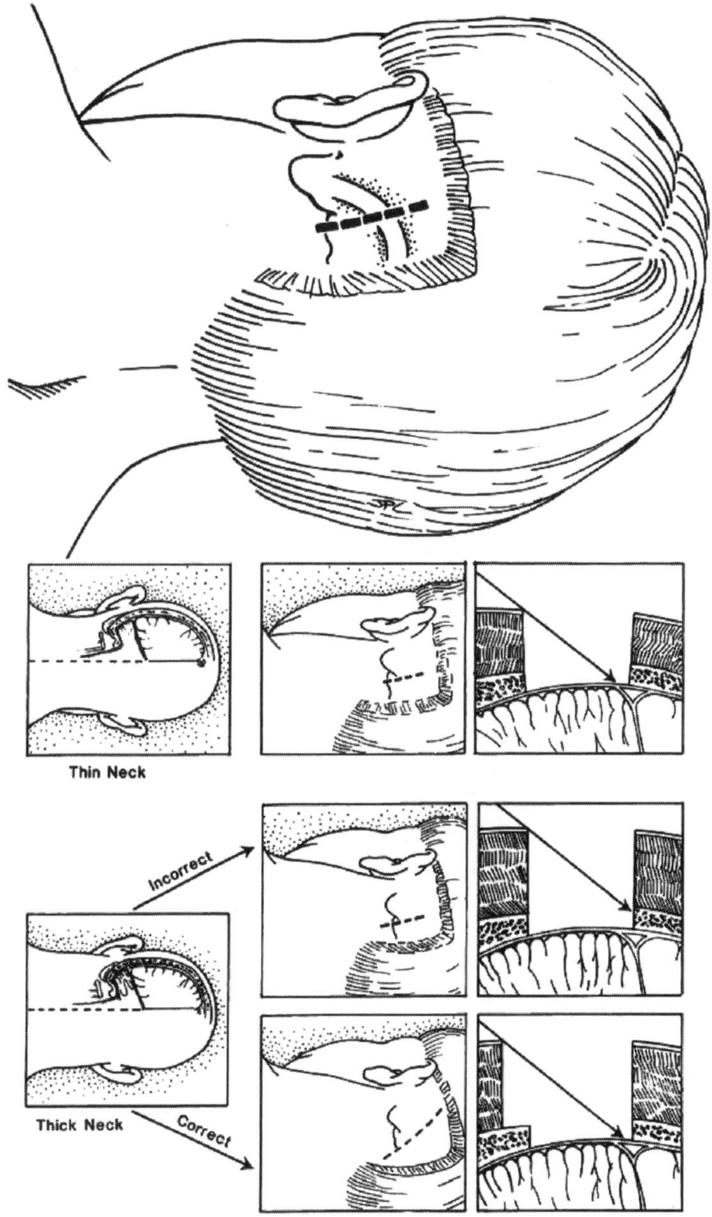

Figure 14.2 Junction of transverse and sigmoid sinuses.

Upper: Drawing showing how the intersection of the digastric groove and the iniomeatal line defines the junction of the transverse and the sigmoid sinuses. With a "mind's eye" view of optimal burr hole placement and craniectomy, an incision is drawn centered over the planned craniectomy. *Lower*: Drawings showing different surgical incisions based on the size of the patient's neck. Short- and thick-necked patients require a more posteriorly placed and (medially) directed incision. This angled incision positions the thicker neck musculature more posteriorly (medially) and out of the operative field. This small adjustment is critical in allowing freer movement of the surgeon's hands and instruments while performing the microsurgery.

STEP 4: BONE REMOVAL

The junction of the transverse and sigmoid sinuses must be visualized before the dural opening.

Before burr hole placement, landmarks should be well exposed. The digastric groove should be clearly visualized, and the soft tissue should be dissected slightly anterior to this landmark. Often the external aspect of the emissary vein does not lie directly over the sinus; rather, the vein meanders in a rostrolateral direction before entering the proximal sigmoid sinus. Therefore, the mastoid emissary vein is a good landmark for the underlying junction of the transverse and sigmoid sinuses. The asterion location is variable and, thus, is not a reliable landmark for the sinus junction. The burr hole should be placed over or inferomedially to the mastoid emissary vein by using a perforator or high-speed drill. The goal of bone exposure should be to identify the edge of the junction of the transverse and sigmoid sinuses first. For a trigeminal approach, the craniectomy should be shaped as an isosceles triangle, with the apex at the junction of the transverse and sigmoid sinuses (Fig. 14.3).

In a dolichocephalic patient, it is important to remove a portion of the posterior mastoid air cells if they protrude over the sigmoid sinus, so that no bone overhang will limit the dural opening. Mastoid air cells should be thoroughly waxed. The dura mater is opened away from the venus sinus. We us a No. 15 blade and suction, followed by toothed forceps to elevate the cut edge, and fine dural scissors. A curvilinear incision works well and may be extended (T) toward the junction of the transverse and sigmoid sinuses as necessary. The dura becomes thicker before one enters

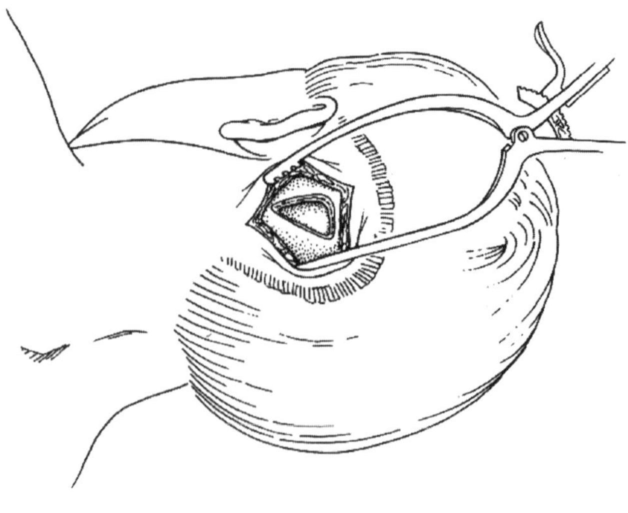

Figure 14.3 Bone exposure should demonstrate the junction of the transverse and sigmoid sinuses.

Surgical exposure can then be tailored according to the cranial nerve approach desired.

a venous sinus. Small bites with a fine scissors ensure that a small sinus opening can be treated easily by using bipolar coagulation. This incision should expose the most superior and lateral corner of the dura adjacent to the junction of the transverse and sigmoid sinuses to allow a direct corridor along the petrotentorial junction. The bone work must be anterior (lateral) enough to allow dural incision and reflection and subsequent closure. The dura is sutured with stay sutures to the galea aponeurotica to facilitate the superolateral route to the junction of the petrous bone and tentorium cerebelli. The self-retaining microsurgical retractor, with the cerebellar cortex protected by a rubber dam-covered cottonoid is placed into a superolateral direction, gently compressing the cerebellum.

STEP 5: TURNING THE CORNER

Turning the corner is the most dangerous stage of the operation and must be executed with patience and the utmost care.

After the dura is sutured back, the binocular operating microscope with a 250 mm objective lens is brought into the field. "Turning the corner" to expose the cerebellopontine angle may be difficult and hazardous. The approach is generally supralateral over the cerebellum. One must at times slide over the superior surface of the cerebellum or down the lateral surface a bit. One must be patient in turning the corner, so that the subarachnoid space can be entered and CSF drained, with resultant falling away of the cerebella and room to work. Impatience may cause bridging veins to be torn, especially at the dural (sinus) junction or injury to the cerebellum. Be patient; the time spent slowly working into the rostral cerebellopontine angle seems like forever, but takes only a few minutes and is well worth it. Occasionally, gentle advancement of a cottonoid with a rubber dam is required to drain CSF from the cerebellopontine angle before placement of a retractor. All cottonoids are moistened with saline and are paired with an appropriately sized (0.5 × 2 inch) piece of rubber cut from a sterile glove.

When the subarachnoid space is entered, the cerebellum falls away rapidly. The arachnoid is opened with sharp dissection, making certain no blood vessels are at risk. One or more branches of the superior petrosal vein may cover part of the trigeminal nerve. The eighth nerve is seen and preserved. Any retraction must elevate and support the ala as much as compress the cerebellum. The pulse rate should be audible to the surgeon throughout.

The rubber prevents adhesion to the cerebellum and allows easy advancement of cottonoids over the cortex to the cerebellopontine angle. A lumbar drain is not necessary. After the CSF has been drained, the cerebellum will begin to fall away from the petrotentorial junction. A tapered retractor blade, bent proximally to a 30- to 60-degree angle, and not curved, is placed over the previously placed rubber dam/cottonoid combination.

The blade and cottonoid are placed over the supralateral aspect of the cerebellar surface, and the ala of the cerebellum is gently elevated. The goal of retraction is to elevate the cerebellum slightly toward the surgeon and not simply to compress it medially. This facilitates CSF drainage, thereby minimizing the need for cerebellar retraction. The petrosal vein complex is identified and placed on gentle traction with the retractor. The relationships of the vein to the trigeminal nerve must be clarified, as this may be the cause of the neuralgia. If necessary, the vein complex is coagulated using micro-bipolar electrocautery, and partially divided to verify adequate hemostasis. The complex is then coagulated a second time and transected completely.

On entering the cerebellopontine angle, the first cranial nerves visualized will usually be the CN VII-VIII complex, located superficially and caudal to the trigeminal nerve. The trigeminal nerve is located in the most superior and deepest position. The petrosal vein complex usually consists of a confluence of two or three veins draining into the tentorial edge. If bleeding is encountered from this complex, it usually comes from a partial separation at the dural sinus. Occasionally, this can even occur during gentle cerebellar exposure before division of the vein. Bleeding can be controlled by gentle pressure and packing of the tentorial side by using Surgicel and a small cottonoid. The retractor can be used to exert gentle pressure while the surgeon looks for the free end of the avulsed vein. Once the vein is identified and coagulated, the procedure can continue. If bleeding is severe, a larger-bore suction tip can be used to allow visualization of the field. Additionally, placing the patient in the reverse Trendelenburg position will decrease venous pressure and bleeding. In the senior author's experience, bleeding can always be controlled, but it may require tamponade for as long as 10–20 minutes.

STEP 6: NERVE DECOMPRESSION

The pathology lies at the brainstem side of the nerve, but may be more lateral and as distal as the rim of Meckel's cave. Decompression is relatively straightforward if the surgeon keeps two principles in mind at all times: (1) There must be at minimum one offending vessel, and it is your job to find it; and (2) the dorsal root entry or exit zone can be variable in length, particularly in the case of the trigeminal nerve, and may extend to a more distal portion of the nerve. Therefore, the nerve should be inspected from its origin at the brainstem laterally to its exit from the cerebellopontine angle, and all vessels should be treated (Fig. 14.4).

The entire trigeminal nerve should be visualized as well as possible before starting the vascular decompression. The superior petrosal vein branches are taken if they are compressing the nerve and are therefore part or all of the pathology (section before visualization is one reason for the "negative" exploration) and if mobilization of an arterial loop cannot be performed adequately because the bridging vein is in the way of the new arterial position. It is better to take a vein in a controlled fashion than to tear it.

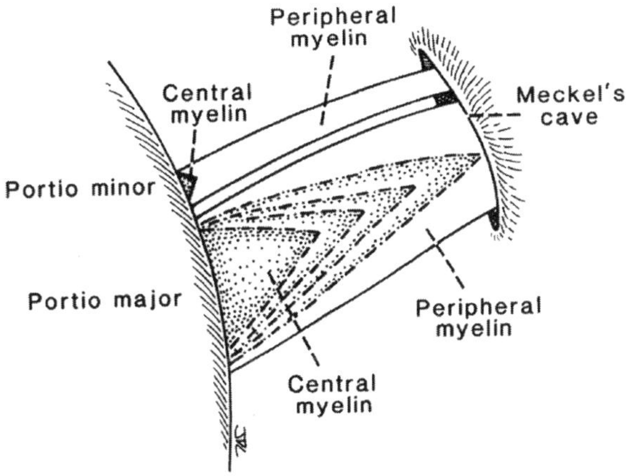

Figure 14.4 Dorsal root entry zone.

Diagram showing that the dorsal root entry zone of the trigeminal nerve can be variable in length and may extend to a more distal portion of the nerve.

Thorough visualization of potential pathology includes the area under the ala of the cerebellum, which may partially cover the proximal nerve at the brainstem. Elevation of the ala may separate an offending blood vessel from the nerve. The anterior axilla of CN V may be seen through a small malleable handled mirror. The distal nerve at the dura may be partly covered by an enostosis. A bridging vein hidden by this bone is easily seen caudal to the nerve and laterally by use of the mirror.

Multiple blood vessels are common. Since release of CSF may cause separation of blood vessels from the nerve and because aging may continue to elongate arteries and cause caudal slippage of the brainstem, all regional vessels should be treated. Polytetrafluoroethylene (PTFE, Teflon) felt is shredded, and various sizes of implants rolled up like cigars. An unshredded piece of felt may act as a secondary missile, transmitting pulsation from a blood vessel to a nerve. Surface veins should be decompressed rather than taken, if at all possible, to prevent recollateralization. Veins passing across and through the nerve seem especially prone to recollateralize and cause recurrence and should be decompressed if possible. Recollateralization and recurrence can occur as early as 6 weeks postoperatively. For some reason, taking a recollateralized vein coursing across and through the nerve is very prone to result in severe numbness. We postulate that a small venous infarction of the nerve could be the cause.

Microvascular decompression of the trigeminal nerve requires sharp dissection of all arachnoid around the trigeminal nerve and superior cerebellar artery. The most common vessel found is a rostroventral superior cerebellar artery loop, which compresses the trigeminal nerve either at the brainstem or distally or both. After the arachnoid is dissected and the vessel

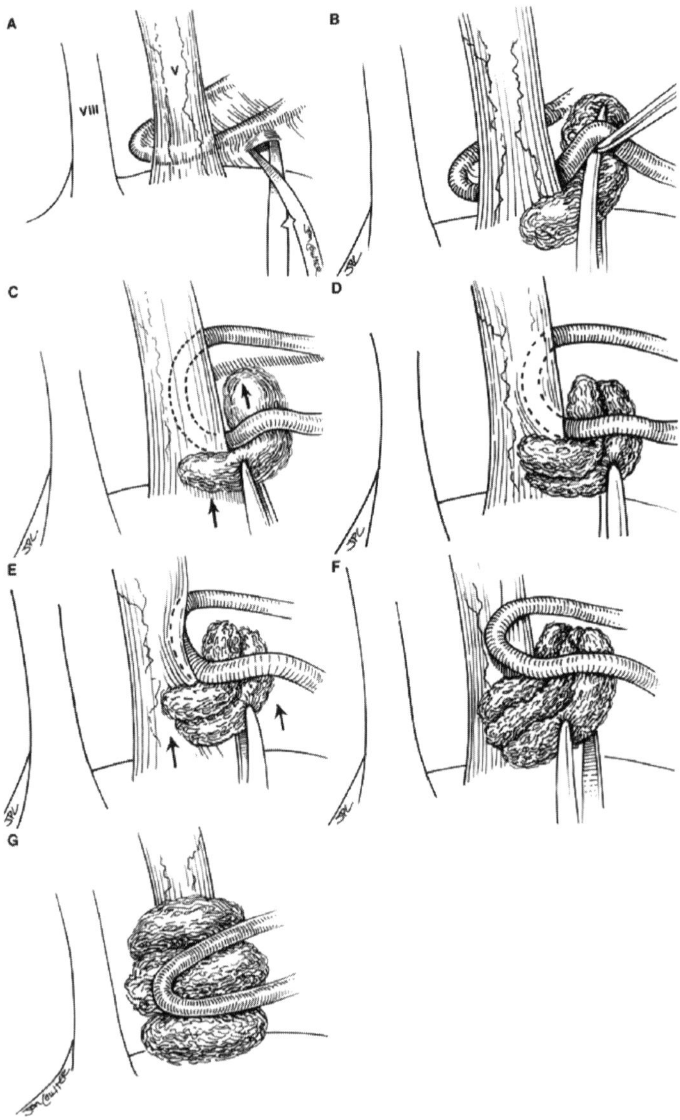

Figure 14.5 Diagrams depicting how dissection and mobilization of the arterial loop depend on the anatomy of compression.

This figure demonstrates the microsurgical movements that are performed when a typical superior cerebellar artery loop is found compressing the trigeminal nerve. The concepts of Teflon felt placement and proximal-to-distal sweeping movements of the felt along the nerve apply for lower cranial nerve decompressions as well. (A) Before the vessel can be moved, the arachnoid must be sharply dissected over the entire length of the loop proximally and distally. (B) After the vessel is freed, the vascular loop is lifted off the brainstem at the rostral aspect of the nerve and a medium-sized cigar-shaped piece of Teflon felt is placed between the vessel and the nerve. It is very important to position the distal portion of the felt with the tips of the forceps. The Teflon felt should not be pushed into position by holding its proximal portion. (C) After the Teflon felt is placed

Figure 14.5 (Continued)

under the loop, the pledget is gently pushed in a proximal-to-distal fashion along the nerve toward Meckel's cave. This movement elevates the arterial loop and causes it to begin to rotate outward from the ventral surface of the nerve. (D) A second Teflon felt, approximately the same size, is placed where the first felt was originally positioned. Using the same proximal-to-distal sweeping motion, the felt should be advanced over the length of the nerve toward Meckel's cave. (E) As the Teflon pledgets are advanced, the vascular loop progressively rotates from the ventral aspect of the nerve to the dorsal side. (F) A third Teflon pledget is placed where the first felt was originally positioned and, again, a proximal-to-distal sweeping movement along the trigeminal nerve flips the vascular loop to the dorsal aspect of the nerve. (G) After the vascular loop is flipped to the dorsal surface of the nerve, pledgets are placed between the vessel and the nerve.

is freed, the loop is mobilized to a horizontal position rostral to the nerve and shredded Teflon felt is placed between the vessel and the nerve (Fig. 14.5). Various neurovascular abnormalities are seen in rostral compression by the superior cerebellar artery is the primary pathology in V_3 or V_{2-3} pain (Fig. 14.6 a and b, 14.7) but may cause V_1, V_2, and V_3 pain. Isolated V_2 pain is frequently caused by a distal crossing vein and isolated V_1 pain by a caudal vessel, often a dolichocephalic vertebral artery.

STEP 7: OPERATIVE CLOSURE

Wax the bone edges on the way in and on the way out.

At the conclusion of the decompression procedure, several Valsalva maneuvers are performed to ensure hemostasis. The retractor is then removed, and the cerebellar surface is carefully inspected. Valsalva maneuvers are repeated to verify hemostasis. The area is gently irrigated with warm saline bulb irrigation, and the durotomy is closed over a strip of Gelfoam. We are aggressive in performing dural closure in which facia/muscle grafts from the inferior portion of the incision are used as necessary to ensure watertight closure. The bone edges are thoroughly waxed for a second time. A small pad of Gelfoam is then placed over the durotomy, and cranioplasty is performed using titanium wire mesh. The deep and superficial muscles are approximated with interrupted 2.0 or 3.0 absorbable sutures, and the fascia is closed with the same type of sutures. The fascial closure must be watertight to prevent any CSF leakage. Interrupted sutures lend strength to the facial closure. A second Valsalva maneuver may reveal further egress of CSF through the fascia, necessitating reinforcement of the closure. The subcutaneous tissues are approximated with No. 5.0 interrupted absorbable sutures. Well-approximated subcutaneous and subcuticular layers will help afford protection from CSF leakage. Water-soluble glue is placed over the incision. A small piece of gauze is placed over this while still wet.

Patients spend 2–4 hours in the recovery room. Incisional pain, headache, and nausea, if present, are treated as necessary. Patients are then sent to a room on the neurosurgical floor. The intensive care unit is utilized only

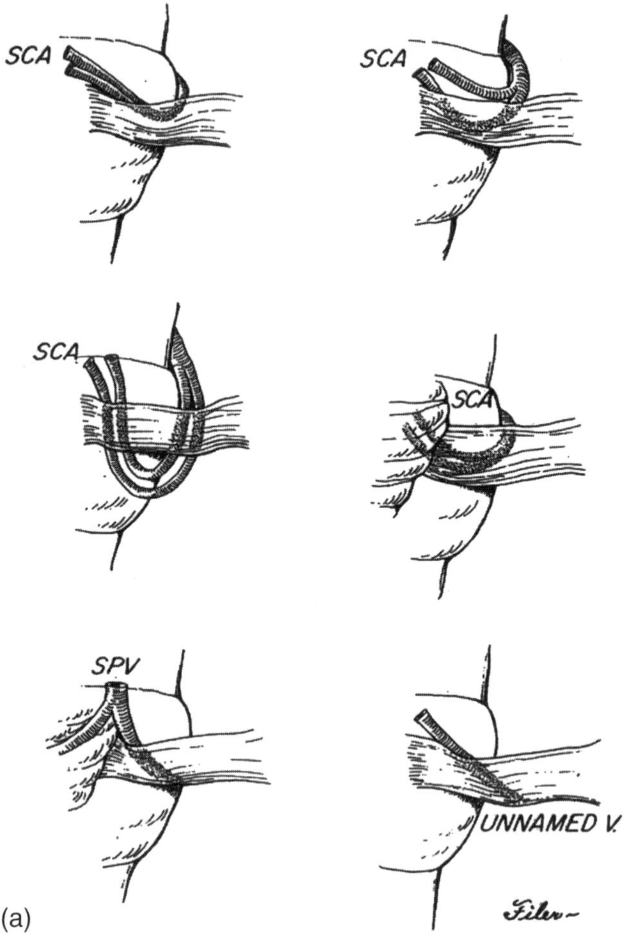

(a)

Figure 14.6a Right trigeminal nerve.

Common types of obvious vascular compression in trigeminal neuralgia.

in patients with special needs. Patients are ambulated on the evening of operation. We routinely use invasive arterial pressure monitoring in the perioperative period. Intravenous antemetic medications are administered liberally to minimize postoperative nausea and emesis.

Early mobilization of our patients is encouraged, beginning on the evening of operation or the next morning. Provided the postoperative course is uneventful, patients are discharged at 24–48 hours. Most patients have some degree of frontal headache or incisional pain; however, the presence of severe headache unresponsive to low-dosage narcotic medications necessitates obtaining a computed tomography (CT) scan to rule out the

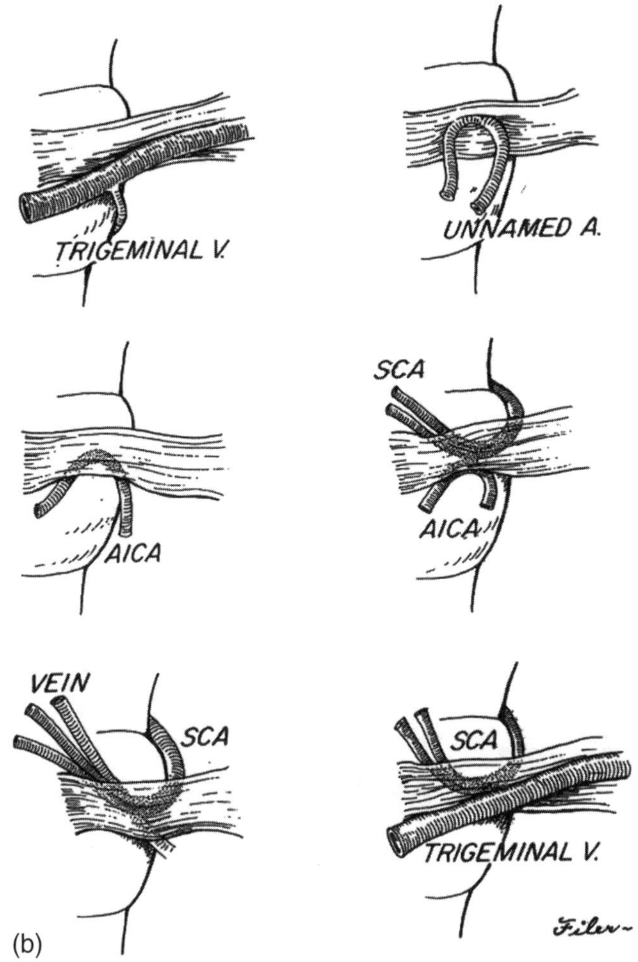

Figure 14.6b Rostral compression generally is found with lower facial neuralgia, lateral or medial compression with V_2 neuralgia, and caudal compression with V_1 neuralgia.

very rare hemorrhage. If the scan is negative for hemorrhage, we routinely perform a lumbar puncture and slowly drain CSF until the closing pressure is halfway down to 100 mm of water. We have found that many postoperative headaches are due to temporarily high opening pressures and are definitively treated with one lumbar puncture and one dose of adrenal cortical steroids (i.e., dexamethasone 10 mg). Gram stain is performed on the CSF before giving the steroid.

Rarely does a patient need readmission. Mild analgesics are prescribed, along with instructions to call us or come to the emergency room if they

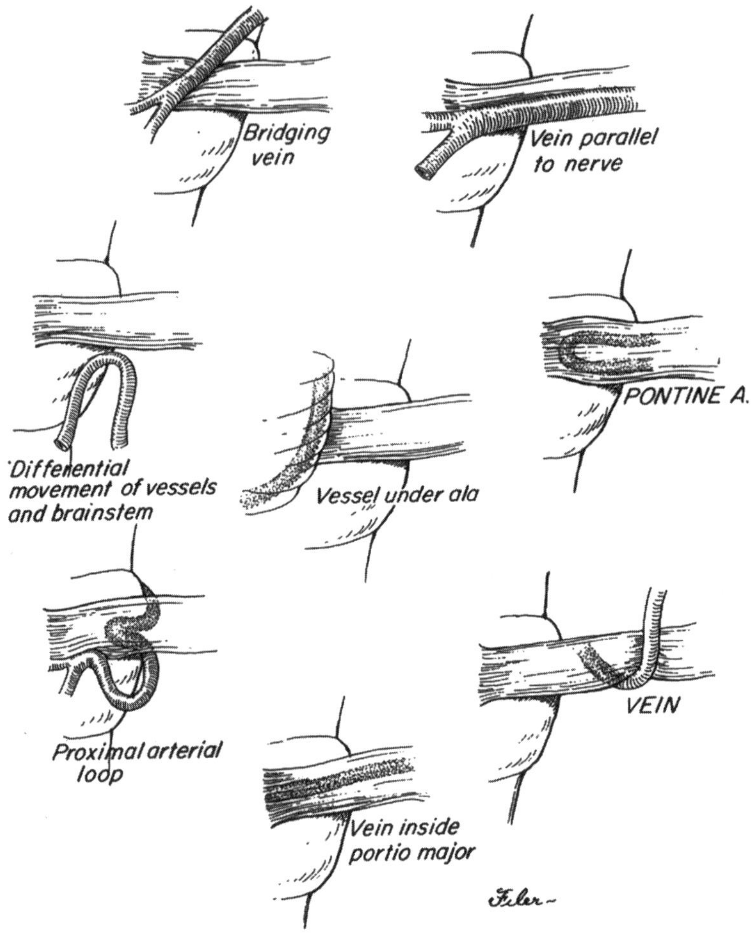

Figure 14.7 Right trigeminal nerve.

More subtle types of vascular compression of the trigeminal nerve. These findings may be the sole cause of trigeminal neuralgia or may be found in combination with more obvious compression (Fig. 14.6).

Table 14.1 Incidence of complications during microvascular decompression of cranial nerves

Complications	Before 1990 (2420 ops)	Since 1990 (1995 ops)	Total (4415 ops)
cerebellar injury	21 (0.87%)	9 (0.45%)	30 (0.68%)
eighth nerve injury	48 (1.98%)	16 (0.80%)	64 (1.45%)
CSF leak	59 (2.44%)	37 1.85%)	96 (2.17%)

Table 14.2 Incidence of hearing loss following microvascular decompression of cranial nerves*

Decom	Before 1990	Since 1990	Total
CN V	22 of 1659 (1.33%)	9 of 1537 (0.59%)	31 of 3196 (0.97%)
CN VII	26 of 692 (3.76%)	6 of 377 (1.59%)	32 of 1069 (2.99%)
CN IX/X	0 of 69 (0.0%)	0 of 81 (0.0%)	0 of 150 (0.0%)
total	48 of 2420 (1.98%)	15 of 1995 (0.75 %)	63 of 4415 (1.43%)

*CN = cranial nerve; decom = decompression procedure.

have any problems. We see patients in the Cranial Nerve Center on the fourth or fifth postoperative day, and they then return to their homes.

COMPLICATION AVOIDANCE

We studied trends over time with respect to the three complications thought to be directly related to operative technique during MVD. The complications evaluated were cerebellar injury, hearing loss, and CSF leakage. These three complications are by no means comprehensive, but are easily defined and determined objectively through routine postoperative clinical, radiographic, and neurophysiological evaluations (McLaughlin et al. 1999).

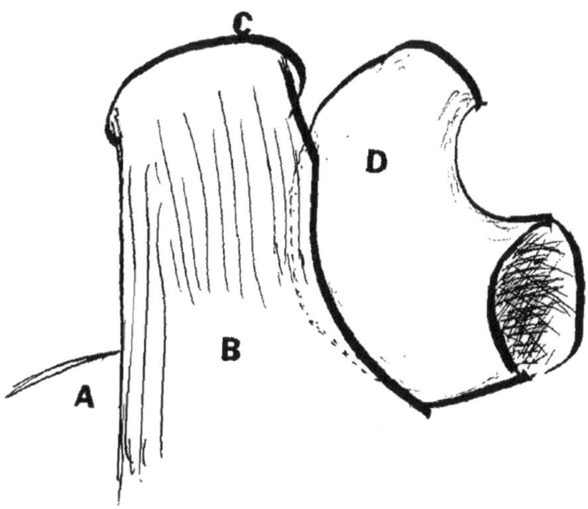

Figure 14.8 Right trigeminal nerve.

Dolichoectatic vertebral artery compressing caudal side of nerve. V_1 distribution of pain. Smaller arteries or veins may be pushed into nerve by a larger artery and must be treated. (A) Pons. (B) Proximal vein. (C) Meckel's cave. (D) Dolichoectatic vertebral artery.

Other rare complications of the procedures, such as facial weakness or anesthesia, lower cranial nerve dysfunction, or recurrent symptoms, were not evaluated because of their relative infrequency and because they have been reported in detail in previous communications (Barker et al. 1995, 1996; Resnick et al. 1995). By evaluating cerebellar injury, hearing loss, and CSF leakage, decreases in their occurrence could be detected in operations performed since 1990. Of the 4,415 operations for TN, hemifacial spasm, or glossopharyngeal neuralgia performed since 1972, there have been 30 cerebellar injuries (0.68%), 64 hearing deficits (1.45%), and 96 CSF leaks (2.17%) (Table 14.1). When operations performed before 1990 were compared with those performed since 1990, we found that these rates have decreased. The largest decline was in hearing loss (1.98% compared with 0.8%, $p < 0.01$; test for equality of distributions, Table 14.1). Although brainstem evoked responses (BSER) were used before 1990, the rate of hearing loss includes many operations performed early in our series, when use of BSERs was experimental. Thus, use of intraoperative BSERs appears to have contributed significantly to the observed decline in postoperative hearing deficits.

Other factors have also contributed to this decline, the most important of which is increased operative experience.

OTHER OPERATIVE NUANCES

Decompression of the fifth cranial nerve requires some support of the cerebellum by a self-retaining retractor, which can put tension on the seventh and eighth nerves and, hence, may lead to hearing loss. If, during a fifth nerve decompression, the BSERs begin to decline, it may be related to tethering of the arachnoid to the seventh–eighth nerve complex. When delays are encountered, the surgeon should continue sharp arachnoidal dissection down to, and slightly below, the seventh–eighth nerve complex. This maneuver frequently will relieve the tension on the cochlear nerve and cause improvement in the BSERs.

Bradycardia may occur with manipulation of an offending blood vessel at the site of compression but is usually self-limited. If cardiac arrest occurs, the implant should be quickly removed. I call this phenomenon "two hearts beating as none." Prolongation of the brainstem auditory evoked potentials should be treated by moving or removing the retractor, and sectioning away arachnoid around CN VIII, which may be secondarily distracting the nerve. I found by bitter experience that the third prolongation of the evoked potentials may be associated with permanent hearing loss. Last, if a caudal-to-rostral coursing vein is taken around CN V, it is important to see that the proximal caudal portion has not dilated, compressing either CN VII or VIII. If so, it should be taken caudal to these nerves. A Valsalva maneuver is performed several times as a check for potential arterial or venous bleeding.

As has been so succinctly stated by Apfelbaum (1977), the cerebellopontine angle is "an unforgiving area." Preventing trouble is much easier than treating trouble.

When BSERs change during the procedure, it is usually due to retraction. The first response of the surgeon should be to reduce or remove retraction, or at least change the position of the retractor. We have found this usually improves the BSERs. Constant surveillance of the retractor is imperative because it often shifts and is frequently only millimeters from the eighth cranial nerve. Occasionally, the BSERs will change after decompression and are not corrected with alterations in retraction. In these cases, inspection of the entire length of the eighth nerve may disclose impingement from a Teflon implant or displaced blood vessel. Appropriate alterations should then be made. Finally, a change in BSERs may occur on closure of the dura. Although this happens very rarely, the dura should always be reopened. Opening the dura usually causes the BSERs to return to baseline. In this situation, reexploration of the decompression and the eighth cranial nerve should be performed. Manipulation of any impingements on the eighth nerve and closure of the dura can then be safely completed. We have also observed that small amounts of blood or cold saline irrigation on the cochlear nerve may adversely affect BSERs.

Injury of the cerebellum, usually minor, including hemorrhage and contusion, have also occurred with less frequency since 1990 (0.8% compared with 0.45%, $p < 0.01$; Table 14.1). Limitation of the degree and duration of retraction remains essential in avoiding cerebellar injury. The entire decompression procedure (from skin incision to skin closure) generally takes less than 2 hours and requires only a small corridor of exposure between the cerebellum and petrous temporal bone. This corridor is kept to a minimum by adequate exposure of the sigmoid sinus by mastoid bone removal prior to durotomy. This allows a dural incision very close to the sigmoid sinus, rather than a more posterior durotomy that requires more cerebellar retraction to permit visualization along the petrous temporal bone. We place rubber dams made from latex gloves on the cerebellar side of all cottonoids so that smooth, gentle advancement can be performed. Also, the approach superiorly and inferiorly allows CSF drainage from cisterns prior to significant retraction. An approach that leads straight in requires more cerebellar tissue to be retracted and exposes the seventh–eighth nerve complex, rather than a CSF cistern, which can allow further relaxation of the cerebellum.

Avoidance of CSF leaks remains problematic after transgression of mastoid air cells and exposure of multiple overlapping tissue planes. Our incidence of CSF leaks has declined since 1990 from 2.44% to 1.85% ($p < 0.01$). Mastoid air cells are frequently opened to obtain adequate visualization of the margin of the sigmoid sinus. Copious amounts of bone should be applied before durotomy and after dural closure. The nuchal musculature does not extend above the digastric groove. Therefore, good surgical technique should be applied, and the muscular layers approximated before fascial closure. Care should be taken not to include the galea in the deep muscle closure at the inferior aspect of the wound, so that a single layer of fascia is left to close along the entire length of the incision. This should be closed with interrupted sutures. An inverted, interrupted No. 3.0 absorbable closure of the subcutaneous tissues should also be watertight and should not be placed until a Valsalva maneuver reveals a watertight galeal closure. Postoperative CSF leaks usually resolve with lumbar drainage, although a minority of cases require operative intervention, including reexploration of the dural closure and careful inspection of the mastoid air cells.

CONCLUSION

Over time, the technique of MVD has progressed, with changes designed to improve safety and efficacy. Implementation of neurophysiological monitoring and meticulous attention to the microsurgical anatomy of the posterior fossa have improved complication rates for cerebellar injury and hearing loss to less than 1%. We believe this seven-step approach, combined with the surgical wisdom gained from a large experience, remains the key to successful outcome.

REFERENCES

Apfelbaum RI. A comparison of percutaneous radiofrequency trigeminal neurolysis and microvascular decompression of the trigeminal nerve for the treatment of tic douloureux. *Neurosurgery* 1977;1(1):16–21.

Barker FG II, Jannetta PJ, Bissonette DJ, et al. Microvascular decompression for hemifacial spasm. *J Neurosurg* 1995;82:201–210.

Barker FG, et al. The long-term outcome of microvascular decompression for trigeminal neuralgia. *N Engl J Med* 1996;334(17):1077–1083.

Bennett MH, Jannetta PJ. Trigeminal evoked potentials in humans. Electroencephalogram. *Clin Neurophysiol* 1980;48(5):517–526.

Bennett MH, Jannetta PJ. Evoked potentials in trigeminal neuralgia. *Neurosurgery* 1983;13(3):242–247.

Dandy WE. The treatment of trigeminal neuralgia by the cerebellar route. *Ann Surg* 1932;96:787–795.

Dandy WE. Concerning the case of trigeminal neuralgia. *Am J Surg* 1934;24:447–455.

Erulkar SD, Sprague JM, Whitsel BL, et al. Organization of the vestibular projections to the spinal cord of the cat. *J Neurophiol* 1966;29:626–644.

Frazier CH. A surgeon's impression of trigeminal neuralgia based on experiences with three hundred and two cases. *JAMA* 1918; 70:1345–1350.

Frazier CH. Subtotal resection of sensory root for relief of major trigeminal neuralgia. *Arch Neurol Psychiat*; 1925;13:376–384.

Gardner WJ, Milkos MV. Response of trigeminal neuralgia to decompression of sensory root. *JAMA* 1959;170:1773–1776.

Jannetta PJ. And Rand RW,SMicroanatomy of the trigeminal nerve. *Anatomical Record* 1966; 54(2):362.

Jannetta PJ. Gross (mesoscopic) description of the human trigeminal nerve and ganglion. *J Neurosurg* (1967):26;109–111.

Lewy F, Grant F. Physiopathological and pathoanatomic aspects of major trigeminal neuralgia. *Arch Neurol Psychiat* 1938;40:1126–1134.

McLaughlin MR, Jannetta PJ, Clyde BL, et al. Microvascular decompression of cranial nerves: lessons learned after 4400 operations. *J Neurosurg* 1999;90:1–8.

Nylen CO. The microscope in aural surgery, its first use and later developments. *Acta Otolaryngol Suppl.* 1954:116:226–240.

Resnick DK, Jannetta PJ, Bissonette D, et al. Microvascular decompression for glossopharyngeal neuralgia. *Neurosurgery* 1995;36:64–69.

15

Endoscopic Vascular Decompression

Hae-Dong Jho, Diana H-J Jho, and David H. Jho

In recent years, interest in adopting the use of an endoscope for intracranial surgery has increased. During microscopic cerebral aneurysm surgery, an endoscope is utilized as an adjunctive instrument introduced into the surgical corridor in order to inspect the hidden corners of the operating area. In a similar way, an endoscope is introduced into the cerebellopontine angle during microscopic vascular decompression (MVD) surgery to visualize hidden corners of the neurovascular compression while the operation is mainly performed under the operating microscope (Magnan & Sanna 1999). Although the use of an endoscope during the surgical treatment of Jannetta's neurovascular compression disorders has not yet demonstrated improved surgical outcomes, it has been claimed that the endoscope demonstrates a higher rate of neurovascular compression than the operating microscope alone. Thus, an endoscope has been sporadically adopted as a tool to assist with microscopic surgery (endoscope-assisted MVD surgery). (Chen et al. 2008; Jarrahy, Berci, & Shahinian 2000; Magnan & Sanna 1999; Rak et al. 2004; Teo, Nakaji, & Mobbs 2006). Noting the safe feasibility of purely endoscopic intracranial surgery with our increasing experiences, we adopted purely endoscopic techniques with Jannetta's neurovascular decompression surgery for neurovascular compression disorders at the cerebellopontine angle. Although endoscopic vascular decompression surgery has been performed for other cranial nerve neurovascular decompression disorders, in this chapter we describe the surgical tools and techniques for endoscopic vascular decompression surgery for trigeminal neuralgia (TN). In addition, alternative endoscopic techniques for Jannetta's vascular decompression surgery are described.

SURGICAL TOOLS AND TECHNIQUES

Surgical Instruments

The required surgical instruments are endoscopes with 0-, 30-, and 70-degree lenses and their appendages, including a video-imaging system, light source and its connections, an endoscope lens-cleansing device, a rigid endoscope holder, and various other surgical instruments specifically designed for endoscopic surgery.

Endoscopes

The endoscopes we use are rod-lens devices that are 4 mm in diameter and 18 cm in length. Being originally developed for paranasal sinus surgery, the physical shape of these endoscopes is not ideal for intracranial surgery. One set consists of five endoscopes; a 0-degree lens endoscope, a 30-degree lens angled away from and toward the light source, and a 70-degree lens angled away and toward the light source (Fig. 15.1). A 0-degree lens endoscope is our basic tool; however, a 30-degree lens endoscope whose lens is angled away from the light source is used when an angled view is required toward the brainstem. A 30-degree lens endoscope whose lens is angled toward the light source is used when an angled view is required toward Meckel's cave or away from the brainstem.

Endoscope Lens-Cleaner

An endoscopic lens-cleansing device is required so that the surgeon can continually operate without interruption (Fig. 15.2). The device consists of an electric-powered motor and a disposable irrigation tube, which is passed through the electric-powered motor. An endoscope is placed through a tubular irrigating sheath, which is connected to the irrigating tube. The irrigation tube is connected to a saline bag, which is hung on a pole, and this motor-powered irrigation device is controlled by a foot pedal to flush

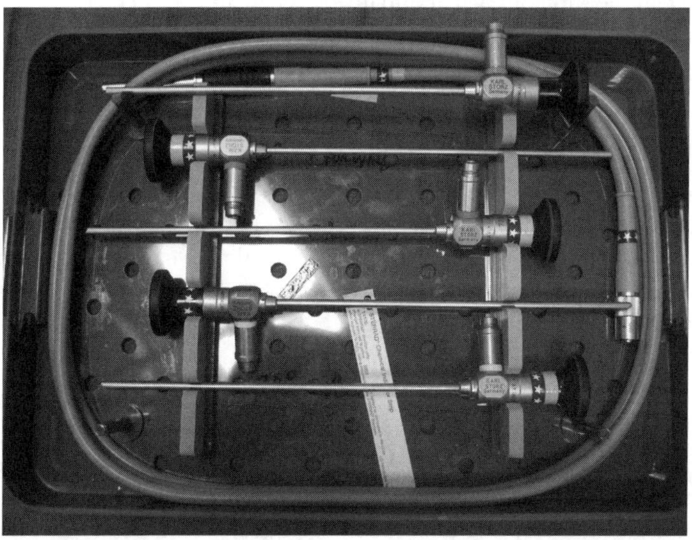

Figure 15.1 Endoscopes. One set of our endoscopes consists of five endoscopes: a 0-degree lens endoscope, 30-degree lens angled away from and toward the light source, and 70-degree lens angled away and toward the light source.

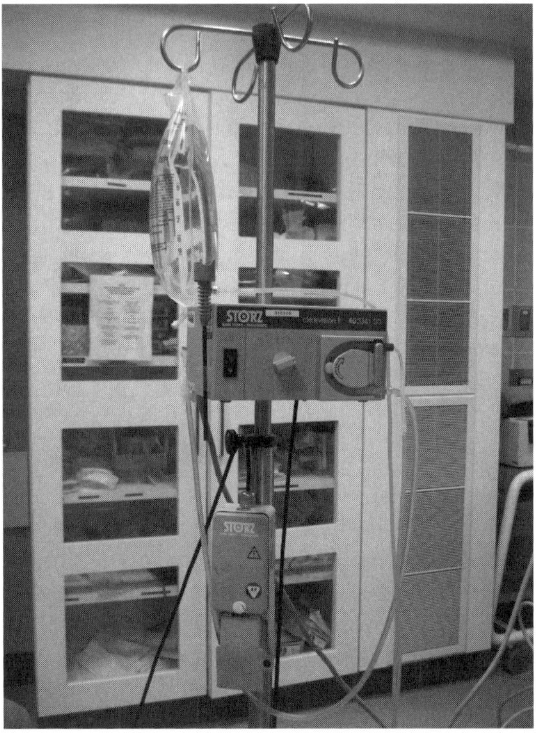

Figure 15.2 An endoscopic lens-cleansing device is required to cleanse the lens so that the surgeon can continually operate without interruption.

The device consists of an electric-powered motor, a foot-control pedal, and a disposable irrigation tube, which is passed through an electric-powered motor.

saline forward. When the foot pedal is released, the motor reverses its rotary direction and draws the saline back from the tip of the endoscope for 1–2 seconds. The forward flow of irrigating saline cleans the lens, and the reverse flow clears water bubbles at the tip of the endoscope. Although this device is not yet ideal, it helps the surgeon significantly in the task of keeping the endoscope lens clean.

Endoscope Holder

An appropriate endoscope holder is another piece of essential equipment required to perform this operation efficiently. An endoscope holder is mounted to the operating table or to various neurosurgical head-holding devices. It not only provides steady video-imaging on a video monitor, but also allows a surgeon to use both hands freely. The holder must provide rigid fixation of the endoscope, and its holding terminal must be compact and slender, to provide adequate operating space around the endoscope shaft allowing the surgeon to maneuver surgical instruments.

Two different types of endoscope holders are currently available, neither of which are ideal. One is a simple manual holder with multiple joints that can be tightened by hand. The other is a holder with joints that are powered by nitrogen gas and controlled by a single button. Manual holders are inconvenient to maneuver with releasing, repositioning, and tightening. They also have limitations in flexibility to reach the various positions. Nitrogen-gas powered devices are better than manual types, but are not as good as the operating microscope to release and lock at various positions. For cranial endoscopic surgery, we use a Mitaka endoscope holder (distributed by Karl Stortz) or an Asculop holder (Fig. 15.3A, B). The Mitaka holder still has very narrow accessibility and needs improvement. The Asculop holder has limitation in distal maneuverability. A few millimeters of sagging after release of the power-button is another problem with the nitrogen-powered holders.

Endoscopic Surgical Instruments

Among various surgical instruments, a monopolar suction coagulator (No. 8 or No. 9 French cannula), a bipolar suction coagulator (No. 8 or No. 9 French cannula), and a single-bladed bipolar coagulator are useful tools for hemostasis. They are all disposable, and the monopolar suction coagulator is malleable and insulated. The bipolar suction coagulator and single-bladed bipolar coagulator have two cables at the single blade for producing bipolar function; the single-bladed bipolar has one electrode at the core and the other at the shell. Various bipolar forceps such as straight, curved-up, and curved-down are used. The two blades of the bipolar forceps are almost parallel to each other. When approximated, the bipolar blades resemble a one-bladed tool. Other two-blade instruments are also modified to a similar shape in order to accommodate the endoscopic surgical environment. Jannetta's microdissectors are modified in their tip curvatures, so that their tips can reach the surgical target area freely in front of an endoscope. (Fig. 15.4) Other surgical instruments utilized are those also used in microscopic surgery.

Surgical Techniques

Positioning of the Patient

The position of the patient is the same as in microscopic surgery. The head of the patient is held in a lateral position; however, the body can be supine, or lateral, or prone (Fig. 15.5). When the patient has a long and supple neck, he or she can be in the supine position with the shoulder raised. Then, the head is turned laterally. The head can be fixed and secured with adhesive tapes or a three-pin head holding system. When the patient's neck is short

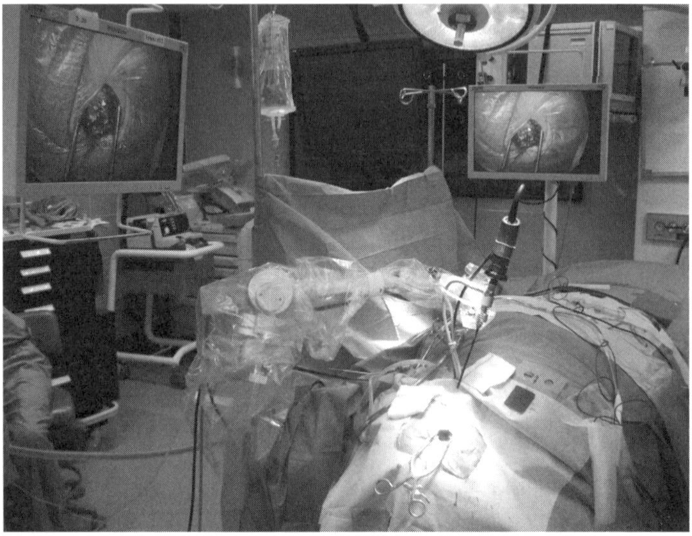

(a)

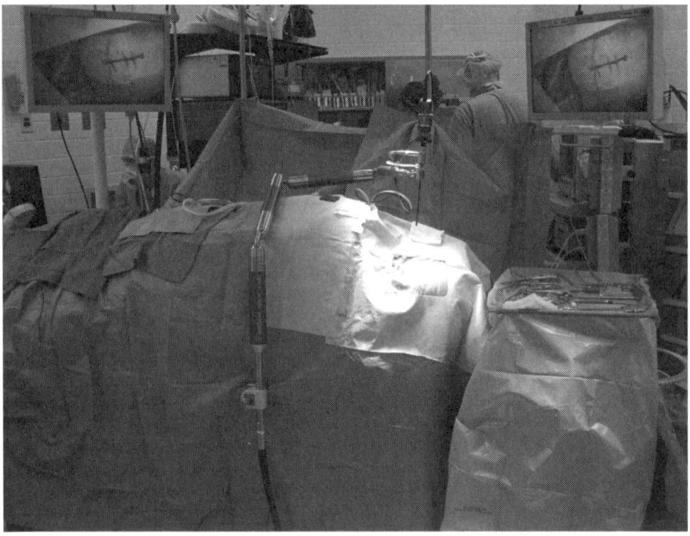

(b)

Figure 15.3 Gas-powered endoscope holders.

For cranial endoscopic surgery, we use a Mitaka endoscope holder (distributed by Carl Stortz) (A); or an Aesculap holder (B).

and has a limited range of motion, the body is positioned laterally, as well as the head. The head is fixed with a three-pin head holding system. When a patient has large shoulders and a very short neck, the superior shoulder in the lateral position will interfere with surgical access to the cerebellopontine angle. In that case, the patient can be positioned a three-quarter-prone position with the head in a lateral position.

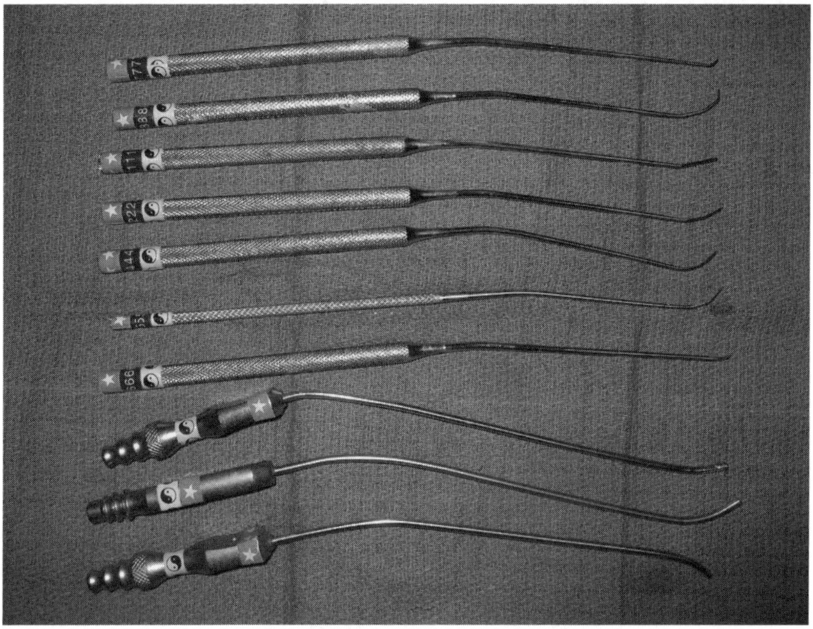

Figure 15.4 Microdissectors and cannulas.

Jannetta's microdissectors and suction cannulas are modified in their tip curvatures, so that their tips can reach the surgical target area freely in front of an endoscope.

Operative Technique

A video monitor is placed in front of the patient's head, so that the surgeon can directly face the video monitor when an endoscope is placed into the cranial cavity. Another video monitor is placed at the patient's leg area, so that the scrub nurse can face the video monitor. While the surgeon stands behind the patient's head, the scrub nurse stands obliquely facing the surgeon at the top of patient's head (Fig. 15.6). The endoscope holder is anchored to the operating table.

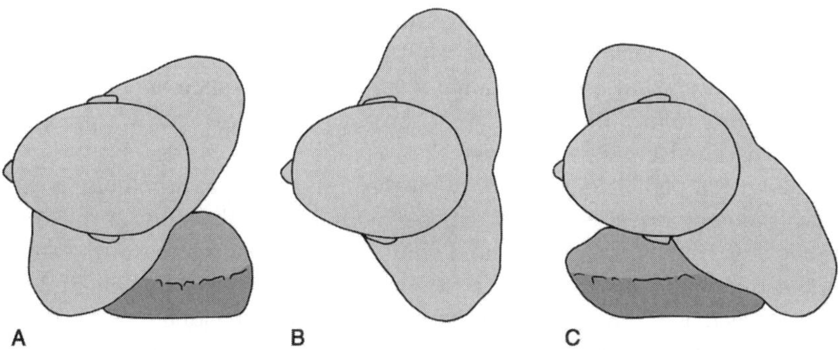

Figure 15.5 Patient positioning. The head is held in lateral; however, the body can be supine (A), or lateral (B), or prone (C).

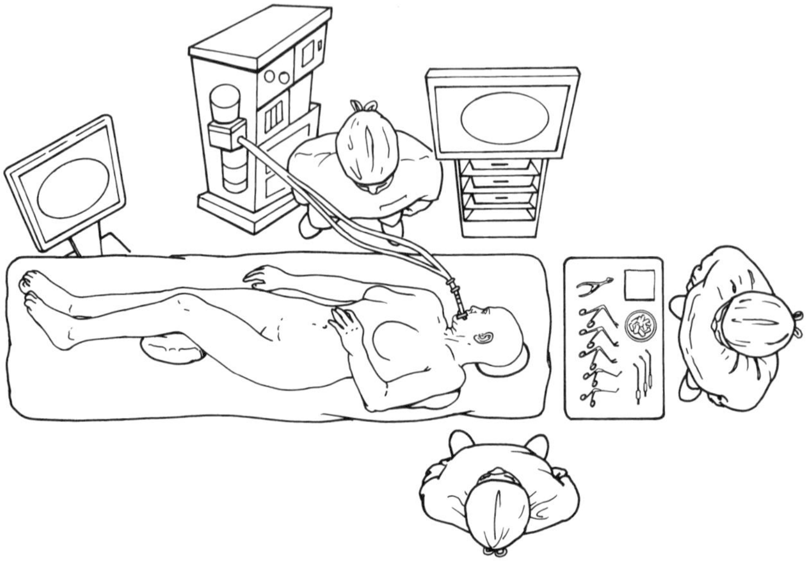

Figure 15.6 Operating room arrangement for endoscopic vascular decompression surgery.

While the surgeon stands behind the patient's head, the scrub nurse stands obliquely facing the surgeon at the top of patient's head.

Two different operative techniques can be used: one is the formal endoscopic surgery through a retromastoid craniectomy or craniotomy, similar to microscopic surgery; the other is the working-channel endoscopy. Formal endoscopic vascular decompression surgery is similar to microscopic surgery (Fig. 15.7). The details of operative techniques are described in Chapter 14. Briefly, approximately a 5 cm oblique skin incision is made 3 cm behind a mastoid tip. The target site of the surgical skull opening is at the junction of the sigmoid and transverse sinus for trigeminal nerve surgery. The target site of skull opening will be just behind the sigmoid sinus when the facial, vestibulocochlear, or glossopharyngeal and vagus nerves are operated on. Traditionally, a burr hole is made and a 2 × 3 cm craniectomy hole is made with Kerrison rongeurs. However, we prefer to perform a small craniotomy rather than a craniectomy. A small bone flap is made with a pediatric craniotomy bit through an 8 mm burr hole. Either way, the bony opening should expose the margin of the sinus at the junction of the transverse and sigmoid sinus. When the curvature of the sinus at the junction of the transverse and sigmoid sinus is clarified, a linear dura incision is made; however, when the angle of the sinus junction is acute, a T-shaped dura incision is made. When the dura is open, the cerebellum should not be allowed to herniate out and be strangulated at the dura opening. Particularly in a young adult, the cerebellum has to be kept inside the dural

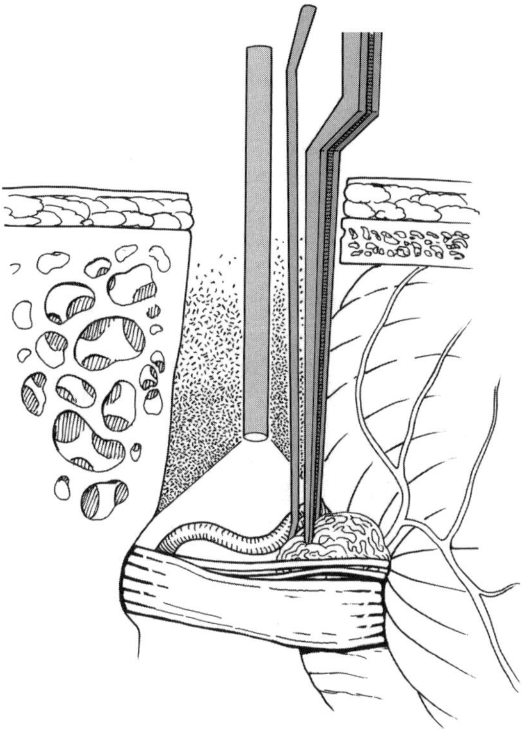

Figure 15.7 A formal endoscopic vascular decompression surgery.

Similar to microscopic surgery, through a small retromastoid craniotomy or craniectomy hole, an endoscope is inserted into the cerebellopontine angle and anchored to the endoscope holder. Neurosurgeon introduces surgical tools with two free hands, as in microscopic surgery.

plane in order not to damage the cerebellum. The cerebellum is covered and protected with a rubber dam and cotton pad.

Endoscopic neurovascular decompression surgery involves two-step endoscopic techniques. The first step is a free-hand technique, and the second step is two-hand technique with the endoscope anchored to the endoscope holder. The endoscope is held in the nondominant hand and a suction cannula in the dominant hand. A suction cannula is advanced between the tentorium and the cerebellum, and the endoscope follows to visualize the tip of the suction cannula and the upcoming anatomy. Once the arachnoid membrane has been identified, it is opened with a suction cannula or microscissors. Cerebrospinal fluid (CSF) is drained until the cerebellum becomes well relaxed. Once the CSF is drained and the cerebellum is well relaxed, the endoscope is attached to the endoscope holding system. Then, the endoscope is carefully placed inside the cranial cavity, visualizing the petrotentorial junction. The endoscope is advanced to visualize the trigeminal nerve and the rostral portion of the vestibulocochlear nerve. The petrosal vein can be kept intact or sacrificed with a bipolar coagulation, as needed. To avoid damage to the vestibulocochlear nerve, the nerve should be within the endoscopic view. An endoscope will visualize the trigeminal nerve from the Meckel's cave orifice to the trigeminal nerve root entry to the pons. At this point, the endoscope will be anchored to the endoscope holder. Using the two-free-hands technique similar to that utilized in microscopic surgery, the arachnoid membrane is dissected off the trigeminal nerve. The blood vessels are separated from the nerve and padded with Teflon felt implants. The operative technique of neurovascular decompression is the same as that of microscopic surgery; however, surgical instrument manipulation requires endoscopic skills in order to navigate around the shaft sitting at the center of the surgical corridor. In the event of unexpected bleeding, often venous in origin, the suction cannula must be kept at the bleeding area in order to continually clear the surgical area until the bleeding is controlled. Once vascular decompression is accomplished, the closure of the operative site is the same as in microscopic surgery. The bone flap is placed back with titanium sutures. Muscles are closed in two layers at the caudal incision and in one layer at the rostral incision. The fascia is then closed in a watertight fashion, placing continuous sutures over interrupted sutures, so that CSF or any body fluid will not leak through the operative incision. The skin is closed with subcuticular sutures, and skin glue is applied for skin surface approximation.

The other operative technique utilizes the working-channel endoscopy (Fig. 15.8) The 3 mm rod lens endoscope with a 1 mm working channel can be used. A 0-degree lens endoscope can be used, but a 30-degree lens endoscope is preferable. Patient positioning is the same as that described earlier; however, a head-holding device has to be applied for the image-guiding system. With the image-guiding system, the junction of the transverse sinus and sigmoid sinus is identified. Through a 1-inch incision, a burr hole is made at the margin of the sinus junction between the transverse sinus and sigmoid sinus. Once the dura mater is exposed at the retromastoid area, an intraoperative cisternal puncture is performed with a 21-gauge spinal needle at the C1–C2 level under fluoroscopic guidance. Approximately 20–30 mL of CSF is drained, until the dura mater at the retromastoid area is sunken in. The spinal needle is then removed. The dura mater at the retromastoid area is opened. The cerebellum is protected with a piece of rubber dam and cotton pad ($1/2 \times 3$). Then, a 3 mm working channel endoscope, preferably equipped with a 30-degree lens, is inserted under the tentorium, aiming to visualize the petrotentorial junction. The petrosal vein can be sacrificed if it is in the way. Through a working channel, a monopolar coagulator is used for coagulation of the petrosal vein. It is then divided with a single-blade flexible scissors. The trigeminal nerve can then be identified. With dissectors and scissors, the trigeminal nerve is exposed from the Meckel's cave orifice to the nerve root entry area at the pons.

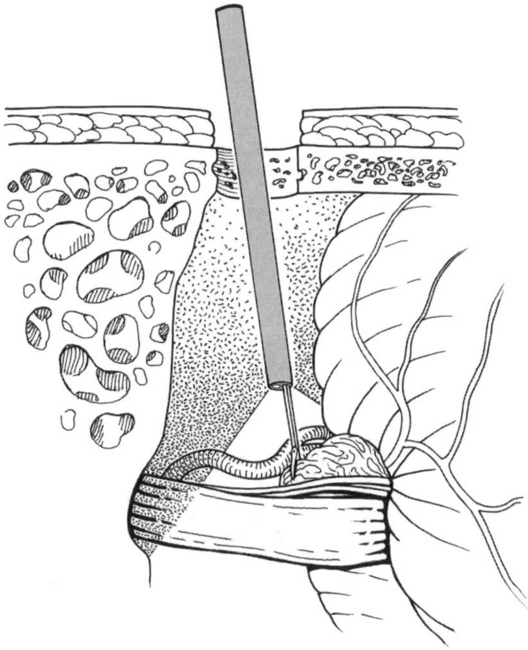

Figure 15.8 Working-channel endoscopy.

Once cerebrospinal fluid is drained with a C1–C2 puncture under the fluoroscopic guidance, a working-channel endoscope is inserted through a burr hole. Dissection and vascular decompression is carried out with one instrument inserted through a working channel.

Compressing vessels are separated off the nerve, and shredded Teflon felt implants are placed through the 1 mm working channel. Once the neurovascular decompression is finished, the cistern is filled with saline solution. The burr hole site is filled with compressed Gelfoam and repaired with a titanium burr hole cover. Periosteum, galea, and skin are closed as described earlier. The authors prefer formal endoscopic techniques to working-channel endoscopy.

We have explored the possible use of a flexible endoscope for neurovascular decompression as a percutaneous technique of endoscopy in cadavers (Fig. 15.9). A flexible endoscope was introduced into the cisterna magnum percutaneously at the C1–C2 interlaminar space or between the foramen magnum and C1 lamina. Endoscopic navigation was carried out through the cisterna magna cephalad. The landmarks for endoscopic navigation start with the vertebral artery. When the endoscope is advanced intracranially, following the vertebral artery, the hypoglossal nerve fascicles are encountered. The endoscope is advanced lateral to the hypoglossal nerve, and the vertebral artery is followed. The vagus and glossopharyngeal nerves are encountered lateral to the vertebral artery. For hemifacial spasm

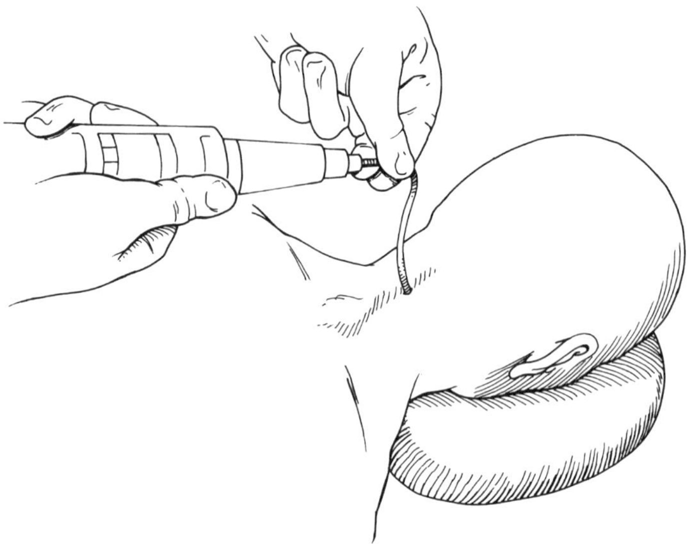

Figure 15.9 Experimental work in percutaneous flexible endoscopy.

A flexible endoscope is inserted at the C1–C2 or C1–cranium and navigated cranially for neurovascular decompression.

surgery, the facial nerve root entry area is visualized medial to the glossopharyngeal–vagus nerve root entry area. Teflon felt implants are placed between the facial nerve entry area and the offending vessels. (Sekula and Jho, 2005) For TN surgery, the endoscope is advanced medial to the facial and vestibulocochlear nerves. The trigeminal nerve is visualized. Neurovascular decompression is performed with Teflon felt implants that are delivered through a 1 mm working channel. (Sekula and Jho, 2005) We have not yet applied this technique in live surgery.

ADVANTAGES OF ENDOSCOPIC VASCULAR DECOMPRESSION SURGERY OVER MICROSCOPIC SURGERY

Optical Advantages of an Endoscope

Wide-angled View

While the operating microscope provides a magnified view of a limited portion of the anatomy through a narrow corridor, an endoscope can physically enter into the cerebellopontine angle and provide a wide-angled panoramic view with zooming capabilities (Fig. 15.10). The operating microscope renders a tubular parallel beam view at the surgical site with desired magnifications. The microscope beam must be directed exactly perpendicular to the surgical target in order to visualize the desired locale. In order to render a straight corridor for the microscopic beam from the lens to the surgical target area, the cerebellum must be retracted. However, an endoscope

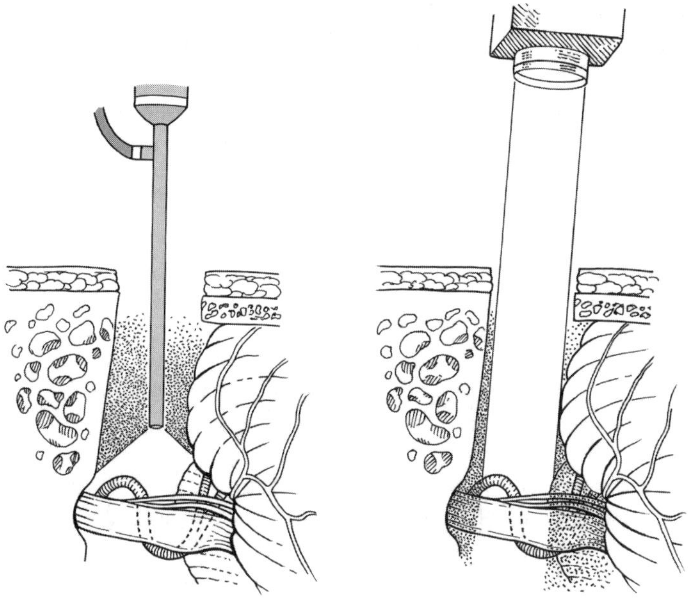

Figure 15.10 Difference between a microscopic and an endoscopic view at the trigeminal nerve area.

Instead of a limited view at a portion of the trigeminal nerve, as the operating microscope renders, an endoscope discloses a full spectrum of the trigeminal nerve from the nerve root entry area at the pons to Meckel's cave orifice.

directly enters into the cerebellopontine angle cistern through a narrow space, thus, cerebellar retraction is not necessary.

Another advantage is that an endoscope depicts a diverging flask-shaped, wide-angled view. The trigeminal nerve will be visualized from the Meckel's cave to the nerve root entry area at the pons. This wide-angled panoramic view is particularly useful for Jannetta's neurovascular decompression surgery at the cerebellopontine angle. Instead of a limited view at a portion of the trigeminal nerve, as the operating microscope renders, an endoscope discloses a full spectrum of the trigeminal nerve from the nerve root entry area at the pons to Meckel's cave orifice. However, it must be recognized that the endoscopic view renders a fish-eye effect, with maximum magnification at the center and relative contraction at the periphery. Thus, the endoscope's optical distortion has to be overcome by a neurosurgeon in order to perceive the true anatomy of the surgical site.

Angled-lens View

The angled-lens endoscopic view provides direct visualization at the anatomical corners, such as at the Meckel's cave, nerve-root entry areas at the brainstem, or the internal view of the auditory meatus. When a 30-degree angled endoscope is inserted into the cerebellopontine angle cistern and rotated through a full revolution, it can visualize the entire circumference of the cistern. These views can be of great assistance even if an endoscope is used only as an adjunctive tool during conventional microscopic surgery. The hidden vein under the petrous prominence that is not disclosed by the operating microscope can be easily visualized. This angled endoscopic view has been used when a neurosurgeon uses an endoscope as an adjunctive tool during microscopic vascular decompression surgery. However, operating solely under an angled-lens endoscope requires specially designed surgical tools and advanced endoscopic surgical skills, particularly for the 70-degree lens endoscope.

Close-up View

Advancing close to the surgical target, an endoscope will progressively magnify its image. This close-up view, in conjunction with digital zooming of the camera, enhances the magnification of the surgical site. The magnification comes with the combined effect of optical and digital magnification. This close-up view can provide the details of vascular compression at the trigeminal nerve root entry area at the brainstem, particularly arteriolar or venular compression. However, during this close-up visualization, surgical view is very limited to the focal area, leaving the vast area of the surgical corridor blind. In particular, surgical instruments passing in and out of the blind surgical corridor can damage neurovascular structures. When the Jannetta decompression surgery is performed solely under an endoscope, the device is anchored to the endoscope holder and placed to visualize that portion of the vestibulocochlear nerve, while producing a view of the entire portion of the trigeminal nerve. In this way, the neurosurgeon can continually watch the surgical instruments in relation to the vestibulocochlear nerve while they are placed in and out of the surgical area.

Physical Advantages of an Endoscope

The slender physical shape of the endoscope shaft with the visualizing lens at the tip allows navigation through narrow anatomical spaces and eliminates the need to retract the cerebellum. Frequently, microscopic surgery requires cerebellar retraction in order to provide a straight tubular surgical corridor. Although the rod-lens endoscope shaft still requires straight entry, it can be placed without the use of cerebellar retraction. Once it enters into the cistern, it visualizes the surgical area well. However, a flexible endoscope can navigate the curved surgical corridor. Endoscopes can be subdivided into two categories: fiber-optic flexible endoscopes (including the recently developed videoscope) and rod-lens rigid endoscopes. The number of fiber-optic fibers in most flexible endoscopes is approximately 10,000, although new flexible endoscopes carrying up to

50,000 fibers are being developed. Thus, the image quality of the flexible endoscope is still inadequate for magnified delicate surgery, and its use is limited to occasional inspection at deep curved anatomical regions. Recently developed videoscopes have provided improved image quality. A 5 mm videoscope with a 1 mm working channel is commercially available. A 3 mm videoscope without a working channel will be available soon. These videoscopes have a good potential in endoscopic surgery because their image quality is better than that of the fiberscope. However, the videoscope image quality is still not as good as that of the rod-lens endoscope's high-definition image. Thus, rod-lens endoscopes are the main tools for neurovascular decompression surgery. Three or 4 mm rod-lens endoscopes can be used for primary visualization; 4 mm rod-lens endoscopes provide full-screen, high-quality images in contrast to the smaller, inferior quality images provided by 3 mm rod-lens endoscopes. The basic endoscopes used by the authors are 4 mm rod-lens endoscopes with 0-, 30-, or 70-degree lenses.

DISADVANTAGES OF ENDOSCOPIC VASCULAR DECOMPRESSION SURGERY OVER MICROSCOPIC SURGERY

The major disadvantage of endoscopic surgery over microscopic surgery is the snake-eye effect of an endoscope. While microscopic view renders views from the surface of the cranial opening to the surgical target inside the cranial cavity, an endoscope provides a view only in front of the endoscopic lens. The surgical corridor along the endoscopic shaft is a completely blind area. While being placed in and out of the surgical corridor, the surgical instruments can damage the surrounding anatomy at the endoscopically blind corridor. Thus, the surrounding blind anatomical area, such as the cerebellum, has to be well protected. Particular care must be exercised while surgical instruments are passed in and out of the surgical corridor. Another disadvantage is mechanical obstruction by the endoscopic shaft placed at the surgical corridor. The endoscopic shaft becomes a continual hindrance for the placement of the two surgical instruments, one in each hand. Thus, surgical instruments have to be modified in order to adapt to the mechanical restraints of the endoscopic shaft. In addition, the surgeon must be trained to become familiar with this mechanical limitation imposed by the endoscopic shaft. The third disadvantage is the flat two-dimensional view through an endoscope. Although a three-dimensional endoscope is available, most endoscopes currently being used render a monocular view. The in-and-out of a surgical instrument in front of an endoscope lens provides the neurosurgeon with relative depth perception at the surgical target area. Also, when bleeding occurs, it can occlude the surgical view. Thus, any potential venous bleeding has to be taken care of in advance. Last, neurosurgeons have to be well trained to work under endoscopic visualization before performing live operations.

CONCLUSION

The use of an endoscope for trigeminal nerve surgery was first described by Doyen in 1917 (Doyen 1917). He described an endoscopic trigeminal rhizotomy through a retrosigmoid approach. Since then, various endoscopic anatomical explorations in cadaver specimens have been reported (O'Donoghue & O'Flynn 1993). When microsurgery was developed in the 1960s, anatomical visualization was drastically improved with good magnification and illumination. Although there have not been any single prospective randomized clinical trials on the benefits of microscopic surgery over conventional naked-eye surgery, microscopic surgery has completely replaced traditional naked-eye surgery in neurosurgical practice. However, microscopic visualization requires a direct, straight surgical corridor to the surgical target area in order to adequately visualize the whole spectrum of the microsurgical anatomy. Endoscopy has been applied to those body organs where a natural tunnel or cavity is present. Thus, in neurosurgical practice, the use of an endoscope was adopted mostly on intraventricular surgery, such as third ventriculostomy and choroid plexus removal. When the Hopkin's rod lens endoscope system was introduced, rapid advances followed in endoscopic surgery in other surgical specialties. The endoscope was applied to compensate for the visual limits with the operating microscope. (Fukushima 1978; Magnan & Sanna 1999; Oppel 1978; Prott 1974). The terminology "endoscope-assisted microsurgery" was coined. Chen et al. reported that the offending blood vessels were discovered by the operating microscope alone in 85% of 167 patients. The use of an endoscope allowed them to discover neurovascular conflict in an additional 15% of the patients (Chen et al. 2008). Teo et al. (2006) reported that the endoscope enhanced visualization of the neurovascular conflict in an additional 33% of 114 patients. Similar experiences were reported by others (Jarrahy, Berci, & Shahinian 2000; Rak et al. 2004). However, the addition of the use of an endoscope during microscopic surgery has not proven to improve the operative outcome of vascular decompression surgery for the trigeminal nerve.

REFERENCES

Chen MJ, Zhang WJ, Yang C, et al. Endoscopic neurovascular perspective in microvascular decompression of trigeminal nerve. *J Cranio-Maxillofacial Surg* 2008; 36:456–461.

Doyen E. Surgical therapeutics and operative techniques. London: Balliere, Tindall and Cox, 1917; 599–602.

Fukushima T. Endoscopy of Meckel's cave, cisterna magna and cerebello-pontine angle. Technical note. *J Neurosurg* 1978;48:302–306.

Jarrahy R, Berci G, Shahinian HK. Endoscope-assisted microvascular decompression of the trigeminal nerve. *Otolaryngol Head Neck Surg* 2000;123(3):218–223.

Magnan Jr, Sanna M, eds *Endoscopy in neuro-otology*. New York: Thieme: 7–23, 1999.

O'Donoghue GM, O'Flynn P. Endoscopic anatomy of the cerebello-pontine angle. *Am J Otol* 1993;14:122–125.

Oppel F. Endoscopy of the cerebello-pontine angle: its diagnostic and therapeutic possibilities. In: *Advances in neurosurgery*, vol. 5. Berlin: Springer 269–275, 1978.

Prott W. Cisternoscopy endoscopy of the cerebello-pontine angle. *Acta Neurochir* 1974;31;105–113.

Rak R, Sekhar LN, Stimac D, et al. Endoscope-assisted microsurgery for microvascular compression syndrome. *Neurosurgery* 2004;54:876–883.

Sekula RF, Jho HD: Experimental Endoscopic Vascular Decompression of Facial Nerve via C1-2 puncture: Proof of Concept Cadaver Study, American Association Neurological Surgeons, Annual Meeting, New Orleans, Louisiana, 2005 [POSTER]

Sekula RF, Jho HD: Experimental Endoscopic Vascular Decompression of Trigeminal Nerve via C1-2 Puncture: Proof of Concept Cadaver Study, American Association Neurological Surgeons, Annual Meeting, New Orleans, Louisiana, 2005 [POSTER]

Teo C, Nakaji P, Mobbs RJ. Endoscope-assisted microvascular decompression for trigeminal neuralgia: Technical case report. *Neurosurgery* 2006;59(ONS Suppl 4): 489–490.

16

Future Medical Therapy

Joanna M. Zakrzewska

Medical therapies for trigeminal neuralgia (TN) are rapidly changing as we enter the era of genetics, increased interest in pain mechanisms, and evidence-based medicine. Patients also are increasingly demanding more information, so that they can learn to control their chronic conditions more effectively.

GENETIC FACTORS

The discovery of the human genome and the subsequent development of new biotechnologies have opened up whole new fields of research. It is now known that variations in DNA sequences may have consequences for whether an individual has an increased or decreased risk of developing a particular disease (e.g., risk of carbamazepine-induced Stevens-Johnson syndrome is strongly associated with the presence of the HLA-B*1502 allele in certain racial groups). However, it needs to be appreciated that the environment interacts with genes and must be taken into account, as it is possible that genes either modulate the effect of environmental exposures or that the effect of the exposure to an environmental pathogen is conditional upon a person's genotype. Thus, to manifest a certain characteristic or effect, it may be that an individual needs to have vulnerable genes, genes that amplify an existing polygenic risk and genes that will have a negative effect on the risk factor, which could be either environmental or behavioral. It is also possible that genetic heterogeneity exists in that different genes cause clinically indistinguishable presentations.

It is highly probable that a large number of genes are involved in TN, and so it is difficult to link symptoms and clinical signs to a particular cell type and hence gene. Although it may be that classical TN patients are a phenotypically homogenous group, it is well known that some patients cannot be fitted into this category, and they are classified as atypical TN (Nurmikko & Eldridge 2001). Are these phenotypically heterogenous group really all the same clinical disorder, which merely expresses itself differently in different subjects?

Several sodium channels have been identified as playing a significant role in neuropathic pain, and these could be abnormal in patients with TN. Genes associated with sodium channel expression include SCN1A, discovered to be the cause of familial hemiplegic migraine, and SCN9A, which is important in neuropathic pain. Other genes have also been identified in modulating pain, including GTP cyclohydrolase (GCH1), which modulates sensitivity to pain in normal individuals and liability to chronic pain, and catechol-O-methyltransferase (COMT) and the cytochrome P450 variant allele CYP3A5, which modulate the genetic response to opioid medications in humans.

These genetic studies may therefore enable an etiology for TN to be determined, which in turn could affect pharmacological activity.

PHARMACOGENETICS (PHARMACOGENOMICS)

Pharmacogenetics (also known as pharmacogenomics) is a growing area of research whose goal is to predict a patient's genetic response to a specific drug, not only in terms of efficacy but also tolerability. As Fishbain et al. (2004) point out, pharmacogenomics have a very wide range of potential uses which include:

- Identifying novel drug targets
- Predicting efficacy in drug development
- Predicting drug toxicity in drug development
- Improving the efficiency of drug development by decreasing the numbers of patients required to show drug efficacy in early clinical trials
- Defining the mechanisms of action of new compounds
- Screening for the direct influence of an agent on a specific pathway
- Identifying drug responders, drug nonresponders, and drug toxic responders in a population (individualized therapy)

It is being increasing recognized that gene polymorphisms may result in variations in individual response to drug efficacy, leading to a need for higher doses, lower doses, or to complete lack of efficacy. Polymorphism could also explain differences in methods of metabolism and pharmacokinetics of drug handling and variations in adverse reactions and drug interactions. It is therefore possible that the efficacy of drug therapy and a reduction in adverse reactions could be improved through genomic testing for enzymes of drug metabolism prior to administration of a drug.

More than 50 phase I trials are currently under way worldwide, assessing specific pain receptor blocking agents, a novel and potentially revolutionary method for preventing pain, and these may in the future apply to TN patients. This is why Woolf (Woolf et al. 1998) as far back as 1998 proposed that a mechanism-based approach to the treatment of pain may be more effective in the long term. For example, two randomised controlled trials have reported the use of lamotrigine in a range of neuropathic pain disorders, including TN, in which outcome measures have been based on (among others parameters) quality of pain (McCleane 1999; Silver et al. 2007).

RANDOMIZED CONTROLLED TRIALS

In these days of evidence-based medicine, it is increasingly important that drugs are tested in randomized controlled trials (RCTs), which also include reporting side effects and adverse events.

An increasing number of drugs are being used for TN, but there remain few high-quality RCTs with large numbers of participants testing the efficacy of drugs on TN pain relief (Jorns & Zakrzewska 2007).

Difficulties in conducting Randomized Controlled Trials in Trigeminal Neuralgia

Several featues of TN increase the difficulties of conducting standardized RCTs on treatments for it.

- Trigeminal neuralgia is a rare condition that makes sample size limited by subject availability. Randomized controlled trials on TN treatment have been done with patient numbers ranging from three to 341 patients; the usual is around 10. Only a few centers have enough patients to enter into trials of sufficient size to show a significant treatment effect.
- The spontaneous remissions and duration of the condition may affect results. It is known that pain relief periods are longer initially and that, with time, the pain-free intervals decrease. However, there is as yet no way of predicting the length of these phases. Patients, therefore, may be recruited at different stages of the disease and may go into spontaneous remission during the trial. In neurosurgery, it has been suggested that duration of disease affects outcomes, and this may be true in drug responses as well (Zakrzewska 2002b).
- The diagnostic criteria have not been validated by case-controlled studies, so a variety of patients may be recruited whose etiology differs (Zakrzewska 2002a). It is clear that atypical TN does exist, and it is not clear if this is the progression of a previously classical TN or an altogether different form (Nurmikko & Eldridge 2001).
- It has been suggested that, provided the pain has the characteristics of neuropathic pain (e.g., burning), then all patients can be treated the same (McCleane 1999). However, not all patients with TN have all the characteristics of neuropathic pain, and many neuropathic pains have not been characterized well enough for this to be feasible at present (Finnerup, Sindrup, & Jensen 2007).
- No standardized outcome measures have been agreed upon and, although pain relief seems an obvious primary outcome measure, sometimes quality-of-life issues predominate in long-term outcomes (Zakrzewska & Lopez 2003). Some of the outcome measures

used in gamma knife evaluation (e.g., the Barrow) have not been validated and assessed for reliability (Rogers et al. 2000).

- When using new drugs, it is difficult to estimate the dosages that are required, and so pilot studies should be conducted and reported. It may be necessary to use sliding scales rather than fixed dosage schemes, as some patients may not respond until larger doses are used.
- Intention to treat analysis (which includes even patients who have dropped out of trials) has rarely been done and yet can affect results.
- A number of ethical issues surround the use of placebo-controlled trials. The pain of TN is often excruciating, and so use of placebo may not be indicated. Use of active controls is difficult, as the gold standard drug, carbamazepine, has long carryover effects and inevitable side effects that make it easy to recognize.

Design of Trials in Trigeminal Neuralgia

It is important that, in the future, a more systematic and unified approach is taken to trials of new drugs in TN. Trials are needed to compare traditional and novel drugs, and single-drug versus add-on therapies.

The following aspects should be considered when designing future trials, bearing in mind that currently there are no universally successful trial designs in chronic pain management (Katz 2005; Rowbotham 2005).

Selection of Patients for Trials

In selecting patients for RCTs, several features need to be taken into consideration:

Diagnostic Criteria

The diagnostic criteria for classical TN of the International Classification of Headache Disorders (ICHD) should be used as a minimum (Anonymous 2004). Those patients who do not strictly meet the ICHD criteria can be enrolled in RCTs of TN but need to be analyzed separately. It is important to include as broad a range of patients as possible, who are representative of the community and which includes the elderly (i.e., those >80 years, who are often excluded from trials). Patients between attacks should not be enrolled in trials, but it is important to recruit patients with varying duration of disease. Those who have undergone surgical procedure for the treatment of TN or who have multiple sclerosis (MS) can be included in trials, but would need to be analyzed separately. This could only be done if the studies are large enough.

Character and Intensity

Most trials of chronic pain specify that patients should have a baseline pain intensity of 4 cm on a Visual Analogue Scale (VAS) of 1–10 cm before being recruited into a trial. This is measured over a period of 1–2 weeks, and allows for a clinically meaningful improvement to be noted (Farrar et al. 2000, 2001; Dworkin et al. 2005). Before recruiting a well-controlled TN patient or one who suffers severe side effects, previous medication should be reduced until the baseline intensity of 4 cm on a VAS is achieved, to ensure that the patient has not gone into remission. In severe cases of TN, a baseline period of observation may not be necessary. The pain should be described as a sharp shooting pain and not a dull, nagging type.

Periodicity, Timing, Duration, and Onset

Patients should have paroxysmal evoked or spontaneous attacks, and these should be followed by periods of complete freedom from pain. For the evoked attacks, a note should be made of the provoking factors, as these could be used as an outcome measure. All patients must record several attacks of pain a day, either evoked or spontaneous. Patients should have had a previous successfully treated episode which, at the time of the trial, has relapsed, as remissions are one of the diagnostic features.

Age at Entry

Age at entry should be determined by medication safety, and patients should be over 18 years of age. It would be preferable not to have an upper limit, as many elderly patients suffer from TN. When enrolling younger patients, it is important to ascertain whether they may not be symptomatic sufferers (e.g., with MS or tumors).

Gender and Ethnicity

Both male and female patients are required but, because of the epidemiology of TN, it may be harder to recruit males. It is important not to exclude patients from ethnic minority groups, even if they need support from advocates to help them understand the study and help in completing outcome measures. There is, however, the problem that validated questionnaires have not always been translated into the required language. It is now increasingly evident that genetic and racial variations can also affect the way patients handle drugs (as has been made very clear with carbamazepine).

Escape Medication

Patients taking other medication that may interact with the active drug or *escape medication* should be excluded. Escape therapy such as carbamazepine or oxcarbazepine should always be available.

Trial Designs

From the both earlier discussion and the Cochrane reviews of trials in TN (He, Wu, & Zhou 2006; Wiffen et al. 2005; Wiffen & Rees 2007), the standard double-blind randomised placebo-controlled trial, even with cross-over, is not entirely suitable for TN except when used in an "*N*-of-1" design. In an *N*-of-1 (sample size of 1) trial design, the study drug and placebo are administered in pairs and ordered randomly in the same patient. The advantages of this design over the standard parallel RCT are economic and that the variation in effect within an individual is much less than the variation between different individuals, thus estimates of the treatment effect are usually more precise. Reported *N*-of-1 RCTs have been used in evaluating treatments for chronic pain such as glossopharyngeal neuralgia (Eide & Stubhaug 1997).

In the future, it may be that the Enhanced Enriched Randomised Withdrawal (EERW) design may become the most popular (McQuay et al. 2008). Patients are openly titrated with the new drug and are randomised only when satisfactory efficacy and lack of severe side effects is established. The time patients take before drop-out from the trial is used to analyze the efficacy of the study drug.

This first phase prior to the randomization is in fact an open-label pilot study. During this phase, the nonresponders may have some phenotypic differences in response to medicines or susceptibility to the adverse effects in comparison with the responder group.

Finnerup et al. (2005) have shown that the enrichment can shift the overall numbers needed to treat (NNT) from 5.4 to 4.2. The extent of the shift will be determined by the proportion of responders to nonresponders, but there is clearly a balance between the degree of clinical need and proportion of responders. If the number of responders is less than 30%, it raises a question of whether the phase III trial should be continued. It does, however, indicate what proportion of patients with the disease are likely to respond to the drug (Fig. 16.1).

This type of design has been used previously in neuropathic pain studies (although it was not explicitly stated), and it suggests that there are both complete and partially enriched enrollment designs. A recent review by Straube et al. (2008), who looked at these designs in neuropathic pain using gabapentin and pregabalin did not show that this type of design enhanced treatment effect.

One of the problems of this design is that in the randomised part of the trial, patients may recognize the drug they are taking by the effects it causes if they have used it previously. The pilot part of this study enables the power of the study to be calculated more accurately, as data are available on responders and nonresponders. Randomization is essential and if it is anticipated that it may be difficult to randomize, then block randomization can be done, which ensures that the groups are similar should the trial be ended early. Randomization also allows for stratification, which could be

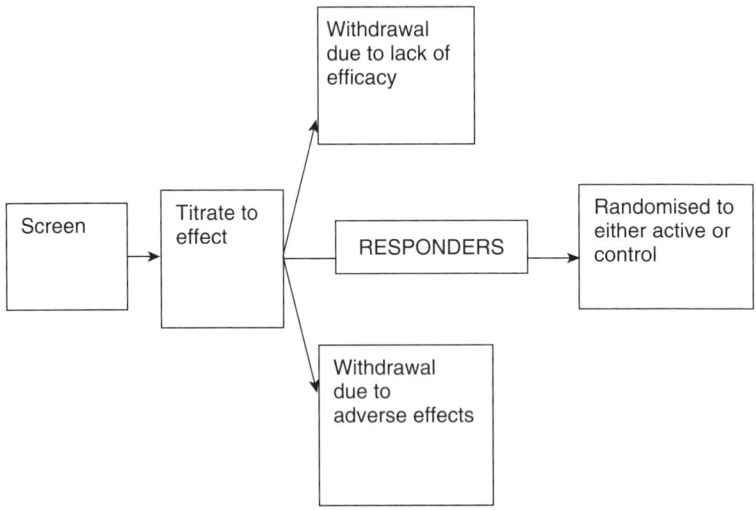

Figure 16.1 Enhanced Enriched Randomised Withdrawal trial (EERW) design.

done for important prognostic factors (e.g., presence of dull background pain, frequency of attacks, number of pain-free periods, and total duration of condition).

Dosage

In assessing any new drug for TN trial, a wide range of possible doses should be tested to define the dose–response relationship. In a randomized, fixed-dose, dose–response study, patients are randomized to one of several fixed-dose groups. Patients may either be placed on their fixed dose initially, or be raised to that dose gradually, but the intended comparison is between the groups on their final dose. In a concentration-controlled trial, treatment groups are titrated to several fixed concentration windows. The use of mg/kg basis is recommended as elderly low-weight patients will need different dosages from younger heavier patients.

Duration of Trial

A variety of factors must be taken into account when deciding on the duration of a trial: need for a period of baseline observations, speed of dosage escalation, and end of study observations to ensure that a patient has not gone into natural remission. Pharmacokinetics of the study drug and the length of escalation period also need to be taken into account. Outcome measures should be based on at least a 2-week steady dose period. As TN is a long-term condition, consideration needs to be taken into a reassessment 6–12 months later.

Evaluation of Results

Analyses should be performed for two populations. The first is the ITT analysis, which includes the number of and reasons why patients do not complete the trial. The second is the *preferred subgroup*, which will comprise all patients who completed the study and complied with the protocol.

Outcome Measures

Outcome measures must follow the proposals of the international workforce on an Initiative on Methods, Measurement, and Pain Assessment in Clinical Trials (IMMPACT) (Dworkin et al. 2005, 2008).

The outcomes of clinical trials are based on the mean responses of large numbers of subjects and fail to take into account interindividual differences which, as discussed earlier, may be due to genetic and environmental differences. Interindividual variations will also be found in relation to pain perception, response, gender, ethnicity, and temperament. Dionne et al. (2005) suggest that a responder index should be designed to use in clinical trials to better detect analgesic activity across patient groups and within subgroups, and to identify molecular-genetic mechanisms that contribute to individual variation.

Outcome measures used must be simple to administer, reliable, valid, precise, acceptable, and amenable to statistical analysis. As well as pain intensity/severity, the timing of attacks needs to be taken into account as TN is an intermittent pain. The reduction of the frequency of paroxysms and duration of attacks, both evoked and spontaneous, and the number of pain-free days are all important outcome measures. The daily pain diary measured on VAS 0–10 cm and a short McGill Pain Questionnaire (MPQ) would be suitable for evaluating the primary and secondary endpoints selected for study.

All pain causes mood changes, and patients with TN are prone to depression, especially when the pain is severe. Zakrzewska et al. (1999) have shown how depression is present prior to surgical treatment, and how this drops dramatically after surgery. The Hospital Anxiety and Depression scale often is used in patients with TN, but other instruments to measure depression include the Beck Depression Inventory. It may be sufficient, however, to ask patients just two questions:

1. During the past month have you often been bothered by feeling down, depressed, or hopeless?
2. During the past month have you often been bothered by having little interest or pleasure in doing things?

If patients answer "yes" to either question, then the specificity of screening can be further increased by asking them whether they want help with their problem (Whooley, Avins, Miranda, & Browner 1997).

It is essential to assess the impact of the new therapy on the quality of life and psychosocial functioning of the patients by assessing aspects of their daily activity. The Brief Pain Inventory scale can be used, as a minimum, to report quality of life in TN patients, as it has proved to be sensitive enough to measure changes in patients with pain and has been used by many pain units in the United Kingdom (Griffiths et al. 2003). The SF36 or shorter SF12 is used widely in neuropathic pain trials, and so could be used to enable comparisons to be made more easily. In the future, it would be useful to work with patients with TN to try to define those outcomes other than pain relief that they consider important.

Most trials ask patients to give a global evaluation of the whole trial, but patients should be helped in defining more clearly what is meant by the overall global satisfaction score. Patients could be asked to prepare a list of four or five activities that they are experiencing difficulty in performing during their pain attacks, for example, brushing teeth, eating, washing or shaving, speaking, and which they have graded from 1 to 5. These activities should then be monitored during the course of the trial.

A review of the RCTs in TN show that previous TN trials were not specific in reporting side effects, their grade and frequency as compared to placebo, or escape medication. These need to be compared to the active controls and placebos, as well as the standard drugs in use. The number and reasons for withdrawal from the trial must be recorded very carefully, and every patient must be accounted for. Patients need to be alerted about how to deal with unexpected adverse events, as well as expected ones, and what can be done to prevent side effects. Side effects should not only be graded against severity but also whether they are reversible or permanent. Trial participants must be aware that there can be marked variation in side effects, and they need to take into account idiosyncratic responses. Different side effects can affect quality of life in a variety of different ways, and this may need to be measured (e.g., dizziness vs. fatigue). Some patients may find the side effects unacceptable, others may tolerate them if their primary objective of pain relief is obtained.

The expectation of therapeutic benefit and of clinical improvement has emerged in recent times as a very important variable that is capable of influencing the response to a therapy even more powerfully than placebo response. The healthcare professional can also be influenced. Thus, patients and clinicians should be asked at the end of the trial what they thought had been given, the studied drug or placebo.

Outcomes are most frequently collected as daily diaries using pen and pencil; this, however, can become unmanageable and electronic formats, such as those that can be loaded into personal digital assistant (PDA) devices, mobile phones, or specially made watches (e.g., the Actiwatch) can be used. The use of electronic devices means that data can be entered quickly into spreadsheets (Dale & Hagen 2007).

Statistics

The primary endpoint in TN treatment can be analyzed using standard statistical methods. In calculations of sample size, the investigator should estimate the placebo response and the difference to be detected. Standard statistical methods can be used for analysis of assessment parameters in both cross-over and parallel trials. Both carry-over and period effect should be dealt with appropriately. Confidence intervals for differences are recommended in order to fully inform the reader of the results of the trial.

Drug Use and Patient Information

With patients taking increased control of their diseases comes a concomitant increased demand for information (Muir Gray 2002). Patients are being asked to take a more active role in decision-making about their therapy, so it is vital to ensure that patients with TN understand how the drugs they use are working. To do this, they need to keep some form of diary, as detailed earlier. The diary allows for a much more comprehensive history to be obtained, as patients can record their pain levels and drug-taking times in real time. Feedback from the diaries can then be used to teach patients how quickly they themselves respond to drug dose changes and whether they are going into remission and therefore need lower doses.

Novel Drugs

New drugs being developed must have some or all of these properties:

- Rapid onset of action
- Specific action
- A twice-daily dosing regimen
- Ease of use and administration (preferably orally, in liquid and tablet form)
- Allow for rapid escalation and abrupt stoppage
- Excretion through the kidneys, without hepatic metabolism
- Few drug interactions
- High tolerability, with low risk of severe side effects
- Safety in pregnancy
- No drug interactions

In order to assess pain control more objectively, functional magnetic resonance imaging (fMRI) is being explored as a surrogate marker for drug efficacy (Lu et al. 2008; Pattinson et al. 2007).

As antiepileptic drugs (AEDs) have been so successful in treating TN, these are always prime candidates for testing. There has been a great increase in the number of these drugs on the market and it is of special interest to choose those drugs with multiple mechanisms of action, such as lacosamide, which has both antinociceptive and anticonvulsant effects.

Neurogenic inflammation may play a role in ectopic discharges, and this has led to a randomised controlled trial on the use of sumatriptan, a drug used to treat migraine (Kanai, Suzuki, Osawa, & Hoka 2006). The success of this trial could lead to use of other triptans to relieve TN pain.

Botulinum toxin has been used in an open-label study in TN, as it may act both peripherally to reduce impulses and also prevent central desensitization (Piovesan et al. 2005). We await further randomised controlled trials.

There is clinical evidence that human pooled intravenous immunoglobulin (IVIG) is effective in some neurological diseases. Intravenous immunoglobulin was originally administered to patients with humoral immunodeficiency but recently it has also been suggested as an effective therapy in patients suffering from chronic pain. A prospective, multiple-dose, open-label cohort study of 130 patients with chronic pain syndromes including TN (Goebel et al. 2002) demonstrated in a subgroup of patients an excellent clinical response to IVIG treatment. One of these subgroups were patients with TN, and six out of ten TN patients reported marked improvement. All patients had been refractory to standard medical therapy. Pain relief was exceptionally long lasting in four of these six responders, between 2 weeks and more than 1 year following one or two doses of IVIG, suggestive of a long-lasting immune modulating effect of IVIG. It is thought that in primary TN both cytokines secreted peripherally at the site of nerve injury and centrally produced mediators may contribute to nociception, and may be targeted by immunoglobulins. Thus, this may be the mechanism of action of IVIG in TN. A trial is now being planned in TN patients (Goebel et al. 2003).

Other novel approaches include drugs that repair myelin (vitamin B has been advocated for many years). Even drugs to control hypertension could play a role in decreasing the effect that vascular compression has on the trigeminal nerve. Calcitonin has also been recently reported.

CONCLUSION

With the increasing interest of researchers in neuropathic pain and the emphasis on translational research, it is possible that in the near future new therapies will be available for managing TN.

REFERENCES

Anonymous. The International Classification of Headache Disorders, 2nd edition. *Cephalalgia* 2004;24(Suppl 1):9–160.

Dale O, Hagen KB. Despite technical problems personal digital assistants outperform pen and paper when collecting patient diary data. *J Clin Epidemiol* 2007; 60:8–17.

Dionne RA, Bartoshuk L, Mogil J, Witter J. Individual responder analyses for pain: does one pain scale fit all? *Trends Pharmacol Sci* 2005;26:125–130.

Dworkin RH, Turk DC, Farrar JT, et al. Core outcome measures for chronic pain clinical trials: IMMPACT recommendations. *Pain* 2005;113:9–19.

Dworkin RH, Turk DC, Wyrwich KW, et al. Interpreting the clinical importance of treatment outcomes in chronic pain clinical trials: IMMPACT recommendations. *J Pain* 2008;9:105–121.

Eide PK, Stubhaug A. Relief of glossopharyngeal neuralgia by ketamine-induced N- methyl-aspartate receptor blockade. *Neurosurgery* 1997;41:505–508.

Farrar JT, Portenoy RK, Berlin JA, et al. Defining the clinically important difference in pain outcome measures. *Pain* 2000;88:287–294.

Farrar JT, Young JP, Jr., LaMoreaux L, et al. Clinical importance of changes in chronic pain intensity measured on an 11-point numerical pain rating scale. *Pain* 2001;94:149–158.

Finnerup NB, Otto M, McQuay HJ, et al. Algorithm for neuropathic pain treatment: an evidence based proposal. *Pain* 2005;118:289–305.

Finnerup NB, Sindrup SH, Jensen TS. Chronic neuropathic pain: mechanisms, drug targets and measurement. *Fund Clin Pharmacol* 2007;21:129–136.

Fishbain DA, Fishbain D, Lewis J, et al. Genetic testing for enzymes of drug metabolism: does it have clinical utility for pain medicine at the present time? A structured review. *Pain Med* 2004;5:81–93.

Goebel A, Moore A, Weatherall R, et al. Intravenous immunoglobulin in the treatment of primary trigeminal neuralgia refractory to carbamazepine: a study protocol [ISRCTN33042138]. *BMC Neurol* 2003;3:1.

Goebel A, Netal S, Schedel R, Sprotte G. Human pooled immunoglobulin in the treatment of chronic pain syndromes. *Pain Med* 2002;3:119–127.

Griffiths DPG, Mitchell Noon J, Campbell FA, Price CM. Clinical governance and chronic pain: towards a practical solution. *Anaesthesia* 2003; 58:243–248.

He L, Wu B, Zhou M. Non-antiepileptic drugs for trigeminal neuralgia. *Cochrane Database Syst Rev* 2006;3:CD004029.

Jorns TP, Zakrzewska JM. Evidence-based approach to the medical management of trigeminal neuralgia. *Br J Neurosurg* 2007;21:253–261.

Kanai A, Suzuki A, Osawa S, Hoka S. Sumatriptan alleviates pain in patients with trigeminal neuralgia. *Clin J Pain* 2006;22:677–680.

Katz N. Methodological issues in clinical trials of opioids for chronic pain. *Neurology* 2005;65:S32–S49.

Lu H, Yang S, Zuo Y, et al. Real-time animal functional magnetic resonance imaging and its application to neuropharmacological studies. *Magn Reson Imaging* 2008;26:1266–1272, 2008.

McCleane G. 200 mg daily of lamotrigine has no analgesic effect in neuropathic pain: a randomised, double-blind, placebo controlled trial. *Pain* 1999;83: 105–107.

McQuay HJ, Derry S, Moore RA, et al. Enriched enrolment with randomised withdrawal (EERW): Time for a new look at clinical trial design in chronic pain. *Pain* 2008;135:217–220.

Muir Gray JA. *The resourceful patient* (pp. 1–154). Oxford: eRosetta Press, 2002.

Nurmikko TJ, Eldridge PR. Trigeminal neuralgia—pathophysiology, diagnosis and current treatment. *Br J Anaesth* 2001;87:117–132.

Pattinson KT, Rogers R, Mayhew SD, et al. Pharmacological fMRI: measuring opioid effects on the BOLD response to hypercapnia. *J Cereb Blood Flow Metab* 2007;27: 414–423.

Piovesan EJ, Teive HG, Kowacs PA, et al. An open study of botulinum-A toxin treatment of trigeminal neuralgia. *Neurology* 2005;65:1306–1308.

Rogers CL, Shetter AG, Fiedler JA, et al. Gamma knife radiosurgery for trigeminal neuralgia: the initial experience of The Barrow Neurological Institute. International *J Radiat Oncol Biol Phys* 2000;47:1013–1019.

Rowbotham MC. Mechanisms of neuropathic pain and their implications for the design of clinical trials. *Neurology* 2005;65:S66–S73.

Silver M, Blum D, Grainger J, et al. Double-blind, placebo-controlled trial of lamotrigine in combination with other medications for neuropathic pain. *J Pain Symptom Manage* 2007;34:446–454.

Straube S, Derry S, McQuay HJ, Moore RA. Enriched enrolment: definition and effects of enrichment and dose in trials of pregabalin and gabapentin in neuropathic pain. A systematic review. *Br J Clin Pharmacol* 2008;66(2):266–276,.

Whooley MA, Avins AL, Miranda J, Browner WS. Case-finding instruments for depression. Two questions are as good as many. *J Gen Intern Med* 1997;12:439–445.

Wiffen PJ, McQuay HJ, Moore RA. Carbamazepine for acute and chronic pain. *Cochrane Database Syst Rev* 2005;CD005451.

Wiffen PJ, Rees J. Lamotrigine for acute and chronic pain. *Cochrane Database Syst Rev* 2007;CD006044.

Woolf CJ, Bennett GJ, Doherty M, et al. Towards a mechanism-based classification of pain? *Pain* 1998;77:227–229.

Zakrzewska JM. Diagnosis and differential diagnosis of trigeminal neuralgia. *Clin J Pain* 2002a;18:14–21.

Zakrzewska JM. Trigeminal neuralgia. In: Zakrzewska JM, Harrison SD, eds., *Assessment and management of orofacial pain* (pp. 267–370). Amsterdam: Elsevier Sciences, 2002b.

Zakrzewska JM, Lopez BC. Quality of reporting in evaluations of surgical treatment of trigeminal neuralgia: recommendations for future reports. *Neurosurgery* 2003;53:110–122.

Zakrzewska JM, Sawsan J, Bulman JS. A prospective, longitudinal study on patients with trigeminal neuralgia who underwent radiofrequency thermocoagulation of the Gasserian ganglion. *Pain* 1999;79:51–58.

Index

Note: Page references followed by "*f*" and "*t*" denote figures and tables, respectively